Hemodialysis – From Basic Research to Clinical Trials

Contributions to Nephrology

Vol. 161

Series Editor

Claudio Ronco *Vicenza*

Hemodialysis – From Basic Research to Clinical Trials

Volume Editors

Claudio Ronco Vicenza
Dinna N. Cruz Vicenza

35 figures, 2 in color, and 14 tables, 2008

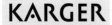

Basel · Freiburg · Paris · London · New York · Bangalore ·
Bangkok · Shanghai · Singapore · Tokyo · Sydney

Contributions to Nephrology

(Founded 1975 by Geoffrey M. Berlyne)

• •

Claudio Ronco
Department of Nephrology
St. Bortolo Hospital
Viale Rodolfi 37
IT-36100 Vicenza (Italy)

Dinna N. Cruz
Department of Nephrology
St. Bortolo Hospital
Viale Rodolfi 37
IT-36100 Vicenza (Italy)

Library of Congress Cataloging-in-Publication Data

Hemodialysis : from basic research to clinical trials / volume editors,
Claudio Ronco, Dinna N. Cruz.
      p. ; cm. – (Contributions to nephrology, ISSN 0302-5144 ; v. 161)
   Includes bibliographical references and indexes.
   ISBN 978-3-8055-8566-8 (hard cover : alk. paper)
  1. Hemodialysis. I. Ronco, C. (Claudio), 1951– II. Cruz, Dinna N.   III.
Series.
   [DNLM: 1. Renal Dialysis–trends.   W1 CO778UN v.161 2008 / WJ 378 H4884
2008]
   RC901.7.H45H448 2008
   617.4′61059–dc22

                                                                    2008015981

© Copyright 2008 by S. Karger AG, P.O. Box, CH–4009 Basel (Switzerland)
www.karger.com
Printed in Switzerland on acid-free and non-aging paper (ISO 9706) by Reinhardt Druck, Basel
ISSN 0302–5144
ISBN 978–3–8055–8566–8

....

Contents

Contents

Contents

....
Preface

The 17th Annual International Vicenza Course on Hemodialysis has yet another exceptional group of speakers and we are excited that this volume of *Contributions to Nephrology* is ready to guide attendees through the event and serve as a valuable tool for the future. All contributions have been collected and published in this volume as a result of the effort of all authors and the team of the Department of Nephrology at San Bortolo Hospital in Vicenza.

Hemodialysis today moves towards innovative techniques, biomaterials and devices with an absolute need for solid evidence around every new treatment or technology. Based on this concept, the course and this book are focused on innovative technology and new therapies from bench to bedside. The continuous effort to improve patient care follows the complex pathway from basic research to clinical trials. We have devoted a good deal of time to the topic of uremic toxins with contributions dealing with this puzzling problem from different points of view. Other emphasized areas include cardiovascular disease examined in its many facets and vascular access. As always, significant attention is placed on the physiological undertakings of treatments. Part of the program deals with practical questions in the dialysis unit. We are privileged to have such a superior group of speakers who can elaborate on these issues and discuss controversies that arise in the world of hemodialysis. Special attention has been placed on the problems of calcium and phosphate disorders, on the management of anemia, and finally on different biological disorders affecting the patients on dialysis. Once more, all these aspects are debated in light of international surveys, objective expert evaluation and recent clinical trials.

We consider this publication to be a useful supplement to the lectures presented at the three-day Vicenza course, but also a useful tool for future consultation by the clinician and all who are involved in the care of hemodialysis patients. We truly appreciate the help of the members of the faculty who have made this possible by submitting their manuscripts in advance.

Our sincere thanks go to Anna Saccardo and Ilaria Balbo who worked in Vicenza on the final arrangement of the course. A special thanks to Karger for the usual outstanding quality of the publication.

We hope that the readers will enjoy the book and will consider it a companion for daily clinical practice as well as for research.

Claudio Ronco Vicenza
Dinna N. Cruz Vicenza

Ronco C, Cruz DN (eds): Hemodialysis – From Basic Research to Clinical Trials.
Contrib Nephrol. Basel, Karger, 2008, vol 161, pp 1–6

....

Water Treatment for Dialysis: Technology and Clinical Implications

Nicholas A. Hoenich[a], Robert Levin[b]

[a]School of Clinical Medical Sciences, Newcastle University, Newcastle
upon Tyne, UK, and [b]Renal Research Institute, New York, N.Y., USA

Abstract

The dialytic process utilizes high volumes of water in the preparation of the dialysis
fluid. Improvements in water treatment equipment have resulted in improvements in chemical quality. Awareness that endotoxin and bacterial fragments present in the water distribution loop within the dialysis, are able to cross the dialyser membrane, has resulted in an
increased focus on this aspect of water quality. Practically, the age of many water treatment
plants, extensions of distribution systems and suboptimal cleaning procedures have prevented the achievement of optimal microbiological quality on a routine basis. When achieved
and maintained, clear benefits to the patient have been demonstrated. Hemodialysis
patients are also subject to increased oxidative stress which may also contribute to their morbidity and mortality. Recent clinical studies using dialysis fluid made with electrolyte-
reduced water have demonstrated benefits to antioxidant status of dialysis patients, offering a
further technological solution to the problem of increased cardiovascular disease in dialysis
patients.

Due to the increased exposure of dialysis patients to water used in the manufacture of dialysis fluid, which originates as drinking water, requires additional
treatment to ensure that it meets a more stringent contaminant level content
than drinking water. The more stringent levels are embodied in national and
international standards that have evolved out of the desire to minimize the complications arising from the use of inappropriate water quality.

For water used in the preparation of dialysis fluid, chemical contaminant
levels are set lower for three groups of chemical contaminants: contaminants to
which exposure is associated with clinical sequelae such as aluminum and fluoride [1, 2], compounds present in the dialysis fluid (e.g. sodium), and trace metals.

Whereas there is general agreement between standards in respect of maximum permitted inorganic chemical contaminants, standards omit requirements for organic chemical contaminants. In contrast, there is a considerable disparity in the standards relating to the maximum level of microbiological contaminants. On the one hand, the United States AASI/AAMI RD 52 suggests levels of 100 CFU/ml for bacteria and 0.25 EU/ml for endotoxin, some dialysis centers in the USA have implemented more stringent limits [3]. European Best Practice Guidelines (EPBG) and the Italian Society of Nephrology, on the other hand, favor the universal use of ultrapure dialysis fluid defined as containing <0.1 CFU/ml for bacteria, and <0.03 EU/ml for endotoxin, the latter representing the sensitivity level of currently used assays. Such fluid is further filtered in online techniques, however, as short DNA fragments (oligodeoxynucleotides (ODN) of 6–20 nucleotides) are able to bind to Toll-like receptors and are stimulatory on immune cells, induce natural killer cell activity and induce IFN-γ, TNF-α, and IL-6 from mononuclear cells, even this level may in the longer term prove to be inadequate.

The purpose of this paper is to review the water treatment technology required to achieve a quality of water stipulated in standards and the implications of achieving these routinely.

Water Treatment Technology

Historically, the treatment of renal failure frequently involved the use of untreated water, however when patients were treated on a repeated basis, by the early 1970s, it was recognized that drinking water was unsuitable for the preparation of dialysis fluid and either softeners or deionizers were used [4]. Today, the treatment that the water undergoes is much more complex as shown in figure 1.

Essential elements of such a system are: pretreatment filtration, softeners, carbon beds, reverse osmosis systems, ultraviolet (UV) irradiators, endotoxin filters as well as monitors for the presence of chlorine or chloramines.

The Problem of the Distribution Loop

Whilst historically there has been emphasis on ensuring that the chemical contaminant levels in the product water meet those specified in the standards, the distribution loop has remained a problem. Early water distribution networks used copper. Subsequently it was demonstrated that a leeching of copper occurred especially in the presence of a low water pH [5]. This meant a move

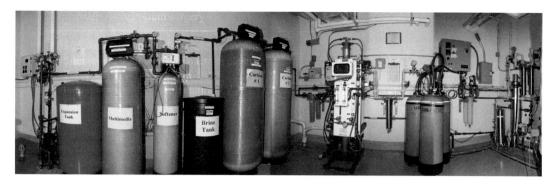

Fig. 1. A panoramic view of a modern water treatment plant.

towards the use of non-toxic materials such as polyvinylchloride. When carbon beds are used in the water treatment, water downstream of such beds does not contain any bacteriostat (chlorine or chloramines) and is vulnerable to bacterial proliferation. Such proliferation is hastened by the presence of low flow and stagnation points within the distribution loop, which coupled with irregular cleaning eventually leads to the formation of a biofilm. In view of this, dialysis centers must have effective and regular quality control programs to ensure that this does not happen. Furthermore, the use of water storage or holding tanks for treated water is best avoided. When used, the tanks should have a conical or bowl-shaped base, should drain from the lowest point of the base, incorporate a tight-fitting lid and be vented through a hydrophobic 0.2-μm air filter. Sight tubes should be avoided due to the possible growth of algae. If an overflow pipe is used it should be fitted with means of preventing contamination. The tank should also be capable of disinfection.

Procedural elements – the timing and type of disinfection procedures used for the waterline system and monitors, the timing and type of water treatment quality control procedures – should be based on action limits and standard operating protocols, the most important aspect being the prevention rather than eradication. Once established the biofilm is difficult to eradicate or remove, and acts as a source of bacterial fragments such as peptidoglycans and endotoxins which have the potential to cross the dialysis membrane and contribute to morbidity and mortality in the patient [6].

To overcome these issues, newer water treatment plants now use heat disinfection, a process that requires little to no rinse time and which may be used daily to clean the distribution loop. Materials such as polyvinylchloride cannot be used safely with heat disinfection and cross-linked polyethylene, polyvinylidene fluoride, or stainless steel (AISI type 316L) are the materials of choice. Such materials also have a smoother internal surface, minimizing attachment of bacterial fragments.

Bacterial proliferation within the distribution loop can be controlled by means other than heat. Ozonation using ozone generators are beginning to be used. Ozone in product water may be harmful to patients, and the product water should not be used until the ozone produced has dissipated. Further approaches to minimize microbiological burden arising from the water use UV irradiation and endotoxin filters. The effectiveness of UV irradiation depends on the dose of radiant energy. A dose of $30 \, mW\text{-}s/cm^2$ will kill $>99.99\%$ of a variety of bacteria, including *Pseudomonas* species, in a flow-through device. Some Gram-negative water bacteria however appear to be more resistant to UV irradiation than others, and the use of sublethal doses of UV radiation, or an insufficient contact time, may lead to proliferation of such bacteria in the water system. UV irradiation at a wavelength of 254 nm converts chloramine (NH_2Cl) to chloride and ammonium ions, easily removed by reverse osmosis, however the positioning of the unit is critical as hard water, high total dissolved solids, or high levels of fluoride, iodine, iron or manganese, may interfere with penetration of UV irradiation through the water and inhibit effectiveness. The radiant energy emitted by the mercury vapor lamps used decreases with time, compromising effectiveness. Prevention of this requires routine monitoring of the radiant energy.

UV irradiators do not eliminate bacteria and when used may even increase endotoxin concentrations. This may be prevented by the use of an endotoxin-retentive filter. Such filters remove endotoxins primarily by size exclusion, although some may also remove some endotoxin by adsorption to the membrane material, should be able to reduce the concentration of bacteria in the feed water to the filter by a factor of at least 10^7 and that of endotoxin by a factor of at least 10^3. Short bacterial DNA fragments may however cross the membranes used in such devices [7].

Practicality of Ensuring the Quality of Water and Clinical Benefits

Water quality is critically dependent upon having the appropriate plant supplemented by standard operating procedures and protocols to ensure a consistent quality. The management as well as the development of such procedures is outside the scope of this article, but guidance relating to the periodicity of testing as well as test procedures may be found in the EBPG [8] and will be available in the form of an international standard currently being developed

(ISO/CD 26722 – Water treatment equipment for hemodialysis applications and related therapies).

Low levels of endotoxins and other bacterial products present in water and dialysis fluid have been implicated as contributing to the low level microinflammation seen in patients undergoing regular dialysis treatment [9]. The use of ultrapure fluids ameliorates microinflammation, reduces the severity of long-term complications of dialysis such as malnutrition, plasma levels of β_2-microglobulin, responsiveness to erythropoietin and slows loss in residual renal function [10–13]. Some remain less convinced, possibly due to the absence of randomized clinical studies exploring these aspects of water quality [14, 15].

Emerging Developments in Water Treatment Technology

Active oxygen species or free radicals cause extensive oxidative damage to biological macromolecules, contributing to disease as well as ageing. Hemodialysis patients are subject to such increased oxidative stress which may contribute to morbidity and mortality. When water is subject to electrolysis, the electrical energy creates oxidized water near the anode and reduced water near the cathode (electrolyte-reduced water). Clinical studies with electrolyte reduced water to produce dialysis fluid have demonstrated a partial restoration of patient antioxidant status, but such technology is only available from a single supplier, and further long-term studies as well as costings are required before the widespread clinical application of this novel approach [16, 17].

Conclusions

Water used in the preparation of dialysis fluid plays an important role in the morbidity and mortality associated with regular dialysis therapy. Historically the emphasis has been on the removal of chemical contaminants, with little attention being paid to the microbiological quality as demonstrated in the findings of several national surveys [18–20]. Although improvement of the microbiological quality of water has yielded a range of benefits, the dialysis patient remains the subject of oxidative stress that can cause oxidation of biologic macromolecules, such as low-density lipoprotein increasing adhesion of monocytes to the endothelium, transformation of macrophages into foam cells and impairment of endothelium-dependent vasorelaxation contributing to atherosclerosis development. The use of electrolyte-reduced water appears to offer a promising resolution of this issue.

References

1 Jaffe JA, Liftman C, Glickman JD: Frequency of elevated serum aluminum levels in adult dialysis patients. Am J Kidney Dis 2005;463:16–19.
2 Bello VA, Gitelman HJ: High fluoride exposure in hemodialysis patients. Am J Kidney Dis 1990; 15:320–324.
3 Hoenich NA, Levin R: The implications of water quality in hemodialysis. Semin Dial 2003;16: 492–497.
4 Ward RA: Water processing for hemodialysis. 1. A historical perspective. Semin Dial 1997;10: 26–31.
5 Matter BJ, Pederson J, Psimenos G, Lindeman RD: Lethal copper intoxication in hemodialysis. Trans Am Soc Artif Intern Organs 1969;15:309–315.
6 Cappelli G, Tetta C, Canaud B: Is biofilm a cause of silent chronic inflammation in haemodialysis patients? A fascinating working hypothesis. Nephrol Dial Transplant 2005;20:266–270.
7 Schindler R, Beck W, Deppisch R, Aussieker M, Wilde A, Gohl H, Frei U: Short bacterial DNA fragments: detection in dialysate and induction of cytokines. J Am Soc Nephrol 2004;15:3207–3214.
8 European Renal Association-European Dialysis and Transplant Association: European Best Practice Guidelines for haemodialysis (Part 1). Nephrol Dial Transplant 2002;17(suppl 7):47–49.
9 Lonnemann G: When good water goes bad: how it happens, clinical consequences and possible solutions. Blood Purif 2004;22:124–129.
10 Lamas JM, Alonso M, Sastre F, García-Trío G, Saavedra J, Palomares L: Ultrapure dialysate and inflammatory response in haemodialysis evaluated by darbepoetin requirements – a randomized study. Nephrol Dial Transplant 2006;21:2851–2858.
11 Furuya R, Kumagai H, Takahashi M, Sano K, Hishida A: Ultrapure dialysate reduces plasma levels of β_2-microglobulin and pentosidine in hemodialysis patients. Blood Purif 2005;23:311–316.
12 Schiffl H, Lang SM, Fischer R: Ultrapure dialysis fluid slows loss of residual renal function in new dialysis patients. Nephrol Dial Transplant 2002;17:1814–1818.
13 Schiffl H, Lang SM, Stratakis D, Fischer R: Effects of ultrapure dialysis fluid on nutritional status and inflammatory parameters. Nephrol Dial Transplant 2001;16:1863–1869.
14 Masakane I: Clinical usefulness of ultrapure dialysate – recent evidence and perspectives. Ther Apher Dial 2006;10:348–354.
15 Bommer J, Jaber BL: Ultrapure dialysate: facts and myths. Semin Dial 2006;19:115–119.
16 Huang KC, Yang CC, Lee KT, Chien CT: Reduced hemodialysis-induced oxidative stress in end-stage renal disease patients by electrolyzed-reduced water. Kidney Int 2003;64:704–5714.
17 Huang KC, Yang CC, Hsu SP, Lee KT, Liu HW, Morisawa S, Otsubo K, Chien CT: Electrolyzed-reduced water reduced hemodialysis-induced erythrocyte impairment in end-stage renal disease patients. Kidney Int 2006;70:391–398.
18 Kulander L, Nisbeth U, Danielsson BG, Eriksson O: Occurrence of endotoxin in dialysis fluid from 39 dialysis units. J Hosp Infect 1993;24:29–37.
19 Arvanitidou M, Spaia S, Askepidis N, Kanetidis D, Pazarloglou M, Katsouyannopoulos V, Vayonas G: Endotoxin concentration in treated water of all hemodialysis units in Greece and inquisition of influencing factors. J Nephrol 1999;12:32–37.
20 De Filippis P, Spitaleri G, Damiani F, Panà A: Microbiological quality of haemodialysis water in various hospitals and private clinics in the Lazio region (Italy): 2000–2004 (in Italian). Ig Sanita Pubbl 2007;63:21–29.

Dr. Nicholas A. Hoenich
School of Clinical Medical Sciences, Newcastle University
Framington Place, Newcastle upon Tyne NE2 4 HH (UK)
Tel. +44 191 6998, Fax +44 191 0721, E-Mail nicholas.hoenich@ncl.ac.uk

Ronco C, Cruz DN (eds): Hemodialysis – From Basic Research to Clinical Trials.
Contrib Nephrol. Basel, Karger, 2008, vol 161, pp 7–11

··········· ············

Dialysate Composition

Sara M. Viganò, Salvatore Di Filippo, Celestina Manzoni,
Francesco Locatelli

Department of Nephrology, Dialysis and Renal Transplantation,
A. Manzoni Hospital, Lecco, Italy

Abstract

The most appropriate dialysate composition is one of the central topics in dialysis treatment. The prescription of a certain dialysate composition could change in order to obtain not only an adequate blood purification but also a high tolerability. Sodium balance represents the cornerstone of cardiovascular stability and good blood pressure control. The goal of dialysis is to remove the amount that has accumulated in the interdialysis period. Potassium removal is adequate when hyperkaliemia is avoided. Bicarbonate in dialysate should be personalized in order to avoid acidosis and end-dialysis excessive alkalosis.

Copyright © 2008 S. Karger AG, Basel

Improvements in the care of dialysis patients and in the practice of renal transplantation have determined a dramatic increase in the number of end-stage renal disease patients referred to renal substitutive treatments over the last decade. The dialysis population is mainly composed of elderly and diabetic patients with a heavy burden of co-morbid conditions, mainly related to systemic vasculopathy and a poor performance status [1]. The choice of dialysate composition is an essential element of hemodialysis (HD) prescription, in order to restore an adequate body electrolytic concentration and acid-base equilibrium.

Sodium

Sodium crosses the dialysis membrane by diffusion and convection. It is well known that the sodium fractions transported by these two mechanisms are not the same [2], and this is important in order to define intra-HD sodium kinetics and to choose the proper dialysate sodium concentration. When dialysate sodium activity corresponds to plasma water sodium activity multiplied by 0.967 (Donnan factor) *('isonatric' dialysate)* and there is no ultrafiltration, the net intra-HD sodium removal is zero. *Hyponatric dialysate* can theoretically be used if the patient should lose sodium by diffusion. Secondary to the loss of sodium by diffusion, plasma osmolarity decreases with two possible side effects: (1) cellular overhydration, caused by osmotic fluid shift from the extracellular to the intracellular compartment, which significantly contributes to the so-called disequilibrium syndrome; (2) intra-HD hypotension, caused by insufficient refilling of the intravascular compartment from the intracellular space. *Hypernatric dialysate* is more frequently used in order to avoid excessive sodium losses due to ultrafiltration and prevent cardiovascular instability. When sodium concentration in the dialysate is higher than the patient pre-HD blood sodium concentration, the patient is supplied with sodium via diffusion for as long as necessary to equalize the difference in concentrations. In this case, the diffusive sodium transport to the patient counteracts the convective sodium removal due to ultrafiltration. Hypernatric dialysis may cause insufficient net sodium removal, and consequently favor the development of refractory hypertension. Moreover, it can trigger an intensive sense of thirst, causing high water intake in the inter-HD interval, which has to be treated with high ultrafiltration rates during HD which, in turn, favors hypotensive episodes. These episodes may prevent dry body weight achievement and prompt the dialysis staff to administer hypertonic saline or to increase dialysate sodium concentration: a vicious circle may be established, resulting in cardiac failure and/or pulmonary edema. To be physiological, sodium mass balance must be zero in patients in dialysis therapy; this means that dialytic sodium removal must be equal to interdialytic sodium load. A zero sodium balance between the intra-HD sodium removal and the inter-HD sodium accumulation can be achieved by individualizing the dialysate sodium concentration for each dialysis, to reach a constant end-dialysis plasma water sodium concentration and applying a rate of ultrafiltration equal to the interdialytic increase in body weight [3]. Unfortunately, this model is unsuitable for routine use because of the need for determination of predialysis plasma water sodium concentration at each dialysis session.

Conductivity Kinetic Modeling

The conductivity kinetic model appears to be more easily applicable, because no blood samples or laboratory tests are needed to determine plasma water conductivity and ionic dialysance, used in place of plasma water sodium concentration and sodium dialysance, respectively. It has also been demonstrated that this model is more accurate and precise in predicting total plasma water sodium concentration as compared with the sodium kinetic model [4].

Potassium

In order to be adequate, potassium removal during dialysis should be equal to the amount accumulated during the interdialytic period. Potassium removal by dialysis is termed satisfactory if predialysis hyperkalemia is avoided, without causing potential dangerous hypokalemia. For stable patients, a dialysate potassium of 2 mmol/l is considered advisable in order to keep pre-HD plasma potassium levels below 6 mmol/l. The safety of dialysate potassium concentration is also related to the avoidance of hypokalemia and dialysis-induced arrhythmias. Post-HD serum potassium concentration is influenced not only by the pre-HD serum potassium concentration and the dialysate potassium concentration, but also by plasma tonicity, changes in plasma tonicity following HD, bicarbonate concentration and glucose in the dialysate.

Dialysate Potassium-Arrhythmia Relationship

The predialysis serum potassium concentration may play a role in certain subsets of patients. Intra-HD serum potassium exchanges are potentially relevant when they induce a certain decrease in serum potassium concentration with each individual having a different arrhythmogenic level. It has been demonstrated that the risk of arrhythmia is lower with a variable removal of potassium during hemodialysis and there is no risk of a destabilizing effect on cardiac cell [5]. Thus, potassium profiling of the dialysate may be an efficient tool to decrease the arrythmogenic effect of HD.

Calcium

Calcium mass balance studies showed that in a patient with a normal serum calcium before HD, dialysate calcium concentrations of 1.25 (low concentration) and 1.75 mmol/l (high concentration) result, respectively, in a negative and a positive intradialytic calcium balance [6], because the use of a 1.75 mmol/l calcium dialysate may constitute a strategy for improving hemodynamic stability in cardiac-compromised patients. In this case, calcium salts and vitamin D products should be used cautiously. Calcium ions play a primary role in the contractile process of both vascular smooth muscle cells and cardiac myocytes. In patients using calcium salts as phosphate binders, it is often advised to use low dialysate calcium concentrations to prevent or treat hypercalcemia [7].

Acid Buffering

The endogenous production of H^+, mainly related to protein ingestion, is ~0.77 mmol/g of protein catabolized [8]. H^+ accumulation in the blood of uremic patients is buffered by plasma bicarbonate, which is used as a surrogate marker of acidemia. A relationship between protein intake and plasma bicarbonate concentration, and between nutritional markers and plasma bicarbonate concentration has been reported [9]. At least on a short-term basis, paradoxically a decrease in plasma bicarbonate level is associated with a more favorable constellation of nutritional markers because of adequate protein intake. A recent study evaluates the associations between baseline predialysis serum bicarbonate and 2-year mortality [10]. They found a lower death risk for those patients with a bicarbonate level values >22 mEq/l.

The bicarbonate flux from the dialysate to the patient is determined by the transmembrane concentration gradient, bicarbonate dialysance and treatment time. The usual average dialysate concentration is 35 mmol/l, obtained from proportioning dialysis stations that mix bicarbonate from solution or dry powder to water and an 'acid' compartment containing a small amount of acetate or lactate and sodium, potassium, calcium and magnesium. Usually, a plateau of plasma bicarbonate is reached after 2 h of HD at an approximate value of 27–30 mmol/l.

Because of the known consequences of metabolic acidosis for the nutritional status of HD patients, higher concentrations of dialysate bicarbonate (39–48 mmol/l), resulting in a significant increase in pre-HD plasma bicarbonate, have been proposed to improve the control of acidosis. This maneuver improved protein turnover and triceps skin fold thickness, and increased serum branched-chain amino acids, but had no effect on serum albumin and total lymphocyte count [11] and could cause postdialysis alkalosis.

In conclusion, acid-base status in HD patients is estimated from plasma bicarbonate. It reflects not only protein catabolism, but also protein intake. As long-term exposure to acidosis may alter nutritional status by enhancing protein turnover, individualization of buffer prescription is desirable in order to avoid metabolic acidosis and post-HD alkalosis. The usual bicarbonate concentration in dialysate is 35 mmol/l. It should be adapted to reach midweek pre-HD plasma bicarbonate values, from an adequately handled sample, ≥22 mmol/l [12].

References

1   Locatelli F, Manzoni C, Del Vecchio L, Di Filippo S: Changes in the clinical condition of haemodialysis patients. J Nephrol 1999;12(suppl 2):82–91.

2   Locatelli F, Colzani S, D'Amico M, Manzoni C, Di Filippo S: Dry weight and sodium balance. Semin Nephrol 2001;21:291–297.

3   Gotch FA, Lam MA, Prowitt M, Keen M: Preliminary clinical results with sodium-volume modeling of hemodialysis therapy. Proc Clin Dial Transplant Forum 1980;10:12–17.

4   Pozzoni P, DI Filippo S, Pontoriero G, Locatelli F: Effectiveness of sodium and conductivity kinetic models in predicting end-dialysis plasma water sodium concentration: preliminary results of a single-center experience. Hemodial Int 2007;11:169–177.

5   Buemi M, Aloisi E, Coppolino G, Loddo S, Crascì E, Aloisi C, Barillà A, Cosentini V, Nostro L, Caccamo C, Floccari F, Romeo A, Frisina N, Teti D: The effect of two different protocols of potassium haemodiafiltration on QT dispersion. Nephrol Dial Transplant 2005;20:1148–1154.

6   Argiles A, Mourad G: How do we have to use the calcium in the dialysate to optimise the management of secondary hyperparathyroidism? Nephrol Dial Transplant 1998;13(suppl 3):62–64.

7   Argiles A, Kerr PG, Canaud B, Flavier JC, Mion C: Calcium kinetics and the long-term effects of lowering dialysate calcium concentration. Kidney Int 1993;43:630–640.

8   Weiner IM, Blanchard KC, Mudge GH: Factors influencing renal excretion of foreign organic acids. Am J Physiol 1964;207:953–963.

9   Messa P, Mioni G, Maio GD, et al: Derangement of acid-base balance in uremia and under hemodialysis. J Nephrol 2001;14(suppl 4):S12–S21.

10 Wu DY, Shinaberger CS, Regidor DL, McAllister CJ, Kopple JD, Kalantar-Zadeh K: Association between serum bicarbonate and death in hemodialysis patients: is it better to be acidotic or alkalotic? Clin J Am Soc Nephrol 2006;1:70–78.

11 Oettinger CW, Oliver JC: Normalization of uremic acidosis in hemodialysis patients with a high bicarbonate dialysate. J Am Soc Nephrol 1993;3:1804–1807.

12 K/DOQI, National Kidney Foundation: Clinical practice guidelines for nutrition in chronic renal failure. Am J Kidney Dis 2000;35(suppl 2):1–140.

Prof. Francesco Locatelli
Department of Nephrology, Dialysis and Renal Transplantation
A. Manzoni Hospital, Via dell'Eremo 9/11
IT–23900 Lecco (Italy)
Tel. +39 0341 489 850, Fax +39 0341 489 860, E-Mail f.locatelli@ospedale.lecco.it

Ronco C, Cruz DN (eds): Hemodialysis – From Basic Research to Clinical Trials.
Contrib Nephrol. Basel, Karger, 2008, vol 161, pp 12–22

....

Challenge for the Interventional Nephrologist: Monitoring the Arteriovenous Fistula

Rodrigo Campos[a], *Miguel C. Riella*[a,b]

[a]Department of Medicine, Renal Division, Evangelic School of Medicine and
[b]Catholic University of Paraná, Paraná, Brazil

Abstract

Arteriovenous fistula (AVF) has been recommended as the first choice for hemodialysis vascular access. This is supported by its superior patency and lower complication rates over grafts and catheters. The increasing incidence of end-stage renal disease patients and consequently higher prevalence of AVF in hemodialysis units have augmented the necessity for a better understanding of AVF peculiarities. As for grafts, the K/DOQI Work Group recommends the routine use of techniques for monitoring AVF to detect dysfunctional access with stenosis and its consequent correction in an attempt to reduce thrombotic episodes, cost and improving quality of life of these patients. All members of a vascular access team should be able to recognize a dysfunctional vascular access and determine the exact moment to intervene. Particularly for the interventionist, these techniques may be used to assist percutaneous transluminal angioplasty, providing information about the success of the procedure and access patency. The present article discusses the methods of AVF surveillance that are routinely performed for hemodialysis patients with the purpose to detect stenosis, reduce thrombosis and assist procedures.

Copyright © 2008 S. Karger AG, Basel

The native arteriovenous fistula (AVF) is regarded as the vascular access of choice for hemodialysis (HD) because of its superior patency and lower complication rates once it has fully matured. Because of that it is recommended as the first choice in order of placement as vascular access for HD [1, 2]. Vascular access dysfunction is a common and daily major problem in HD units. These complications account for 15–24% of hospitalizations in end-stage renal disease HD patients [3] and are directly related to increased mortality because of inadequately delivered dialysis doses [4]. Associated to that, a thrombosed access frequently requires an implantation of tunneled and non-tunneled catheters, in such case increasing the risk of sepsis and morbidity [5].

As recommendation of the last two K/DOQI guidelines [1, 2], AVF prevalence in this decade has increased in the United States [6] and it was already the most prevalent access in Europe and Japan [7]. This implication in AVF use will produce clinical benefits for patients and savings in vascular access costs [8]. Despite this known superiority over arteriovenous graft (AVG) it too suffers from frequent development of stenosis and thrombosis. For this reason, the K/DOQI recommends programs for detection of stenosis and its consequent correction in an attempt to reduce the event of thrombosis.

Once the AVF has matured and the patient is receiving maintenance HD, the responsibility of AVF care and stenosis detection is referred to the dialysis staff. However, this access care should not be transferred to only one individual, such as the nurse. Best results in detection of stenosis and prolonging access patency are obtained when a multidisciplinary relationship among vascular surgeons, nephrologists, nurses, interventional radiologists and interventional nephrologists is developed [9]. The interventional nephrologist should know how to perform and interpret methods of AVF surveillance, such as physical examination (PE), intra-access pressure (IAP), access recirculation and access blood flow. This knowledge promotes a correct recognition of a dysfunctional vascular access, determines the exactly moment to correct the stenosis and aids in the success of the procedure. The present review discusses the methods of surveillance that are routinely performed for AVF in HD patients.

Detection of Access Dysfunction

The fundamental idea of vascular access monitoring and surveillance is that stenosis develops over variable intervals in the great majority of AVFs and if detected and corrected timely, maturation can be promoted, underdialysis minimized or avoided and thrombosis avoided or reduced [10]. As defined in the K/DOQI vascular access guidelines, 'monitoring' of vascular access makes use of PE and clinical signs to identify the access with dysfunction and the term 'surveillance' is referred to tests that may involve special instrumentation [2]. It is important to emphasize that dysfunctional vascular access is not defined only by the presence of a significant stenosis (reduction >50% of normal vessel diameter) and it should not be repaired merely because they are present. Stenosis must be accompanied by a hemodynamic or clinical abnormality [2]. Another important point involved in the process is that every protocol must involve multiple techniques for the detection of stenosis and in each technique multiple repetitive measurements must be carried out, so that inappropriate referrals to correct stenosis are not made [10].

Monitoring

Some indirect findings may suggest the presence of stenosis. Unexplained decreases in delivered dialysis dose, as measured by Kt/V or urea reduction ratio, may be associated with vascular access dysfunction. An AVF which does not support a pump flow >350 ml/min, because of decreased blood flow, will become ineffective and recirculation problems will occur. Prolonged bleeding after removal of the needles from punctures sites may occasionally be an indicator of elevated IAP (in the absence of excessive anticoagulation). These indirect findings may be influenced by other factors and both are identified too late.

PE is the main part of vascular access monitoring. This method is easily performed, non-invasive and costless. It is not useful only after maturation of AVF, since there is evidence that proves its ability in the prediction of AVF maturation [11, 12]. As soon as a non-matured AVF is identified, it can be promptly corrected and becomes possible to puncture [13]. Evaluation of a fistula should be performed weekly after surgery and if it fails to mature by 6 weeks, an imaging study should be obtained to determine the cause of the problem as recommended by the current K/DOQI Vascular Access Work Group [2].

Once it is matured, PE must be performed at least monthly and be part of any protocol of surveillance [14]. In one study that utilized a detection protocol of stenosis for graft and AVF, PE was included as one of the examination methods. The authors reported an isolated specificity of 95% for PE. It was not possible to identify the isolated sensitivity. The occurrence of thrombosis with treatment by percutaneous transluminal angioplasty (PTA) was reduced from 48 to 17% after the initiation of the protocol. Only 18% of the accesses were AVF [15]. Similarly, in another study with AVF and vascular grafts, the whole protocol specificity was elevated (92.8%), however with low sensitivity (35.8%). This study did not identify isolated sensitivity and specificity for PE [16]. In another report, the accuracy in the diagnosis of stenosis in vascular grafts was found to be 91.8% utilizing PE [17]. Recently, Asif et al. [18] examined the accuracy of PE exclusively in suspected dysfunctional AVF referred for angiography and found a sensitivity and specificity for the outflow and inflow stenosis of 92 and 86% and 85 and 71%, respectively. Our group evaluated the accuracy of PE in the detection of stenosis exclusively in AVFs without a prior screening test and found a sensitivity of 96% and specificity of 76% [19].

AVF PE begins by the anastomosis. The two most important components of anastomosis examination is the thrill, which is an indicator of flow, and the pulse, which is an indicator of downstream resistance. Another component that can be evaluated is the bruit. Normally the thrill and bruit are prominent near the anastomosis and they are both present in systole as well as early diastole (continuous). The presence of stenosis reduces the blood flow and this, in turn, reduces the strength of the thrill. If stenosis is present at a point away from the anastomosis, the intra-access resistance rises and the flow may occur only during systole. In this situation the thrill and bruit will be found only in systole (not continuous). With regard to the pulse, it must be soft. If it is forceful, like a 'water-hammer' pulse, this often suggests the presence of stenosis. The intensity of the hyperpulsatility is proportional to the severity of the stenosis. Another step is to examine the entire length of the AV fistula. Moving up the vein away from the anastomosis, the thrill and bruit gradually diminish. An increase in the strength of the thrill or a new palpable thrill downstream from the anastomotic site suggests the presence of a stenosis. The pulse should be soft and compressible as in the anastomosis. The pulse becomes hard in the presence of a body stenosis. An important maneuver to evaluate the pulse is to elevate the arm above the level of the heart. Normally, the pulse may collapse with arm elevation. If it does not, the IAP must be high and a significant stenosis may be the cause. In this case only the segment upstream from the stenosis does not collapse but the downstream segment does. This is a good clue to find the location of the stenosis.

An important cause of AVF maturation failure is the presence of accessory veins. They must be distinguished from collateral veins, which are pathological and develop in the presence of stenosis. The development of AV fistula depends on the inflow pressure and the resistance of draining veins. This resistance is decreased in the presence of side branch vessels (accessory veins), thus limiting the maturation of the AV fistula. Accessory veins may be single or multiple, but not all apparently decrease blood flow. When the fistula is occluded proximally, the thrill at the fistula should disappear. If it does not, an accessory vein may be providing an outflow channel. In this setting, palpation of the main vein below the site of the manual occlusion will reveal a thrill at the site of the accessory vein.

Another step is to check for pulse augmentation. With one hand, the body of the AV fistula is manually occluded proximally and with the other hand the pulse is palpated next to the anastomosis. With this maneuver, the pulse must become hyperpulsatile. If the pulse augments poorly, it is an indicator of low inflow. In this case, the arteries, anastomosis and juxta-anastomotic region should be evaluated. In cases where the pulse is already hyperpulsatile, the maneuver of pulse augmentation can be used to assess the severity of the stenosis. If there is no increase in pulse intensity, it means that the stenosis is severe, comparable to total occlusion. In contrast, when the intensity increases, the stenosis must be of lesser degree. Other physical signs such as swelling in the access arm and multiple subcutaneous collateral veins at the neck, shoulder and upper chest are highly suggestive of central vein stenosis.

PE may assist the interventionist during PTA. Findings as non-soft palpable pulse and non-continuous thrill at anastomosis may change after a successful procedure. In one report the authors concluded that the presence of a thrill or slightly pulsatile thrill at the venous part of a dialysis graft was a good predictor of outcome after percutaneous intervention [20]. Although this study was performed only with AVG, this information may be translated also for AVF interventions.

Surveillance

Intra-Access Static Pressures

In AVF, the IAP falls to about 20% of the systemic arterial pressure in the initial segment used for arterial needle puncture because of venous vessels capacitance. However, in a well-functioning AVG, the systemic arterial pressure is dissipated across the two anastomoses: 45% at the arterial and 25% at the venous end. In dysfunctional AVF, the IAPs tend to be lower than in grafts, making it more difficult to detect an appropriate increase. Notwithstanding the differences in pressure profiles between AVF and AVG, access flow rates tend to be quite similar when compared at similar anatomical locations [21]. When a stenosis develops in an AVF, the IAP may be stable because collateral channels (accessory or collateral veins) permit exit of the inflowing blood. Consequently the flow in the upstream segment may not change. Thus, it is important to identify these side branch veins in PE. By contrast, when stenosis develops in any segment of AVG the flow invariably decreases, because there are no collateral channels to dissipate the inflowing blood. As discussed above, theoretical considerations suggest that the measurement of IAP in AVF may not be as useful as for AVG.

For a reliable measure of IAP it must be normalized for mean arterial pressure [22]. It should be measured both in the arterial puncture site (aIAP) and venous puncture site (vIAP), because vIAP alone may fail to detect lesions located between the needles and in the juxta-anastomotic area and it is well known that in >70% of cases stenosis is located in these areas [23]. However, the last K/DOQI Vascular Access Work Group does not support the use of aIAP for use in AVF. We recently compared the results of aIAP in AVF with Doppler ultrasound. The measurement of aIAP did not demonstrate having a good relationship with the presence of stenosis (a sensitivity of only 60%) [19], nevertheless it is important to note that measurement of aIAP was performed at a single moment and not as multiple measurements as recommended. We believe that IAP, measured in arterial and venous sites, is extremely important when performed periodically and associated with other methods as PE and blood flow [24]. Thus, IAP monitoring cannot be recommended as the only method for surveillance of AVF at this time. Perhaps a hybrid program with other methods may be the choice [25]. IAP performed during AVF procedural and soon after may be useful to demonstrate a functional improvement after a successful PTA. In AVG, IAP measurements have proved to assist in hemodynamic assessment during angioplasty procedure [26].

IAP can be measured directly or indirectly. The indirect technique for measuring IAP uses HD machine equipment [22]. This technique uses the pressures from arterial pre-pump and venous post-pump drip chambers when the blood pump is turned off. The height distance from the AVF to the upper meniscus of the blood drip chamber is measured, converted into mm Hg and then added to the IAP value. Nevertheless, this methodology is time-consuming, requiring eleven separated steps to assure accuracy [1]. To simplify the process, the IAP can be measured directly with an aneroid pressure meter or a digital one.

Recirculation

Measurements of recirculation become a more useful screening tool for AVF than in AVG because blood flow in AVF, unlike AVG, can decrease to a level less than the prescribed HD machine pump flow ($<$300 ml/min), while maintaining access patency [27]. Because of that, this technique is not recommended as a surveillance test in grafts [2]. However, up to one third of dysfunctional AVF will show an increase in recirculation that may be manifested as a decrease in urea reduction ratio or Kt/V, but this occurs late [28, 29]. Measurement of access recirculation can be conducted using the urea-based method or one of the non-urea methods. Nevertheless, even with ideal sample timing and correct vein puncture, laboratory variability in urea-based measurement methods will produce variability in calculated recirculation [30]. Therefore, individual recirculation values $<$10% by using urea-based methods may be clinically unimportant. The K/DOQI Work Group does not recommend further evaluation. Values $>$10% by using urea-based recirculation measurement methods require investigation [2]. Other non-urea methods seem to be more accurate in determining the exact value of recirculation as ultrasound dilution technique [30], potassium and glucose-based dilutional methods [31, 32].

Blood Flow

An adequate AVF blood flow is a necessary part for a successful HD delivery dose. The volume of AVF blood flow represents the quality of a matured fistula. It is important to emphasize that the quality and physical dimensions of the artery and vein will determine the initial AVF function. If the artery is healthy, the flow capacity of the AVF will be determined by the characteristics of the vein used in access construction. Too small a vein will limit the flow [10]. AVFs constructed with proximal arteries have the capacity to deliver flows higher than distal AVFs. In general, forearm radiocephalic AVFs have flows of 600–1,000 ml/min, whereas proximal fistulas (brachiobasilic and brachiocephalic) have flows of 1,000–2,000 ml/min [33]. As an adequate blood flow predicts the high quality of a matured AVF, an inadequate flow may predict its dysfunction. It is important to emphasize that the successful maturation of AVF may be restricted by anatomical and acquired variables as: site of anastomosis, presence of lager diameter accessory veins, presence of disease in feeding artery and presence of fibrotic veins, absence of patient's ability to augment cardiac output in response to the new AVF. Nevertheless, the most important factor that blocks fistula maturation, reduces blood flow in a matured fistula and predisposes to thrombosis is the development of stenosis.

In native AVFs, inadequate flow through the access, originally caused by stenosis, is the primary functional defect that produces underdialysis and increases the probability of thrombosis. Although there is agreement that blood flow surveillance identifies stenosis in patients with AVF, the threshold value to conduct an intervention is debated. The K/DOQI Work Group recommends performing intervention when AVF blood flow is $<$500 ml/min [2]. In a study with 340 AVFs comparing different values of blood flow, the best threshold for significant stenosis diagnosis was 500 ml/min [34]. However, two other reports found higher values for stenosis detection [35] and for prediction of AVF thrombosis [36]. Thus, it seems that a single value may vary in different groups. A report which measured blood flow twice monthly found that younger patients, non-diabetics, higher systolic blood pressure and proximal AVFs were significantly associated with higher blood flow values [37]. Probably, multiple measurements and percent declines related to basal values offer a more realistic prediction of fistula thrombosis.

Blood flow measurements can be performed during HD as dilution ultrasound and other indirect techniques or by direct techniques as duplex Doppler ultrasound and magnetic resonance imaging [2]. However, because these last two methods are operator-related and have equipment-related limitations, sequential measurements have been used to detect and refer patients for interventions or predict the risk for thrombosis [38, 39]. In addition to flow measurements, both duplex Doppler ultrasound and magnetic resonance imaging provide anatomic assessment and direct evidence for the presence, location, and severity of access stenosis. However, the current cost of these methods, as well as the inability to make measurements during HD, limits their use. The current K/DOQI Work Group indicates that there is insufficient literature evidence to prefer one surveillance blood flow technique over the other [2].

Some studies have demonstrated the importance of blood flow surveillance to prolong AVF patency. One study compared AVF survival in a group followed by measurements of blood flow to another which was not. AVF thrombosis was lower in the group of blood flow surveillance (p = 0.024) [40]. Two other studies by the same group reported that prophylactic PTA in low blood flow AVF with diagnosis of significant stenosis improved survival of the access [41, 42]. Some information related to blood flow seems to be important for the interventionist. The degree of improvement in blood flow after PTA was the only variable associated with AVF patency in the same study mentioned before [42]. Following that, blood flow should be measured before and soon after an angioplasty, preferably by Doppler ultrasound, thus promoting valuable information about success of the procedure. Recently, one report of 580 PTAs in 190 AVFs found a significant negative correlation between the degree of stenosis and the preangioplasty blood flow. The only variable that correlated negative with postangioplasty blood flow was the number of stenosis in the same access [43].

Despite the recommendation of surveillance in AVF with the aim of reducing thrombosis, based on the above studies [2], some controversy has questioned the beneficial use of blood flow to reduce costs. One study noted that healthcare costs in HD patients with permanent access was reduced after implementation of blood flow surveillance, nevertheless the benefit was seen only for patients with AVG [44]. Another similar study demonstrated a reduction in cost, thrombosis, hospitalization and catheter placement for AVG as well as for AVF [45]. A report that tried to find the most economic blood flow threshold noted no benefits for both values when compared to no screening scenario [46]. However it is important to keep in mind that any preventive exposure to catheters will improve HD patients' healthcare and reduce morbidity.

Conclusion

Routine use of monitoring and surveillance methods for AVF such as PE and measurements of IAP and blood flow will reduce thrombosis and will improve quality of life in HD patients. All members of vascular access teams mostly recognize and interpret the findings of these techniques. Specifically, interventionists should interpret these methods just before and soon after the execution of PTA procedures. This action adds to successful procedures and prolongation of vascular access life.

References

1   NKF-K/DOQI Clinical Practice Guidelines for Vascular Access: Update 2000. Am J Kidney Dis 2001;37(suppl 1):S137–S181.
2   NKF-K/DOQI Clinical Practice Guidelines for Vascular Access: Update 2006. Am J Kidney Dis 2006;48(suppl 1):S176–S276.
3   Sehgal AR, Dor A, Tsai AC: Morbidity and cost implications of inadequate hemodialysis. Am J Kidney Dis 2001;37:1223–1231.
4   Hakim RM, Breyer J, Ismail N, Schulman G: Effects of dose of dialysis on morbidity and mortality. Am J Kidney Dis 1994;23:661–669.
5   Oliver MJ, Rothwell DM, Fung K, Hux JE, Lok CE: Late creation of vascular access for hemodialysis and increased risk of sepsis. J Am Soc Nephrol 2004;15:1936–1942.
6   Lok CE: Fistula first initiative: advantages and pitfalls. Clin J Am Soc Nephrol 2007;2:1043–1053.
7   Rayner HC, Pisoni RL, Gillespie BW, Goodkin DA, Akiba T, Akizawa T, Saito A, Young EW, Port FK: Creation, cannulation and survival of arteriovenous fistulae: data from the Dialysis Outcomes and Practice Patterns Study. Kidney Int 2003;63:323–330.
8   Schon D, Blume SW, Niebauer K, Hollenbeak CS, de Lissovoy G: Increasing the use of arteriovenous fistula in hemodialysis: economic benefits and economic barriers. Clin J Am Soc Nephrol 2007;2:268–276.
9   Allon M, Bailey R, Ballard R, Deierhoi MH, Hamrick K, Oser R, Rhynes VK, Robbin ML, Saddekni S, Zeigler ST: A multidisciplinary approach to hemodialysis access: prospective evaluation. Kidney Int 1998;53:473–479.
10   Besarab A, Asif A, Roy-Chaudhury P, Spergel LM, Ravani P: The native arteriovenous fistula in 2007. Surveillance and monitoring. J Nephrol 2007;20:656–667.
11   Robbin ML, Chamberlain NE, Lockhart ME, Gallichio MH, Young CJ, Deierhoi MH, Allon M: Hemodialysis arteriovenous fistula maturity: US evaluation. Radiology 2002;225:59–64.
12   Asif A, Cherla G, Merrill D, Cipleu CD, Briones P, Pennell P: Conversion of tunneled hemodialysis catheter-consigned patients to arteriovenous fistula. Kidney Int 2005;67:2399–2406.
13   Beathard GA, Arnold P, Jackson J, Litchfield T: Aggressive treatment of early fistula failure. Kidney Int 2003;64:1487–1494.
14   Beathard GA: Physical examination of the dialysis vascular access. Semin Dial 1998;11:231–236.
15   Safa AA, Valji K, Roberts AC, Ziegler TW, Hye RJ, Oglevie SB: Detection and treatment of dysfunctional hemodialysis access grafts: effect of a surveillance program on graft patency and the incidence of thrombosis. Radiology 1996;199:653–657.
16   Malik J, Slavikova M, Malikova H, Maskova J: Many clinically silent access stenoses can be identified by ultrasonography. J Nephrol 2002;15:661–665.
17   Beathard GA: Physical examination of AV grafts. Semin Dial 1996;5:74.
18   Asif A, Leon C, Orozco-Vargas LC, Krishnamurthy G, Choi KL, Mercado C, Merrill D, Thomas I, Salman L, Artikov S, Bourgoignie JJ: Accuracy of physical examination in the detection of arteriovenous fistula stenosis. Clin J Am Soc Nephrol 2007;2:1191–1194.
19   Campos RP, Chula DC, Perreto S, Riella MC, Nascimento MM: Accuracy of physical examination and intra-access pressure in the detection of stenosis in hemodialysis arteriovenous fistula. Semin Dial 2008 (in press).
20   Trerotola SO, Ponce P, Stavropoulos SW, Clark TW, Tuite CM, Mondschein JI, Shlansky-Goldberg R, Freiman DB, Patel AA, Soulen MC, Cohen R, Wasserstein A, Chittams JL: Physical examination versus normalized pressure ratio for predicting outcomes of hemodialysis access interventions. J Vasc Interv Radiol 2003;14:1387–1394.
21   Besarab A: Advances in end-stage renal diseases 2000. Access monitoring methods. Blood Purif 2000;18:255–259.

22   Besarab A, Frinak S, Sherman RA, Goldman J, Dumler F, Devita MV, Kapoian T, Al-Saghir F, Lubkowski T: Simplified measurement of intra-access pressure. J Am Soc Nephrol 1998;9: 284–289.

23   Turmel-Rodrigues L, Pengloan J, Rodrigue H, Brillet G, Lataste A, Pierre D, Jourdan JL, Blanchard D: Treatment of failed native arteriovenous fistulae for hemodialysis by interventional radiology. Kidney Int 2000;57:1124–1140.

24   Campos RP, Do Nascimento MM, Chula DC, Do Nascimento DE, Riella MC: Stenosis in hemodialysis arteriovenous fistula: evaluation and treatment. Hemodial Int 2006;10:152–161.

25   Besarab A: Preventing vascular access dysfunction: which policy to follow. Blood Purif 2002; 20:26–35.

26   Asif A, Besarab A, Gadalean F, Merrill D, Rismeyer AE, Contreras G, Leclercq B, Lenz O, Wallach J, Wallach J, Levine MI: Utility of static pressure ratio recording during angioplasty of arteriovenous graft stenosis. Semin Dial 2006;19:551–556.

27   Besarab A, Sherman R: The relationship of recirculation to access blood flow. Am J Kidney Dis 1997;29:223–229.

28   Besarab A, Lubkowski T, Frinak S, Ramanathan S, Escobar F: Detecting vascular access dysfunction. ASAIO J 1997;43:M539–M543.

29   Besarab A, Lubkowski T, Frinak S, Ramanathan S, Escobar F: Detection of access strictures and outlet stenoses in vascular accesses. Which test is best? ASAIO J 1997;43:M543–M547.

30   Hester RL, Curry E, Bower J: The determination of hemodialysis blood recirculation using blood urea nitrogen measurements. Am J Kidney Dis 1992;20:598–602.

31   Brancaccio D, Tessitore N, Carpani P, Gammaro L, Losi B, Zoni U, Maschio G, Gallieni M: Potassium-based dilutional method to measure hemodialysis access recirculation. Int J Artif Organs 2001;24:606–613.

32   Magnasco A, Alloatti S, Bonfant G, Copello F, Solari P: Glucose infusion test: a new screening test for vascular access recirculation. Kidney Int 2000;57:2123–2128.

33   Begin V, Ethier J, Dumont M, Leblanc M: Prospective evaluation of the intra-access flow of recently created native arteriovenous fistulae. Am J Kidney Dis 2002;40:1277–1282.

34   Tonelli M, Jhangri GS, Hirsch DJ, Marryatt J, Mossop P, Wile C, Jindal KK: Best threshold for diagnosis of stenosis or thrombosis within six months of access flow measurement in arteriovenous fistulae. J Am Soc Nephrol 2003;14:3264–3269.

35   Tessitore N, Bedogna V, Gammaro L, Lipari G, Poli A, Baggio E, Firpo M, Morana G, Mansueto G, Maschio G: Diagnostic accuracy of ultrasound dilution access blood flow measurement in detecting stenosis and predicting thrombosis in native forearm arteriovenous fistulae for hemodialysis. Am J Kidney Dis 2003;42:331–341.

36   Basile C, Ruggieri G, Vernaglione L, Montanaro A, Giordano R: The natural history of autogenous radiocephalic wrist arteriovenous fistulas of haemodialysis patients: a prospective observational study. Nephrol Dial Transplant 2004;19:1231–1236.

37   Tonelli M, Hirsch DJ, Chan CT, Marryatt J, Mossop P, Wile C, Jindal K: Factors associated with access blood flow in native vessel arteriovenous fistulae. Nephrol Dial Transplant 2004;19: 2559–2563.

38   Grogan J, Castilla M, Lozanski L, Griffin A, Loth F, Bassiouny H: Frequency of critical stenosis in primary arteriovenous fistulae before hemodialysis access: should duplex ultrasound surveillance be the standard of care? J Vasc Surg 2005;41:1000–1006.

39   Duijm LE, Liem YS, van der Rijt RH, Nobrega FJ, van den Bosch HC, Douwes-Draaijer P, Cuypers PW, Tielbeek AV: Inflow stenoses in dysfunctional hemodialysis access fistulae and grafts. Am J Kidney Dis 2006;48:98–105.

40   Roca-Tey R, Samon Guasch R, Ibrik O, Garcia-Madrid C, Herranz JJ, Garcia-Gonzalez L, Viladoms Guerra J: Vascular access surveillance with blood flow monitoring: a prospective study with 65 patients. Nefrologia 2004;24:246–252.

41   Tessitore N, Mansueto G, Bedogna V, Lipari G, Poli A, Gammaro L, Baggio E, Morana G, Loschiavo C, Laudon A, Oldrizzi L, Maschio G: A prospective controlled trial on effect of percutaneous transluminal angioplasty on functioning arteriovenous fistulae survival. J Am Soc Nephrol 2003;14:1623–1627.

42   Tessitore N, Lipari G, Poli A, Bedogna V, Baggio E, Loschiavo C, Mansueto G, Lupo A: Can blood flow surveillance and pre-emptive repair of subclinical stenosis prolong the useful life of arteriovenous fistulae? A randomized controlled study. Nephrol Dial Transplant 2004;19:2325–2333.
43   Monroy-Cuadros M, Salazar A, Yilmaz S, McLaughlin K: Native arteriovenous fistulas: correlation of intra-access blood flow with characteristics of stenoses found during diagnostic angiography. Semin Dial 2008;21:89–92.
44   Wijnen E, Planken N, Keuter X, Kooman JP, Tordoir JH, de Haan MW, Leunissen KM, van der Sande F: Impact of a quality improvement programme based on vascular access flow monitoring on costs, access occlusion and access failure. Nephrol Dial Transplant 2006;21:3514–3519.
45   McCarley P, Wingard RL, Shyr Y, Pettus W, Hakim RM, Ikizler TA: Vascular access blood flow monitoring reduces access morbidity and costs. Kidney Int 2001;60:1164–1172.
46   Tonelli M, Klaarenbach S, Jindal K, Manns B: Economic implications of screening strategies in arteriovenous fistulae. Kidney Int 2006;69:2219–2226.

Miguel C. Riella, MD, PhD
Renal Division, Evangelic School of Medicine
Rua Bruno Filgueira 369, Curitiba 80240-220 (Brazil)
Tel. +55 41 3342 5849, Fax +55 41 3244 5539, E-Mail mcriella@pro-renal.org.br

Ronco C, Cruz DN (eds): Hemodialysis – From Basic Research to Clinical Trials.
Contrib Nephrol. Basel, Karger, 2008, vol 161, pp 23–29

······················

Preoperative Hemodialysis Fistula Evaluation: Angiography, Ultrasonography and Other Studies, Are They Useful?

William F. Weitzel

University of Michigan, Department of Internal Medicine, Division of Nephrology,
102 Observatory, 312 Simpson Memorial Institute, Ann Arbor, Mich., USA

Abstract

Background: There is increasing emphasis on optimizing fistula use for end-stage renal disease patients. Although early referral and strategies for vein preservation are clearly important, imaging modalities have assumed an ever-increasing role in preoperative vascular access assessment and management. **Methods/Results:** Review of available literature demonstrates angiography and ultrasonography provide anatomic information useful in diagnostic decision-making in many clinical settings. Targeted clinical programs can increase fistula use, and various practice patterns have emerged to achieve this goal depending on the available expertise, center-dependent experience, and differing patient populations. In recent years there have been a series of studies evaluating provocative maneuvers assessing vascular mechanics that attempt to increase the predictive power of imaging modalities. Assessing arterial and venous mechanics may help predict outcomes and assist in preoperative planning. **Conclusion:** In the quest to optimize fistula use, study results examining the value of angiography and ultrasonography demonstrate that there is currently no universal application of specific cut-offs on vessel diameter or even measures of distensibility and vessel mechanics. It is clear, however, that implementing programs that include imaging to increase fistula creation do achieve their goal. Conversely, in other settings, fistula failure rates have increased without significantly increasing the numbers of fistulae. The impact of preoperative diagnostic angiography and ultrasonography rests in part on identifying the underlying disease process involving arteries and veins that may change treatment decisions preoperatively. In many clinical settings where the dialysis population is becoming increasingly elderly, diabetic and with more vascular disease, these additional studies may be very useful. Given the variation in clinical study outcome and variations in patient populations, presently these methods will be used most effectively in the setting of strong quality assurance programs, and wherever feasible under study protocols for the purpose of improving practice patterns.

Copyright © 2008 S. Karger AG, Basel

This work was supported in part by NIH grant DK62848.

There is increasing emphasis on optimizing fistula use for end-stage renal disease (ESRD) patients. Although early referral and strategies for vein preservation clearly play a role, imaging modalities have assumed an ever-increasing role in the preoperative vascular access assessment and management [1]. Angiography and ultrasonography provide anatomic information, and in the last several years there have been an interesting series of studies evaluating provocative maneuvers that attempt to increase the predictive power of imaging modalities. Assessing arterial and venous mechanics may help predict outcomes in fistula creation and assist in preoperative planning, which has been the motivation for much of the recent work in ultrasound-based measurement methods. While targeted clinical programs can increase fistula use [2, 3], various practice patterns have emerged to achieve this goal depending on the available expertise, center-dependent experience, and differing patient populations.

Angiography

Although most programs use combinations of angiography and ultrasonography, vascular access programs have been successful in maximizing fistula creation, even in catheter-dependent patients, when practice patterns rely solely on contrast angiography [3]. In particular, contrast venography has been an extremely helpful tool, providing anatomic information along the course of the vessel both in the extremity and throughout the central vasculature. While respiration-induced peripheral venous flow variations that depend on central anatomy can be diagnosed by ultrasonography [4], angiography has the advantage over ultrasonography in providing detailed anatomic information of the central vessels. Angiography is therefore of the utmost importance in preoperative evaluation of central vessel stenosis. Even though the practice has shifted away from subclavian vein catheter use toward internal jugular catheters, innominate vein stenosis may still be problematic and venography provides accurate diagnostic information [2, 5].

Arteriography typically has been reserved for patients where the suspicion for arterial disease is high. Importantly, at least one study prospectively used arterial imaging in all consenting subjects (81% of 139 subjects) undergoing preoperative evaluation for vascular access [2]. In this series, 30% of subjects were found to have significant forearm arterial occlusive disease, defined as >50% luminal narrowing. Invasive studies (arteriography and venography) led to a change in operative plan based on non-invasive (ultrasound) studies in 19% of subjects, with half of these exhibiting a radial artery unsuitable for fistula creation. Even with this invasive arterial assessment, ischemia developed in 8% of subjects. While clearly arteriography should be used selectively in patients undergoing fistula creation, these findings and others highlight the importance of assessing arterial disease in ESRD [1, 4].

Because predialysis ESRD patients are susceptible to contrast nephropathy, attempts are made to minimize contrast exposure for these studies [1] and alternatives to iodinated contrast, namely carbon dioxide and gadolinium, have been used. However, there is increasing concern over the role of gadolinium-based contrast agents in nephrogenic systemic fibrosis [6]. It should be noted that several recently published reports mention the use of gadolinium as a viable contrast alternative without cautioning about this risk.

Ultrasonography

Over the last decade there has been a groundswell of interest in preoperative ultrasonography for dialysis vascular access. This was stimulated initially by the ease and safety of ultrasonography in providing anatomic information about peripheral vessels. In addition, many practitioners find ultrasound an easy extension of the physical examination process normally carried out at the time of the preoperative encounter. Beyond anatomic information, however, the ultrasound allows rapid assessment of changes in the vasculature anatomy in response to various maneuvers, stimulating tremendous interest in improving diagnostic test performance as part of the preoperative assessment.

Arterial Assessment

Numerous studies have evaluated the radial artery diameter preoperatively to assess the use of this parameter in predicting outcome and therefore potentially using it in preoperative decision-making. For radiocephalic arteriovenous fistulae, many studies have found increased failure of fistulae to mature when the radial artery is less than a threshold value ranging from 1.5 to 2.1 mm [4, 7, 8]. It is important to recognize however that success rates may still be 50% in some populations even with radial arteries <1.5 mm [8] and creating an arteriovenous anastomosis may be appropriate even when success is far from certain in some clinical situations. For example, in a patient with sufficient lead time before initiating dialysis, the arterial and venous dilation resulting from the construction of a wrist fistula, in the event that it is inadequate for dialysis, may be helpful in preparing the patient for a staged procedure or more proximal fistula in the future. Interestingly, one analysis of prospectively collected data found the greatest one year patency of radiocephalic fistulae with preoperative radial artery diameters between 2.1 and 2.5 mm [7]. While the authors concluded that a single radial artery cut-off cannot be recommended, these results highlight the importance of including other factors in conjunction with radial artery diameter in predicting success. It should be noted that other arterial ultrasound characteristics are often reported but less well quantified such as arterial wall echogenicity or irregularity [4]. Perhaps the most appropriate conclusion is that diameter is one factor influencing the success of fistula creation to be used in conjunction with others for individualized treatment decision-making.

In addition to diameter, another interesting diagnostic maneuver that may be helpful is assessing the artery's propensity to dilate in response to clenching the fist [4]. However, another study suggested this maneuver was less predictive in a different population with subgroup analysis showing it to be more predictive in women compared to men [9]. Despite conflicting study results, this type of provocative test is extremely interesting. It is known for example that a dramatic increase in fistula volume flow, perhaps 50% of the eventual volume flow [10], occurs within a day of fistula construction [8, 10]. The diameter changes in response to fistula construction are followed by further changes in fistula flow over the remaining weeks related to subsequent vessel remodeling. While numerous factors influence fistula outcome, arterial mechanics and propensity to dilate appear to be reasonable candidates for further study.

Underlying vascular disease which leads to reduced vascular compliance may potentially be assessed by intima media thickness of the radial artery measured by ultrasound, which was more strongly associated with fistula failure than was the preoperative inner diameter of the radial artery [11]. It has also long been known that arterial mechanics are complex and highly non-linear and in order to fully characterize the non-linear arterial mechanics in health and disease, distensibility should be measured over a range of physiologic pressures [12]. We have been evaluating phase-sensitive ultrasound speckle tracking as a means of analyzing vascular mechanics with high resolution and accuracy [12] and found that non-linear ultrasound strain measurements of brachial arteries differ widely when normal subjects are compared with those with renal failure and diabetes (fig. 1). This method [12] is currently being evaluated in a prospective study to evaluate fistula outcome. Improved arterial assessment may not only predict fistula flow or successful cannulation for dialysis, but may also help stratify risk for ischemic complications, as supported by preoperative digital pressures and digital brachial indices <1.0 being predictive of higher risk of arterial steal [1]. So, while results vary, there are both considerable data suggesting the utility of anatomic information as well as emerging tools to measure arterial mechanics. Additional study will need to focus on the patient populations where these tools are most helpful in clinical decision-making, as well as continuing to test hypotheses that make use of vascular mechanics that may be predictive of clinical outcome.

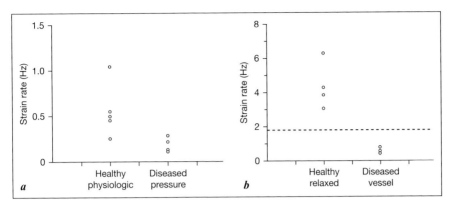

Fig. 1. High-resolution ultrasound speckle tracking is used to measure the peak brachial artery compliance (strain rate) and shows a typical non-linear pattern with vessels being more rigid at maximal distension with lower strain rates (*a*) partly distinguishing normal from ESRD with diabetes. However, the high degree of non-linearity of the stress-strain relationship is demonstrated by complete separation between normal and ESRD with diabetes when the vessel is relaxed and more compliant to achieve higher strain rates (*b*) using methods of pressure equalization.

Venous Assessment

Multiple studies have assessed the vein size as a predictor of fistula outcome, with larger vein diameter associated with improved outcome and thresholds ranging from 2.0 to 3.0 mm [2, 13] with varying attention paid to vein dilation with either blood pressure cuff or tourniquet. The propensity of the vein to dilate may reasonably be expected to be a predictor of outcome, and the occluding pressures used to assess vein dilation have ranged from 40 to 80 mm Hg (or uncertain occluding pressures when a tourniquet is applied). One study analyzed the propensity of the vein to dilate in response to degrees of venous occlusion and suggested outcome could be related to measures of vein distensibility assessed by strain gauge plethysmography [14]. The ratio of changes in forearm volume to cuff pressures ranging from 0 to 60 mm Hg was assessed using a linear regression of the data. Interestingly, examination of vein distesibility [14, 15] shows a non-linear stress strain relationship as expected from theory and practice and seen with detailed assessment of arteries [12]. While this may eventually prove to be very helpful, recent information about the reproducibility of ultrasound vein imaging to assess distensibility of individual veins, even using large pressure ranges from 10 to 80 mm Hg [15], indicates improvements in standardization of these tests is needed for them to be used routinely in clinical practice.

Conclusion

In the quest to optimize fistula use, study results examining the value of angiography and ultrasonography do lead one to conclude that there is currently no universal application of specific cut-offs on vessel anatomy or even measures of distensibility and vessel mechanics. It is clear, however, that implementing programs that include imaging to increase fistula creation do achieve their goal [2, 3]. Conversely, we also must recognize the unintended consequences seen in other settings where failure rates increased without significantly increasing fistula rates [13]. There are many patient-specific medical history and examination findings useful for access planning and the impact of preoperative diagnostic angiography and ultrasonography studies rests in part on identifying the underlying disease process involving arteries and veins that may change treatment decisions prior to surgery. Preoperative evaluation with imaging may include anatomic information and measures assessing both the artery and vein propensity to dilate sufficiently to develop into a functional access. In most clinical settings where the dialysis population is becoming increasingly elderly, diabetic and with more vascular disease, these additional studies may be very useful. Given the variation in clinical study outcome and variations in patient populations, presently these methods will most effectively be used in the setting of strong quality assurance programs, and wherever feasible under study protocols for the purpose of improving practice patterns.

References

1   Tordoir J, Canaud B, Haage P, Konner K, Basci A, Denis Fouque D, Kooman J, Martin-Malo A, Pedrini L, Pizzarelli F, Tattersall J, Vennegoor M, Wanner C, Wee P, Vanholder R: EBPG on vascular access. Nephrol Dial Transplant 2007;22(suppl 2):ii88–ii117.

2   Huber TS, Ozaki CK, Flynn TC, Lee WA, Berceli SA, Hirneise CM, Carlton LM, Carter JW, Ross EA, Seeger JM: Prospective validation of an algorithm to maximize native arteriovenous fistulae for chronic hemodialysis access. J Vasc Surg 2002;36:452–459.

3   Asif A, Cherla G, Merrill D, Cipleu CD, Briones P, Pennell P: Conversion of tunneled hemodialysis catheter-consigned patients to arteriovenous fistula. Kidney Int 2005;67:2399–2406.

4   Malovrh M: Native arteriovenous fistula: preoperative evaluation. Am J Kidney Dis 2002;39: 1218–1225.

5   Karakayali F, Ekici Y, Görür SK, Arat Z, Boyvat F, Karakayali H, Haberal M: The value of preoperative vascular imaging in the selection and success of hemodialysis access. Ann Vasc Surg 2007;21:481–489.

6   Grobner T, Prischl FC: Patient characteristics and risk factors for nephrogenic systemic fibrosis following gadolinium exposure. Semin Dial 2008;DOI: 10.1111/j.1525-139X.2007.00406.

7   Korten E, Toonder IM, Schrama YC, Hop WCJ, van der Ham AC, Wittens CHA: Dialysis fistulae patency and preoperative diameter ultrasound measurements. Eur J Vasc Endovasc Surg 2007;33: 467–471.

8   Parmar J, Aslam M, Standfield N: Preoperative radial arterial diameter predicts early failure of arteriovenous fistula for haemodialysis. Eur J Vasc Endovasc Surg 2007;33:113–115.

9   Lockhart ME, Robbin ML, Allon M: Preoperative sonographic radial artery evaluation and corre-
    lation with subsequent radiocephalic fistula outcome. J Ultrasound Med 2004;23:161–168.
10 Lomonte C, Casucci F, Antonelli M, Giammaria B, Losurdo N, Marchio G, Basile C: Is there a
    place for duplex screening of the brachial artery in the maturation of arteriovenous fistulas? Semin
    Dial 2005;18:243–246.
11 Ku YM, Kim YO, Kim JI, Choi YJ, Yoon SA, Kim YS, Song SW, Yang CW, Chang YS, Bang BK:
    Ultrasonographic measurement of intima-media thickness of radial artery in pre-dialysis uraemic
    patients: comparison with histological examination. Nephrol Dial Transplant 2006;21:715–720.
12 Weitzel WF, Kim K, Rubin JM, Xie H, O'Donnell M: Renal advances in ultrasound elasticity
    imaging: measuring the compliance of arteries and kidneys in end-stage renal disease. Blood Purif
    2005;23:10–17.
13 Patel ST, Hughes J, Mills JL: Failure of arteriovenous fistula maturation: An unintended conse-
    quence of exceeding dialysis outcome quality initiative guidelines for hemodialysis access. J Vasc
    Surg 2003;38:439–445.
14 Van der Linden J, Lameris TW, van den Meiracker AH, de Smet AAEA, Blankestijn PJ, van den
    Dorpel MA: Forearm venous distensibility predicts successful arteriovenous fistula. Am J Kidney
    Dis 2006;47:1013–1019.
15 Planken RN, Keuter XH, Kessels AG, Hoeks AP, Leiner T, Tordoir JH: Forearm cephalic vein
    cross-sectional area changes at incremental congestion pressures: towards a standardized and
    reproducible vein mapping protocol. J Vasc Surg 2006;44:353–358.

William F. Weitzel, MD
University of Michigan, Department of Internal Medicine
Division of Nephrology, 102 Observatory, 312 Simpson Memorial Institute
Ann Arbor, Michigan, USA 48109-5725 (USA)
Tel. +1 734 615 3994, Fax +1 734 615 4887, E-Mail weitzel@umich.edu

Ronco C, Cruz DN (eds): Hemodialysis – From Basic Research to Clinical Trials.
Contrib Nephrol. Basel, Karger, 2008, vol 161, pp 30–38

....

Endovascular Procedures

Arif Asif

Section of Interventional Nephrology, Division of Nephrology, University of Miami
Leonard A. Miller School of Medicine, Miami, Fla., USA

Abstract

Vascular access-related procedures commonly performed by nephrologists include percutaneous balloon angioplasty, intravascular coil and stent insertion, thrombectomy, vascular mapping and tunneled hemodialysis catheter-related procedures. In addition, using vein obliteration and percutaneous balloon angioplasty techniques, nephrologists have recently documented successful salvage of arteriovenous fistulas that had failed to mature, whereas traditionally these fistulas have frequently been abandoned. While the performance of these procedures by nephrologists offers many advantages, appropriate training in order to develop the necessary procedural skills is critical. Recent data have emphasized that a nephrologist can be successfully trained to become a competent interventionalist. In addition to documenting excellent outcome data, multiple reports have demonstrated the safety and success of interventional nephrology. This report focuses on hemodialysis access-related procedures performed by nephrologists and calls for a proactive approach in optimizing this aspect of patient care.

Vascular access dysfunction contributes to the morbidity and mortality of patients who depend on this form of renal replacement therapy [1]. Therefore, the manner in which vascular access procedures are performed has a major effect on the quality of the overall medical care delivered to the dialysis patient. For example, delaying a thrombectomy for an occluded vascular access has adverse consequences. First, with elapsed time the thrombus can become more resistant to thrombectomy [2]. Second, and of greater importance, the necessity for a dialysis treatment during the period of delay may result in the insertion of a temporary catheter. This subjects the patient to an unnecessary procedure, the potentially life-threatening complications associated with catheter use, and the additional costs associated with catheter use, which may include a period of hospitalization.

Over the past decade, significant advances have been made by nephrologists in the performance of hemodialysis access-related procedures [3–15].

Because of their training and experience, nephrologists have a unique clinical perspective on vascular access-related issues, renal disease, renal replacement therapy, and dialysis outcomes. This perspective makes them ideally suited to perform vascular access-related procedures. Recent data have emphasized that nephrologists can assume a greater role in the procedural aspect of vascular access, providing effective, efficient, and safe treatment [3–10, 12–15].

The purpose of this report is to review a variety of vascular access-related procedures performed by nephrologists, including angioplasty for venous stenosis, treatment of thrombosed vascular access, salvage of undeveloped arteriovenous fistulas (AVFs), management of tunneled dialysis catheters, and other related procedures. In addition, it calls for a proactive role by nephrologists in optimizing this aspect of patient care.

Percutaneous balloon angioplasty has become a standard treatment for the management of arteriovenous dialysis access (graft and fistula) stenosis [3, 16, 17]. This is due in part to an improvement in the ability to predict the presence of vascular access stenosis prospectively through access monitoring and surveillance [1, 18]. It is also due to the fact that the technique has been demonstrated to be safe, easily performed, and effective.

Percutaneous Balloon Angioplasty

Percutaneous balloon angioplasty for access stenosis is an outpatient procedure that does not prohibit the immediate use of the access for dialysis. There is minimal to no blood loss, hospitalization is avoided, and there is rarely any postprocedure discomfort for the patient. Lesions in all locations within the access system (venous, arterial, and central) can be easily, effectively, and safely treated. Its only disadvantages are that there are occasional lesions that do not respond to treatment and the results obtained are not permanent.

Both arteriovenous grafts (AVGs) and AVFs may develop vascular stenosis. However, arteriovenous dialysis grafts are prone to problems, early and recurrently. The pathophysiologic mechanisms of stenosis are complex, however neointimal hyperplasia appears to play a pivotal role [19, 20]. Stenosis occurs most frequently at the venous anastomosis (60%), but may occur anywhere within the feeding artery, the arterial anastomosis, graft and the draining veins, both peripheral and central. In addition, in a given patient, stenotic lesions can exist as single or multiple.

Access stenosis should be treated if the stenosis is ≥50% and is associated with clinical or physiologic abnormalities such as a previous thrombotic episode, elevated venous dialysis pressure, abnormal recirculation test, abnormal physical findings, unexplained decrease in the measured dialysis dose, and decreased access flow. The abnormal clinical parameters used to suspect the presence of stenosis should return to within acceptable limits following intervention. In a series of 1,120 cases of venous stenosis treated by angioplasty, the initial success rate was reported to be 94% [21]. Primary (unassisted) patency determined by lifetable analysis was as follows: 1 month, 87.4%; 2 months, 84.8%; 3 months, 77.2%; 6 months, 66.4%; 1 year, 44.5%. These results are comparable to those reported by interventional radiology [22, 23].

Identification of a poorly functioning vascular access and correction of stenoses results in prolonged survival of the access, increased blood flow, and a decrease in access thrombosis, access replacement, hospitalization related to vascular access, access-related missed dialysis days, and decreased cost for thrombosis-related events [9, 24–29]. A nephrologist can effectively establish a surveillance program to monitor vascular access function, identify the failing access, and perform percutaneous intervention to correct stenosis and maintain a healthy vascular access and avoid access failure. Indeed, vascular stenosis is a major cause of thrombosis resulting in access failure and must be corrected promptly [9].

A significant number (10–25%) of AVFs do not adequately develop and fail to sustain dialysis therapy [30–35]. Recent data have classified fistula failure into early and late failure [7]. Early failure refers to the fistula that never develops to the point where it can be used or fails within 3 months of successful use. In contrast, late failure denotes failure after 3 months of successful use. Traditionally these undeveloped fistulas were abandoned. Unpublished data from our center have shown that failed fistulas were frequently not studied properly and either failed or were converted to AVGs.

Recently, Beathard et al. [7] provided invaluable information regarding how to improve the function of an AVF that is not developing properly. In their prospective observational study, 100 patients with early failure underwent evaluation and treatment at six free-standing outpatient vascular access centers. Vascular stenosis and the presence of a significant accessory vein (an accessory vein is described as a branch coming off the main venous channel that comprised the fistula) alone or in combination were found to be the culprits. Venous stenosis was present in 78% of the cases. A majority of these lesions (48%) were found to be close to the anastomosis (a juxta-anastomotic lesion). A significant accessory vein was present in 46% of the cases. Percutaneous balloon angioplasty and accessory vein obliteration using any of the three techniques (percutaneous ligation using 3/0 nylon, venous cutdown, coil insertion) were used to salvage the failed fistulas. Angioplasty was performed with a 98% success rate and vein obliteration with a 100% success rate. After intervention, it was possible to initiate dialysis using the fistula in 92% of the cases. Actuarial lifetable analysis showed that 84% were functional at 3 months, 72% at 6 months, and 68% at 12 months. Other nephrologists have described a percutaneous technique for accessory vein ligation of AVFs that failed to achieve adequate blood flow or size for successful cannulation [6].

By the use of an aggressive approach and employment of two basic techniques – balloon angioplasty and vein obliteration – nephrologists can successfully salvage and subsequently utilize an otherwise failed fistula. The diagnosis of a failed fistula can easily be made during a routine examination for abnormal physical findings seen in vascular stenosis and the presence of accessory veins. It has been suggested that such an examination be performed 4 weeks after fistula creation [3]. Any fistula that fails to mature adequately and demonstrates abnormal physical findings must be studied angiographically and possibly corrected before a plan to create a new access is made. The most common form of permanent dialysis access in the United States is the AVG [36]. The most common complications associated with AVGs are stenosis and thrombosis. Since the most common cause of access thrombosis is stenosis, these should not be considered separate problems. Venous stenosis and access thrombosis share the relationship of cause and effect. Indeed, the frequency of stenosis identified at thrombolysis has been found to exceed 90% [9].

Thrombectomy Procedure

Nephrologists routinely perform thrombolysis procedures for clotted arteriovenous hemodialysis accesses [4, 5, 8, 9]. Both mechanical and pharmaco-mechanical thrombolysis for the treatment of a thrombosed dialysis access can be successfully performed by nephrologists [5, 8, 9]. Although the initial success rate (95%) of thrombectomy procedure of an AVG is similar to the angioplasty procedure, primary patency rates after declotting of a clotted vascular access are markedly reduced when compared to the primary patency following angioplasty of access stenosis. In a prospective analysis of 1,176 cases, 3-, 6-, and 12-month primary patency following mechanical thrombolysis of thrombosed grafts was found to be 52, 39, and 17%, respectively [9]. These results are comparable to those reported by interventional radiology [2, 22, 23]. In addition to an AVG, an AVF can also be declotted. However, initial success is less than what is observed for an AVG.

Thrombosis leading to access failure is a major issue. It often causes unnecessary hospitalization, missed dialysis, frustration on the part of the dialysis staff and patients, and exposes the patient to temporary catheters. Ideally, this complication should be managed rapidly, under local anesthesia, and on an outpatient basis. Recent data have clearly shown that such care is being delivered successfully by nephrologists in many centers on an outpatient basis [3–5, 9]. Nevertheless, aggressive detection and early correction of hemodialysis access stenosis is of utmost importance to decrease graft thrombosis and improve access survival.

Tunneled Hemodialysis Catheter Procedures

Percutaneously placed, cuffed, tunneled hemodialysis catheters and subcutaneous hemodialysis ports have greatly expanded the range of treatment options for the end-stage renal disease patient. Cuffed, tunneled hemodialysis catheters are commonly used as a bridge access to allow time for placement or maturation of a permanent vascular access (AVF, AVG). In addition, they may be used as a temporary access for hemodialysis for patients with acute renal failure. Finally, tunneled catheters may also be used as a permanent vascular access for patients who have exhausted all other options to receive hemodialysis. Traditionally these catheters were placed by surgeons and followed by interventional radiologists [36]. However, nephrologists have recently begun performing this procedure both on an inpatient as well as outpatient basis [10, 12–14]. In addition to catheter insertion, catheter exchange, and catheter removal procedures, nephrologists are also engaged in developing optimal catheter designs to achieve adequate blood flow to sustain dialysis treatment [14].

Tunneled catheters play a major role in the delivery of hemodialysis therapy to a large portion of the dialysis population [36]. However, their use is associated with many complications [15, 37–40]. In addition to catheter-related infection, fibroepithelial sheath formation is associated with these catheters and leads to catheter malfunction and occlusion [15, 40]. A recent study [40] evaluating 947 cases of catheter dysfunction (inability to sustain a blood flow >300 ml/min) documented that fibrin was detected in 368 cases (38.8%). The presence of a fibrin sheath was determined at the time of exchange using radiocontrast material administered through the venous port of the old catheter. In this study, an angioplasty balloon catheter was inserted on a guidewire through the catheter tunnel, and thus through the lumen of the fibrin sheath, and was then inflated to disrupt the fibroepithelial sheath. The investigators used an 8-mm diameter balloon, with a 100% success rate. Removal of the sheath was confirmed by a repeat radiocontrast injection when the new catheter was inserted. Catheter blood flow rates sufficient for dialysis were achieved in 99% of patients.

The presence of a fibrin sheath is a relatively common cause of tunneled catheter dysfunction [15, 40]. Nephrologists can successfully manage this complication on an outpatient basis by using percutaneous balloon angioplasty and over-the-wire catheter exchange techniques.

While the performance of vascular access-related procedures by nephrologists is a significant step toward optimal care of hemodialysis patients, at the same time a critical analysis of procedure-related complications when performed by nephrologists must be included. Indeed, providing procedural care in a timely fashion and minimizing complication rates are the primary goals. Recently, Beathard and Litchfield [41] reported on the complications of endovascular procedures. To date, this is the largest prospective series (n = 14,047) reported for arteriovenous hemodialysis access in which procedures were performed by interventional nephrologists. In this report, data on basic hemodialysis procedures (tunneled hemodialysis catheter insertion and exchange, percutaneous transluminal angioplasty [PTA; grafts and fistulas], and thrombectomy [grafts and fistulas]) were analyzed for safety and effectiveness.

A total of 4,027 tunneled hemodialysis catheter-related procedures were evaluated for complications [41]. In the tunneled hemodialysis catheter insertion procedure group (n = 4,027), complications included minor oozing at the cannulation and exit site (0.36%) and major adverse events like pneumothorax (0.06%). In contrast, both the surgical and radiologic literature have documented a much higher incidence rate of complications, including pneumothorax (2.5%) [42], hemothorax (0–0.6%, bleeding requiring exploration and/or transfusion (0–4.7%), and recurrent laryngeal nerve palsy (0–1.6%) [42–45]. When cases with tunneled hemodialysis catheter exchange were analyzed (n = 2,262), only 1.41% had minor complications, and there were no major complications identified [41].

In 5,121 PTA procedures (fistulas n = 1,561; grafts n = 3,560), the complication rate in cases of fistulas and grafts included 3.35 and 0.76% grade 1 hematomas (stable, does not affect flow), 0.4 and 0.11% grade 2 hematomas (stable, slows or stops flow), and 0.19 and 0.05% grade 3 hematomas (represents a complete vascular rupture, expands rapidly, and leads to access loss), respectively [41]. These results are far superior to those reported previously (1.7–6.6%) [46–49].

Among 4,899 thrombectomy cases (fistulas n = 228; grafts n = 4,671), the complication rate in cases of fistulas and grafts included 5.7 and 3.32% grade 1 hematomas (stable, does not affect flow), 0.88 and 0.83% grade 2 hematomas (stable, slows or stops flow), and 0.43 and 0.41% grade 3 hematomas (represents a complete vascular rupture, expands rapidly, leads to access loss), respectively [41]. Peripheral artery embolism occurred in 0.38% of cases. These complication rates are lower than those reported previously (10–16%) [23, 50, 51].

Conclusion

A variety of endovascular procedures are now being performed by nephrologists. Data clearly indicate safety, success, quality, and excellent outcomes when vascular access-related procedures are performed by nephrologists. The all-too-frequent delays are minimized and procedural care is more efficiently delivered by a nephrologist trained in hemodialysis vascular access procedures. We suggest that nephrologists should play a more proactive role and occupy a pivotal position in the procedural management of hemodialysis vascular access.

References

1   National Kidney Foundation: K-DOQI clinical practice guidelines for vascular access: update 2000. Guideline 10: monitoring, surveillance, and diagnostic testing. Am J Kidney Dis 2000;37 (suppl 1):S150–S164.
2   Vesely TM: Interventional radiology management of hemodialysis access-related problems: the use of mechanical thrombectomy devices. Dial Transplant 1998;27:252–267.
3   Beathard GA: Percutaneous transvenous angioplasty in the treatment of access vascular stenosis. Kidney Int 1992;42:1390–1397.
4   Jackson JW, Lewis JL, Brouillette JR, Brantley RR: Initial experience of a nephrologist-operated vascular access center. Semin Dial 2000;13:354–358.
5   Schon D, Mishler R: Pharmacomechanical thrombolysis of natural vein fistulas: reduced dose of TPA and long-term follow-up. Semin Dial 2003;16:272–275.
6   Faiyaz R, Abreo K, Zaman F, Pervez A, Zibari G, Work J: Salvage of poorly developed arteriovenous fistulae with percutaneous ligation of accessory veins. Am J Kidney Dis 2002;39:824–827.
7   Beathard GA, Arnold P, Jackson J, Litchfield T, Physician Operators Forum of RMS Lifeline: Aggressive treatment of early fistula failure. Kidney Int 2003;64:1487–1494.
8   Schon D, Mishler R: Salvage of occluded autologous arteriovenous fistulae. Am J Kidney Dis 2000;36:804–810.
9   Beathard GA, Welch BR, Maidment HJ: Mechanical thrombolysis for the treatment of the thrombosed hemodialysis grafts. Radiology 1996;200:711–716.
10 Asif A, Byers P, Vieira CF, Roth D: Developing a comprehensive diagnostic and interventional nephrology program at an academic center. Am J Kidney Dis 2003;42:229–233.
11 American Society of Diagnostic and Interventional Nephrology: Available at http://www.asdin.org; accessed 2001.
12 Work J: Hemodialysis catheters and ports. Semin Nephrol 2002;22:211–219.
13 Mankus RA, Ash SR, Sutton JM: Comparison of blood flow rates and hydraulic resistance between the Mahurkar catheter, the Tesio twin catheter, and the Ash Split Cath. ASAIO J 1998;44:M532–M534.
14 Ash SR: The evolution and function of central venous catheters for dialysis. Semin Dial 2001; 14:416–424.
15 Schon D, Whittman D: Managing the complications of long-term tunneled dialysis catheters. Semin Dial 2003;16:314–322.
16 Glanz S, Gordon D, Butt KM, Hong J, Adamson R, Sclafani SJ: Dialysis access fistulas: treatment of stenoses by transluminal angioplasty. Radiology 1984;152:637–642.
17 Schwab SJ, Saeed M, Sussman SK, McCann RL, Stickel DL: Transluminal angioplasty of venous stenosis in polytetrafluoroethylene vascular access grafts. Kidney Int 1987;32:395–398.
18 Schwab SJ, Raymond JR, Saeed M, Newman GE, Dennis PA, Bollinger RR: Prevention of hemodialysis fistula thrombosis, early detection of venous stenoses. Kidney Int 1989;36:707–711.
19 Roy-Chaudhury P, Kelly BS, Miller MA, Reaves A, Armstrong J, Nanayakkara N, Heffelfinger SC: Venous neointimal hyperplasia in polytetrafluoroethylene dialysis grafts. Kidney Int 2001;59: 2325–2334.
20 Sukhatme VP: Vascular access stenosis. Prospects for prevention and therapy. Kidney Int 1996; 49:1161–1174.
21 Beathard GA: Percutaneous angioplasty for the treatment of venous stenosis: a nephrologist's view. Semin Dial 1995;8:166–1670.

22   Gray RJ, Sacks D, Martin LG, Trerotola SO: Reporting standards for percutaneous interventions in dialysis access. Technology assessment committee. J Vasc Interv Radiol 1999;10:1405–1415.

23   Aruny JE, Lewis CA, Cardella JF, Cole PE, Davis A, Drooz AT, Grassi CJ, Gray RJ, Husted JW, Jones MT, McCowan TC, Meranze SG, Van Moore A, Neithamer CD, Oglevie SB, Omary RA, Patel NH, Rholl KS, Roberts AC, Sacks D, Sanchez O, Silverstein MI, Singh H, Swan TL, Towbin RB, et al: Quality improvement guidelines for percutaneous management of the thrombosed or dysfunctional dialysis access. J Vasc Interv Radiol 1999;10:491–498.

24   Fan PY, Schwab SJ: Vascular access: concepts for the 1990s. J Am Soc Nephrol 1992;3:1–11.

25   Schwab SJ, Harrington JT, Singh A, Roher R, Shohaib SA, Perrone RD, Meyer K, Beasley D: Vascular access for hemodialysis. Kidney Int 1999;55:2078–2090.

26   Windus DW: Permanent vascular access: a nephrologist's view. Am J Kidney Dis 1993;21: 457–471.

27   Beathard GA, Marston WA: Endovascular management of thrombosed dialysis access grafts. Am J Kidney Dis 1998;32:172–175.

28   Beathard GA: Angioplasty for arteriovenous grafts and fistulae. Semin Nephrol 2002;22: 202–210.

29   Schwab SJ, Oliver MJ, Suhocki P, McCann R: Hemodialysis arteriovenous access: detection of stenosis and response to treatment by vascular access blood flow. Kidney Int 2001;59:358–362.

30   Kinnaert P, Vereerstraeten P, Toussaint C, Van Geertruyden J: Nine years' experience with internal arteriovenous fistulas for haemodialysis: a study of some factors influencing the results. Br J Surg 1977;64:242–246.

31   Bonalumi U, Civalleri D, Rovida S, Adami GF, Gianetta E, Griffanti-Bartoli F: Nine years' experience with end-to-end arteriovenous fistula at the 'anatomical snuffbox' for maintenance haemodialysis. Br J Surg 1988;69:486–488.

32   Reilly DT, Wood RF, Bell PR: Prospective study of dialysis fistulas: problem patients and their treatment. Br J Surg 1982;69:549–553.

33   Palder SB, Kirkman RL, Whittemore AD, Hakim RM, Lazarus JM, Tilney NL: Vascular access for hemodialysis. Patency rates and results of revision. Ann Surg 1985;202:235–239.

34   Winsett OE, Wolma FJ: Complications of vascular access for hemodialysis. South Med J 1985;78:513–517.

35   Kherlakian GM, Roedersheimer LR, Arbaugh JJ, Newmark KJ, King LR: Comparison of autogenous fistula versus expanded polytetrafluoroethylene graft fistula for angioaccess in hemodialysis. Am J Surg 1986;152:238–243.

36   US Renal Data System: USRDS 2002 Annual Data Report. Bethesda, National Institutes of Health, National Institute of Diabetes and Digestive and Kidney Diseases, 2002, chapt 12.

37   Beathard GA: Catheter management protocol for catheter-related bacteremia prophylaxis. Semin Dial 2003;16:403–405.

38   Beathard GA: Management of bacteremia associated with tunneled-cuffed hemodialysis catheters. J Am Soc Nephrol 1999;10:1045–1049.

39   Saad TF: Bacteremia associated with tunneled, cuffed hemodialysis catheters. Am J Kidney Dis 1999;34:1114–1124.

40   Beathard GA, Arnold P, Litchfield T: Management of fibrin sheath associated with tunneled hemodialysis catheters (abstract). J Am Soc Nephrol 2003;14:241A.

41   Beathard GA, Litchfield T: Effectiveness and safety of dialysis vascular access procedures performed by interventional nephrologists. Kidney Int 1996;66:1622–1632.

42   Lund GB, Trerotola SO, Scheel PF Jr, Savader SJ, Mitchell SE, Venbrux AC, Osterman FA Jr: Outcome of tunneled hemodialysis catheters placed by radiologists. Radiology 1996;198:467–472.

43   Bour ES, Weaver AS, Yang HC, Gifford RR: Experience with the double lumen Silastic catheter for hemoaccess. Surg Gynecol Obstet 1990;171:33–39.

44   McDowell DE, Moss AH, Vasilakis C, Bell R, Pillai L: Percutaneously placed dual-lumen silicone catheters for long-term hemodialysis. Am Surg 1993;59:569–573.

45   Schwab SJ, Beathard G: The hemodialysis catheter conundrum: hate living with them, but can't live without them. Kidney Int 1999;56:1–17.

46   Longwitz D, Pham TH, Heckemann RG, Hecking E: Angioplasty in the stenosed hemodialysis shunt: experiences with 100 patients and 166 interventions (in German). Rofo 1998;169:68–76.

47   Rundback JH, Leonardo RF, Poplausky MR, Rozenblit G: Venous rupture complicating hemodialysis access angioplasty: percutaneous treatment and outcomes in seven patients. Am J Roentgenol 1998;171:1081–1084.

48   Raynaud AC, Angel CY, Sapoval MR, Beyssen B, Pagny JY, Auguste M: Treatment of hemodialysis access rupture during PTA with Wallstent implantation. J Vasc Interv Radiol 1998;9:437–442.

49   Turmel-Rodrigues L, Pengloan J, Baudin S, Testou D, Abaza M, Dahdah G, Mouton A, Blanchard D: Treatment of stenosis and thrombosis in haemodialysis fistulas and grafts by interventional radiology. Nephrol Dial Transplant 2000;15:2029–2036.

50   Haage P, Vorwerk D, Wildberger JE, Piroth W, Schurmann K, Gunther RW: Percutaneous treatment of thrombosed primary arteriovenous hemodialysis access fistulae. Kidney Int 2000;57: 1169–1175.

51   McCutcheon B, Weatherford D, Maxwell G, Hamann MS, Stiles A: A preliminary investigation of balloon angioplasty versus surgical treatment of thrombosed dialysis access grafts. Am Surg 2003;69:663–667.

Arif Asif, MD, Director
Interventional Nephrology, Associate Professor of Medicine
University of Miami Leonard A. Miller School of Medicine
1600 NW 10th Ave (r 7168) Miami, FL 33136 (USA)
Tel. +1 305 243 3583, Fax +1 305 243 3506, E-Mail Aasif@med.miami.edu

Ronco C, Cruz DN (eds): Hemodialysis – From Basic Research to Clinical Trials.
Contrib Nephrol. Basel, Karger, 2008, vol 161, pp 39–47

······················

Optimal Management of Central Venous Catheters for Hemodialysis

Bernard Canaud[a,b], *Leila Chenine*[a], *Delphine Henriet*[a], *Hélène Leray*[a]

[a]Lapeyronie Hospital – Nephrology, and [b]Renal Research and Training Institute, Montpellier, France

Abstract

Good medical practices for optimizing the management of central venous catheters (CVCs) can be summarized in the following ten commandments: (1) the indications of CVC use you will restrict; (2) the choice of the catheter type and site venous you will discuss; (3) an experienced operator you will choose; (4) validated protocols of use and maintenance of catheters you will respect; (5) caring and nursing staff of the dialysis unit you will train and control; (6) the patients you will educate; (7) monitoring and maintenance care of CVC you will apply; (8) the duration of CVC use you will restrict; (9) specific patient risk factors you will evaluate and correct, and (10) a continuous quality improvement care process for CVC you will establish and apply in your dialysis unit.

Vascular access (VA) is a basic need for launching an extracorporeal blood purification (hemodialysis, hemofiltration, hemodiafiltration). The performances of the VA largely condition the effectiveness of the renal replacement therapy (RRT) program. VA morbidity is the first cause of hospitalization among dialyzed patients accounting for about 25% of the annual causes of hospitalization. If native arteriovenous fistula (AVF) and PTFE synthetic graft (PVF) represent the best VA option, in many situations the use of a central venous catheter (CVC) is needed to carry out RRT. Recent studies indicate that CVCs are used in 20–50% of incident (<6 months) chronic kidney disease (CKD-5) patients and still used in 10–20% of prevalent hemodialysis patients (>6 months) [1–3].

Acute untunneled CVC used in emergency situations or as a short bridging solution (<7 days) will not be discussed in this chapter, only chronic tunneled CVC used for mid- or long-term (14 days to 6 months) treatment in acute kidney injury or chronic kidney patients. Obviously, safety rules and recommendations for chronic tunneled use CVCs are applicable to acute CVCs. Most clinical reports have shown that CVCs offer an effective and convenient vascular access in dialysis patients. CVCs allow to maintain CKD patients treated on an ambulatory mode. CVCs provide flow performances close to AVF and AVG permitting to maintain a short treatment time schedule without any changes.

CVC-related complications represent a significant burden on the management of the RRT program and mortality risk for the dialysis patient. The incidence of CVC-related complications is significantly higher than with AVF. Infectious catheter-related risk is 7 times higher than AVF and 3 times higher than AVP [4].

VA recommendations are close to each other and consensual. All international guidelines suggest that CVC indications should be restricted and the duration of use should be reduced to a minimum [5]. CVC management requires maximal precautions and multiple safety barriers for preventing complications [6]. Faced with this unavoidable risk, one would underline the fact that CVC risk is controllable by applying good clinical practice rules.

Ten Commandments for the Best Use of Hemodialysis CVC

Good medical practices for optimizing the management of CVCs can be summarized in the following ten commandments:

(1) The Indications of CVC Use You Will Restrict
Catheter insertion must be restricted to specific cases in which no other VA alternatives exist. Several indications are consensually recognized – they include acute renal failure when dialysis support is needed at short notice and chronic renal failure when no permanent VA is usable (end-stage renal disease patient not equipped with VA, thrombosis or dysfunction of the permanent VA, transfer from peritoneal dialysis or transplant without access).

For CKD patients, AVF construction must anticipated early enough during the course of the disease to facilitate maturation and use when needed. European Best Practice Guidelines recommend to plan an AV fistula creation at stage 4-5 CKD, that is, CKD patients must be referred to a nephrologist and surgeon in a timely adequate manner [7]. Vascular mapping (artery and vein) of the upper limbs by ultrasound Doppler imaging is highly suitable to improve VA outcomes. A multidisciplinary approach involving a nephrologist, surgeon, angiologist and radiologist is required to optimize VA creation. Regular monitoring of VA by non-invasive methods such as ultrasound Doppler imaging and/or online measurement of VA flow performances and recirculation by specific devices (Transonics, CritLine, Dialysis machine monitoring) is also needed as a part of the quality assessment program [8]. These simple measures may have the potential of enhancing AV fistula creation success rate and reducing the incidence of VA thrombosis. Consequently, by improving AV fistula outcomes, resorting to CVC will be reduced.

(2) The Choice of the Catheter Type and Site Venous You Will Discuss

Acute untunneled catheter use will be restricted to short-term use (<14 days) or as salvaging solution in CKD patients without a usable permanent access [9]. Chronic tunneled catheter will be indicated preferentially and as soon as possible [10].

CVC choice will privilege a long-term tunneled and hemocompatible catheter. Catheter design comprising a double lumen or a double catheter made of hemocompatible soft polymer (silicone, polyurethane) with a long tunnel and a subcutaneous anchoring system will be inserted. Such catheter design improves the patient's comfort, reduces the infectious risk and provides blood flow performances for high-efficiency dialysis. The venous site insertion choice will be guided by clinical history and physical examination and if needed by ultrasound Doppler imaging [11]. When possible, the venous catheter insertion will be guided continuously by ultrasound imaging technique at the bedside. In all cases, catheter insertion should be performed by an experienced physician following strict hygienic rules (sterile drape, gloves, mask, gown) in a clean dedicated room equipped with adequate monitoring material. Skin preparation (shaving, cleaning and disinfecting) will be performed 10–20 min before the catheter insertion. A tunneling catheter is an essential step for protecting CVC and for improving the patient's comfort. The right jugular vein is preferred to femoral and subclavian to reduce stenosis and/or thrombosis of the host vein and to reduce the infectious risk.

(3) An Experienced Operator You Will Choose

Implanting a CVC for dialysis should not be considered as a banal act given to an inexperienced fellow [12]. It is a risky procedure that requires an experienced physician and an adequate aseptic environment. The CVC insertion technique affects dialysis performances and treatment quality. Particular attention should be paid to catheter insertion in order to best locate the CVC end tip (right atrium, inferior central vena cava) to ensure best blood flow performances. Catheter location and positioning should be controlled by chest x-ray (or abdomen x-ray), electrocardiography or ultrasound Doppler imaging, immediately after insertion and before use [13]. Lack of traumatic complications should be confirmed by the same imaging technique.

(4) Validated Protocols of Use and Maintenance of
Catheters You Will Respect

Medical practices applied in catheter management have a direct and major impact on CVC performances and long-term outcomes. Regular monitoring of CVC performances (blood flow, resistance, recirculation, dialysis dose delivery) is the only effective way of detecting early catheter dysfunction and preventing further deterioration of dialysis efficacy (reduced dialysis dose delivery). CVC monitoring requires the implementation within the dialysis unit of strict and comprehensive protocols of follow-up under the supervision of a referent nurse [14]. The nursing staff should be trained for best use of CVCs.

Long-term results of CVC are heavily burdened by dysfunction and complications [15]. It is the duty of each dialysis facility to define its own indicators facilitating follow-up and assessment of CVC performances and complications over time. One can cite as an example some parameters that may be followed on a monthly basis: mean effective blood flow, venous pressure, recirculation, dialysis dose delivered (Kt/V), number of infections, number of flow dysfunctions [16, 17]. Protocols of care and CVC maintenance should be adapted to dialysis facility results and to a patient-specific profile. They should comply with local and national recommendations in order to prevention nosocomial infections and to reduce CVC-related risks.

(5) Caring and Nursing Staff of the Dialysis Unit You Will Train and Control

CVC care is usually provided by the nursing staff insuring dialysis connection and disconnection. The incidence of CVC-related complications is clearly associated with nursing staff experience and respect of catheter-handling protocols [18]. For each dialysis facility a specific training program and a protocolized handling procedure should be defined and adapted to their results. Aseptic rules for manipulating CVC at the time of dialysis connection and disconnection should be applied at all times. They include for the nurse, the use of sterile disposable material (drape, gown, gloves) and additive protecting barriers (mask, cap) and resort to an auxiliary caregiver to facilitate connection to the dialysis machine while preventing contamination. A new hope of reducing catheter-related infection has been given by the regular use of an antiseptic/antibiotic catheter-locking solution [19, 20]. Catheter-locking solutions are gaining more clinical acceptance but this approach must be validated in larger clinical trials [21, 22].

Defining dedicated referent nurses facilitating and harmonizing CVC management procedures is highly desirable. An expert referent nurse will educate and train the new or inexperienced nursing staff while ensuring correct application of CVC protocols in the dialysis unit. Several types of CVC protocol should be proposed. They include periodicity and type of CVC performance tests to be performed (effective flow rate, recirculation, dialysis dose delivered).

In addition, it is interesting to mention that some specific acts, such as restoring CVC permeability (fibrinolytic lock solution) or culturing catheter clot (insipient infection) should be programmed according to patient profile, CVC performances and CVC risks. By the way, such an approach has a high potential of reducing CVC-related complications and particularly CVC infection.

(6) The Patients You Will Educate

Patients harboring a CVC are obviously more exposed to complications than those having a native AV fistula. CVC made of foreign inert material offers an excellent media for seeding of bacteria. CVC breaks the skin integrity and facilitates germ access to blood. These two conditions increase risk of CVC-related infection. Moreover, CVC blood contact activates the coagulation cascade and promotes thrombosis both in the catheter and in the host vein. Patients harboring CVC should be informed of this increased risk and nursing staff should be prepared and trained to minimize these risks. Specific body hygienic rules should be given to the patient in order to reduce skin colonization and to prevent CVC contamination such as a permanent carrying of a protective and waterproof plastic bandage for the catheter. Bathing or swimming should be prohibited. Chronic carriers of bacteria (nephrostomy, colostomy, previous history of bacterial infection, nasal carriage…) present an increased risk of infection and should be detected and treated. Regular disinfection of the skin exit and catheter hub and pavilion should be performed regularly at the time of dialysis connection.

(7) Monitoring and Maintenance Care of CVC You Will Apply

Regular inspection of the skin exit and CVC emergence is necessary to detect early local signs of inflammation or infection. Inspection results should be collected and documented in the patient's folder. Any abnormal aspect of the skin exit should be immediately reported and local corrective action should be taken.

Performances of CVC should be regularly evaluated [23]. Multiple indicators of CVC performances have been defined. Some parameters should be selected according to the facility practices: number of dialysis sessions performed without problems, venous and arterial pressures display by the dialysis machine for a set blood flow value, recirculation, dialysis dose delivered with CVC over time.

Cleaning and decontamination of the skin area surrounding the emergence of CVC should be performed regularly. Chest shaving is needed in men. Skin cleaning and disinfection should be performed with non-aggressive and non-irritating agents. A hypoallergenic bandage should be preferred.

Preventive cleaning or reopening CVC with fibrinolytic agents (tPHA, urokinase) or fibrin sleeve stripping should be performed when CVC dysfunction is observed [24, 25]. According to the importance of the CVC dysfunction, fibrinolytic agents should be applied as short- or mid-term locking solution or by continuous transcatheter infusion.

CVC clot and blood culture should be performed as soon as an infection is suspected or when sepsis origin has not been identified.

(8) The Duration of CVC Use You Will Restrict

Infectious complications of CVC are due to hygienic conditions of insertion and handling, but also dependent on staff expertise, practice patterns of the dialysis unit and patient's hygiene [26, 27]. The incidence of CVC-related infection is maximal within the first 3 months following insertion, then reduced over time, although the risk still persists afterwards.

Early infection should be considered as related to the implantation act and/or bacterial contamination of the catheter during handling procedures. Late infection (after 90 days) is mainly due to endoluminal contamination leading to microbial biofilm formation. Preventing penetration and seeding of bacteria within the catheter lumen at the time of dialysis connection is essential, and is achieved by applying strict aseptic rules of catheter handling. Preventing formation of microbial biofilm is also essential, and is obtained by locking the catheter during the interdialytic period with antiseptic/antithrombotic solutions [28].

Stenosis and thrombosis of the central vein secondary to CVC are increasingly reported and usually associated with the duration of insertion and use [29]. Up to 50% of CVCs inserted for >12 months are complicated by host vein stenosis when phlebography is performed after CVC removal [30, 31]. This figure may certainly underestimate the true incidence of CVC-related stenosis. For CVC used as bridging solution, they should be ideally withdrawn within 6 months after insertion. It should also be mentioned that these complications are related to type of catheters, insertion technique and handling management of CVC. Preventing subclinically infectious complications and preventing a chronic inflammatory state is certainly one of the best ways of preventing the occurrence of vein stenosis.

(9) Specific Patient Risk Factors You Will Evaluate and Correct

Uremic patients are not equal to CVC complication risks. Curiously, some patients will harbor CVC for several years without any problems, while others bearing CVC will develop multiple complications soon after CVC insertion. This clinical observation suggests that dialysis patients present with a personal sensitivity which is difficult to quantify in practice.

To illustrate this point, one can take two examples. Dialysis patients presenting with 'high infection risk' (diabetics, chronic bearer of bacteria, previous history of bacteremia, skin infectious disease…) should benefit from specific protocol-reinforcing hygienic rules [32] and using preemptively antiseptic/

antithrombotic (or antibiotic/antithrombotic) catheter-locking solutions [33–36]. Dialysis patients presenting with 'high thrombotic risk' (previous history of thrombosis, inflammation, coagulation disease…) should benefit from preemptive long-term anticoagulation based on a low dose of antivitamin K or antiplatelet agents [37]. In these cases, a personalized monitoring protocol should be indicated to detect early thrombotic or infectious complications [38].

(10) A Continuous Quality Improvement Care Process for CVC You Will Establish and Apply in Your Dialysis Unit

Implementing a continuous quality improvement care process in the dialysis unit is an essential tool for reducing the incidence of VA- and CVC-related complications [39, 40]. Accordingly, it is necessary to follow guidelines and recommendations as defined earlier, to define core indicators assessing quality and performances of CVC, to nominate a care nursing staff referent, to establish, validate and apply protocols for catheter use in the dialysis unit and finally to analyze results of the unit and amend protocols according to outcomes [41].

To conclude, the use of CVCs and implantable port catheter devices is a necessity when treating chronic renal failure patients. It has been one of the most innovative and productive aspects in the field of RRT [42, 43]. Venous access facilitates ambulatory management of the chronic renal failure patient. CVC is a warranty for RRT maintenance when a permanent AV fistula and graft have failed. CVC is a very comfortable VA for patients and nurses.

Unfortunately, CVC use is associated with a higher incidence of complications (infection, dysfunction and thrombosis) compared to native AV fistula. It must now be underlined that optimal use of CVCs should significantly reduce the incidence of these complications [44]. CVC represents an undesirable but unavoidable device for ensuring RRT both in acute and chronic conditions.

References

1   Combe C, Pisoni RL, Port FK, Young EW, Canaud B, Mapes DL, Held PJ, Dialysis Outcomes and Practice Patterns Study: Données sur l'utilisation des cathéters pour hémodialyse. Néphrologie 2001;22:379–384.
2   Rayner HC, Pisoni RL, Bommer J, Canaud B, Hecking E, Locatelli F, Piera L, Bragg-Gresham JL, Feldman HI, Goodkin DA, Gillespie B, Wolfe RA, Held PJ, Port FK: Mortality and hospitalization in haemodialysis patients in five European countries: results from the Dialysis Outcomes and Practice Patterns Study (DOPPS). Nephrol Dial Transplant 2004;19:108–120.
3   Moist LM, Chang SH, Polkinghorne KR, McDonald SP, Australia and New Zealand Dialysis and Transplant Registry (ANZDATA): Trends in hemodialysis vascular access from the Australia and New Zealand Dialysis and Transplant Registry (ANZDATA) 2000–2005. Am J Kidney Dis 2007;50:612–621.
4   Hoen B, Paul-Dauphin A, Hestin D, Kessler M: EPIBACDIAL: a multicenter prospective study of risk factors for bacteremia in chronic hemodialysis patients. J Am Soc Nephrol 1998;9:869–876.

5   NKF-K/DOQI Clinical Practice Guidelines for Vascular Access: Update 2000. Am J Kidney Dis 2001;37:S137–S181.

6   Pastan S, Soucie JM, McClellan WM: Vascular access and increased risk of death among hemodialysis patients. Kidney Int 2002;62:620–626.

7   Tordoir J, Canaud B, Haage P, Konner K, Basci A, Fouque D, Kooman J, Martin-Malo A, Pedrini L, Pizzarelli F, Tattersall J, Vennegoor M, Wanner C, ter Wee P, Vanholder R: European Best Practice Guidelines on Vascular Access. Nephrol Dial Transplant 2007;22(suppl 2):ii88–ii117.

8   Besarab A: Access monitoring is worthwhile and valuable. Blood Purif 2006;24:77–89.

9   Weijmer MC, ter Wee PM: Temporary vascular access for hemodialysis treatment. Current guidelines and future directions. Contrib Nephrol. Basel, Karger, 2004, vol 142, pp 94–111.

10 Weijmer MC, Vervloet MG, ter Wee PM: Compared to tunnelled cuffed haemodialysis catheters, temporary untunnelled catheters are associated with more complications already within twp weeks of use. Nephrol Dial Transplant 2004;19:670–677.

11 Denys BG, Uretsky BF, Reddy PS: Ultrasound-assisted cannulation of the internal jugular vein. A prospective comparison to the external landmark-guided technique. Circulation 1993;87: 1557–1562.

12 Fry AC, Stratton J, Farrington K, Mahna K, Selvakumar S, Thompson H, Warwicker P: Factors affecting long-term survival of tunnelled haemodialysis catheters a prospective audit of 812 tunnelled catheters. Nephrol Dial Transplant 2008;23:275–281.

13 Cavatorta F, Zollo A, Galli S, Mij M, Dolla D: Ultrasound-guided cannulation and endocavitary electrocardiography placement of internal jugular vein catheters in uremic patients: the importance of routine chest X-ray evaluation. J Vasc Access 2001;2:37–39.

14 Sullivan R, Samuel V, Le C, Khan M, Alexandraki I, Cuhaci B, Nahman NS Jr: Hemodialysis vascular catheter-related bacteremia. Am J Med Sci 2007;334:458–465.

15 Beathard GA: Management of bacteremia associated with tunneled-cuffed hemodialysis catheters. J Am Soc Nephrol 1999;10:1045–1049.

16 Canaud B, Leray-Moragues H, Kerkeni N, Bosc JY, Martin K: Effective flow performances and dialysis doses delivered with permanent catheters: a 24-month comparative study of permanent catheters versus arteriovenous vascular accesses. Nephrol Dial Transplant 2002;17:1286–1292.

17 Moist LM, Hemmelgarn BR, Lok CE: Relationship between blood flow in central venous catheters and hemodialysis adequacy. Clin J Am Soc Nephrol 2006;1:965–971.

18 Vanherweghem JL, Dhaene M, Goldman M, Stolear JC, Sabot JP, Waterlot Y, et al: Infections associated with subclavian dialysis catheters: the key role of nurse training. Nephron 1986;42: 116–119.

19 McIntyre CW, Hulme LJ, Taal M, Fluck RJ: Locking of tunneled hemodialysis catheters with gentamicin and heparin. Kidney Int 2004;66:801–805.

20 Allon M: Prophylaxis against dialysis catheter-related bacteremia: a glimmer of hope. Am J Kidney Dis 2008;51:165–168.

21 Saxena AK, Panhotra BR, Sundaram DS, Al-Hafiz A, Naguib M, Venkateshappa CK, Abu-Oun BA, Hussain SM, Al-Ghamdi AA: Tunneled catheters' outcome optimization among diabetics on dialysis through antibiotic-lock placement. Kidney Int 2006;70:1629–1635.

22 Weijmer MC, van den Dorpel MA, Van de Ven PJ, ter Wee PM, van Geelen JA, Groeneveld JO, van Jaarsveld BC, Koopmans MG, le Poole CY, Schrander-Van der Meer AM, Siegert CE, Stas KJ, CITRATE Study Group: Randomized, clinical trial comparison of trisodium citrate 30% and heparin as catheter-locking solution in hemodialysis patients. J Am Soc Nephrol 2005;16: 2769–2777.

23 Bosc JY, Martin K, Leray-Moragues H, Canaud B: Surveillance des accès veineux centraux pour hémodialyse. Néphrologie 2001;22:413–415.

24 Gray RJ, Levitin A, Buck D, Brown LC, Sparling YH, Jablonski KA, et al: Percutaneous fibrin sheath stripping versus transcatheter urokinase infusion for malfunctioning well-positioned tunneled central venous dialysis catheters: a prospective, randomized trial. J Vasc Interv Radiol 2000;11:1121–1129.

25 Oliver MJ, Mendelssohn DC, Quinn RR, Richardson EP, Rajan DK, Pugash RA, Hiller JA, Kiss AJ, Lok CE: Catheter patency and function after catheter sheath disruption: a pilot study. Clin J Am Soc Nephrol 2007;2:1201–1206.

26   Oliver MJ, Callery SM, Thorpe KE, Schwab SJ, Churchill DN: Risk of bacteremia from temporary hemodialysis catheters by site of insertion and duration of use: a prospective study. Kidney Int 2000;58:2543–2545.

27   Mermel LA: Prevention of intravascular catheter-related infections. Ann Intern Med 2000;132: 391–402.

28   De Lancey Pulcini E: Bacterial biofilms: a review of current research. Néphrologie 2001;22: 439–441.

29   Mickley V: Central vein obstruction in vascular access. Eur J Vasc Endovasc Surg 2006;32: 439–444.

30   Oguzkurt L, Tercan F, Torun D, Yildirim T, Zümrütdal A, Kizilkilic O: Impact of short-term hemodialysis catheters on the central veins: a catheter venographic study. Eur J Radiol 2004;52:293–299.

31   MacRae JM, Ahmed A, Johnson N, Levin A, Kiaii M: Central vein stenosis: a common problem in patients on hemodialysis. ASAIO J 2005;51:77–81.

32   Sesso R, Barbosa D, Leme IL, Sader H, Canziani ME, Manfredi S, Draibe S, Pignatari AC: *Staphylococcus aureus* prophylaxis in hemodialysis patients using central venous catheter: effect of mupirocin ointment. J Am Soc Nephrol 1998;9:1085–1092.

33   Canaud B: Reducing infections associated with central vein catheters. Semin Dial 2000;13: 206–207.

34   Sodemann K, Polaschegg HD, Feldmer B: Two years' experience with Dialock and CLS (a new antimicrobial lock solution). Blood Purif 2001;19:251–254.

35   Allon M: Prophylaxis against dialysis catheter-related bacteremia with a novel antimicrobial lock solution. Clin Infect Dis 2003;36:1539–1544.

36   Macrae JM, Dojcinovic I, Djurdjev O, Jung B, Shalansky S, Levin A, Kiaii M: Citrate 4% versus heparin and the reduction of thrombosis study (CHARTS). Clin J Am Soc Nephrol 2008;3: 369–374.

37   Mokrzycki MH, Jean-Jerome K, Rush H, Zdunek MP, Rosenberg SO: A randomized trial of minidose warfarin for the prevention of late malfunction in tunneled, cuffed hemodialysis catheters. Kidney Int 2001;59:1935–1942.

38   Willms L, Vercaigne LM: Does warfarin safely prevent clotting of hemodialysis catheters? A review of efficacy and safety. Semin Dial 2008;21:71–77.

39   Bosch JP, Walters BA: Quality assurance and continuous quality improvement in the management of vascular access. Contrib Nephrol. Basel, Karger, 2002, vol 137, pp 60–69.

40   Wijnen E, Planken N, Keuter X, Kooman JP, Tordoir JH, de Haan MW, Leunissen KM, van der Sande F: Impact of a quality improvement programme based on vascular access flow monitoring on costs, access occlusion and access failure. Nephrol Dial Transplant 2006;21:3514–3519.

41   Canaud B: Haemodialysis catheter-related infection: time for action. Nephrol Dial Transplant 1999;140:2288–2290.

42   Canaud B, My H, Morena M, Lamy-Lacavalerie B, Leray-Moragues H, Bosc JY, et al: Dialock: a new vascular access device for extracorporeal renal replacement therapy. Preliminary clinical results. Nephrol Dial Transplant 1999;14:692–698.

43   Schwab SJ, Weiss MA, Rushton F, Ross JP, Jackson J, Kapoian T, et al: Multicenter clinical trial results with the LifeSite hemodialysis access system. Kidney Int 2002;62:1026–1033.

44   Quarello F, Forneris G, Borca M, Pozzato M: Do central venous catheters have advantages over arteriovenous fistulas or grafts? J Nephrol 2006;19:265–279.

Prof. Bernard Canaud
Nephrology, Dialysis and Intensive Care, Hôpital Lapeyronie
CHU Montpellier, 371, Av du Doyen G. Giraud
FR–34925 Montpellier Cedex 05 (France)
Tel. +33 467 338 955, Fax +33 467 603 783, E-Mail b-canaud@chu-montpellier.fr

Ronco C, Cruz DN (eds): Hemodialysis – From Basic Research to Clinical Trials.
Contrib Nephrol. Basel, Karger, 2008, vol 161, pp 48–54

....

Trends in Medication Use and Clinical Outcomes in Twelve Countries: Results form the Dialysis Outcomes and Practice Patterns Study (DOPPS)

Francesca Tentori

Arbor Research Collaborative for Health, Ann Arbor, Mich., USA

Abstract

The Dialysis Outcomes and Practice Patterns Study (DOPPS) was designed to identify clinical practices of hemodialysis associated with patients longevity. For more than 10 years, DOPPS has been collecting detailed information on patients and facility characteristics from 12 countries across the world. Multiple aspects of clinical care in hemodialysis may be associated with improved outcomes. However, changes in many practices are hard to implement. One practice that can be relatively easier to modify is the physician prescription of medications. The associations between medication prescription and outcomes have been the object of several DOPPS publications. We present here a brief summary of DOPPS findings on prescription of several classes of medications and clinical outcomes.

The Dialysis Outcomes and Practice Patterns Study (DOPPS) is a prospective observational study designed to identify clinical practices of hemodialysis (HD) associated with patients longevity [1, 2]. For more than a decade, DOPPS has been collecting comprehensive information on patients and facility characteristics, processes of care and outcomes across the world. Thanks to the unique design of DOPPS, data collected from study participants are representative of the HD population in each participating country [3]. Currently, more than 144,000 patients in 320 facilities are enrolled in 12 countries, representing ~70% of the world's HD population. This international design greatly enhances DOPPS ability to identify practices associated with positive clinical outcomes because of the large variability in the approaches to HD practices in different countries.

Multiple aspects of clinical care in HD may be associated with improved outcomes. However, due to several reasons, including social, cultural and financial factors, many clinical practices are not readily modifiable. One practice pattern that can be relatively easier to modify is the physician prescription of medications. The associations between prescription of several medications and clinical outcomes have been the object of several DOPPS analyses and publications.

We present here a brief summary of DOPPS findings on use of several classes of medications and associated clinical outcomes.

Methods

Details of the study design, facility sampling, patient sampling, and data collection have been published previously [1]. Briefly, the DOPPS sample contains detailed data on over 39,000 patients (baseline data on over 144,000 patients) from three study phases: DOPPS I (1996–2001), DOPPS II (2001–2004), and DOPPS III (2005-present). Seven countries (Japan, USA, France, Germany, Italy, Spain, UK) participated in DOPPS I. DOPPS II and III included the seven original countries and Sweden, Australia-New Zealand, Belgium, and Canada. In all phases, the study design and data collection instruments were uniform across countries. A nationally representative sample of dialysis facilities was enrolled in each country, followed by selection of a random sample of HD patients at each participating center. Between 20 and 40 randomly selected adult chronic HD patients (age >17 years) participated from each facility, based on the facility size. Study patients who departed from a facility were periodically replaced with patients who started HD treatment at the facility. Consent to collect patient information without patient identifiers was obtained as needed from the local or national Ethics Committee or Institutional Review Board. US facilities started the study in 1997, European facilities in 1998, and Japanese facilities in 1999. The present analysis used data gathered at 4-month follow-up intervals for DOPPS I & III, while data collection occurred once yearly for DOPPS II. For descriptive purposes, the following geographic regions were identified: ANZ (= Australia + New Zealand), Japan, North America (= USA + Canada) and Europe. Results are also shown separately for Italy.

Logistic regression was used to investigate patient characteristics associated with specific medication prescription. Associations between prescription and outcomes were analyzed using Cox proportional Hazards ratios. Models typically adjusted for demographics, 14 summary comorbid conditions, and time on dialysis. Robust estimators were used to account for facility clustering.

Results

Distributions of medication prescription among a cross-section of patients participating in DOPPS II are shown in figure 1. Wide variability in patterns of medication prescription was observed across DOPPS regions. Among antihypertensive agents (AHA), angiotensin-converting enzyme inhibitors (ACEi), angiotensin receptor blockers (ARB) and calcium channel blockers were commonly used in all regions; however these drugs were prescribed less frequently in Italy compared to the other European countries. Similarly, prescription of satins, antidepressant agents and analgesic was lower in Italy. Prescription of multivitamins was most frequent in North America (73.9% of study participants) and relatively rare in Japan (5.9%) and Italy (7.1%).

Several analyses of DOPPS data have addressed the relationship between medication use and clinical outcomes. We present here a brief summary of the major findings of the most relevant publications.

Antihypertensive Agents

Bragg-Gresham et al. [4] recently reported on prescription of diuretics and associated outcomes among participants in DOPPS I. In all DOPPS countries the use of diuretics decreased sharply after the initiation of HD. However, wide variability in diuretic prescription remained after 90 days on HD, with 21.3% of patients in Europe and only 9.2% of patients in the USA reported to be on a diuretic. These rates were slightly lower compared to those observed among participants in DOPPS 2 (26.2% in Europe and 15.5 in the USA), as shown in figure 1. Overall, 10.7% of patients were reported to be on a diuretic after more than 2 years on HD. The strongest predictor of diuretic prescription was diabetes (OR = 1.57; $p < 0.0001$). Among prevalent patients, diuretic use was associated with several positive outcomes, including lower interdialytic weight gain (–0.4%), decreased incidence of dialysis-related hypotension (odds ratio [OR] = 0.55) and of hyperkalemia (OR = 0.49) ($p < 0.001$ for all). Mortality due to cardiac events was significantly lower among patients who were prescribed a diuretic (RR = 0.86; $p = 0.03$). Surprisingly, in analyses stratified by residual renal function, the survival benefit of diuretics was significant only for patients with no residual renal function.

Prescription of AHA has been associated with improved vascular access survival among DOPPS participants [5]. Specifically, prescription of calcium channel blockers was associated with significant decreased risk of arteriovenous grafts (AVG) failure (RR = 0.86), while therapy with ACEi was associated with better arteriovenous fistula (AVF) secondary patency (RR = 0.556).

Sexual dysfunction is a commonly reported side effect of antihypertensive therapy. In a recent DOPPS analysis, increased problems with arousal were reported for use of loop diuretics (OR = 1.24), peripheral α-blockers (OR = 1.29), and central antagonists (OR = 1.19) [6].

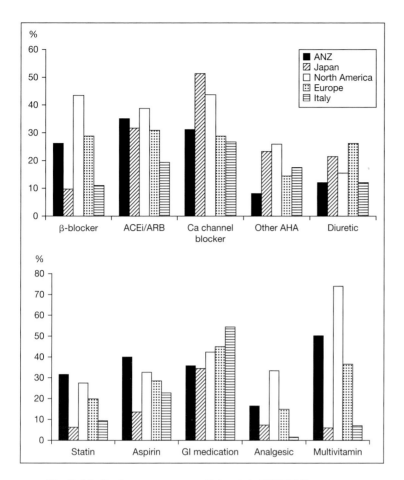

Fig. 1. Medication use among participants in DOPPS II.

Statins (HMG-Coenzyme A Reductase Inhibitors)

An analysis of DOPPS participants in the year 2000 demonstrated that pre-scription of statins was relatively uncommon among HD patients, ranging from 3.5% in Italy to 16.6% in the USA (overall prescription rate = 11.8%) [7]. 81% of participating facilities prescribed statins for <20% of their patients. As shown in figure 1, statins prescription increased among participants in DOPPS II in all countries. Specifically, statins were prescribed for 9.4% of Italian participants.

In DOPPS I, patients on statins had a 23% lower risk for cardiac death and 44% lower risk for non-cardiac deaths. The practice of prescribing statins to more patients within a dialysis unit was also associated with lower patient mortality (HR = 0.95 [0.90–0.99] per 10% increase in facility statins prescription).

Aspirin

Among participants in the first two phases of DOPPS, wide variations in aspirin prescription were observed across DOPPS countries, ranging from 8% in Japan to 41% of patients in Australia and New Zealand. In Italy, aspirin was prescribed for 19.3% of patients in DOPPS I and 22.8% in DOPPS II [8].

Aspirin prescription was associated with decreased risk of stroke (RR = 0.2; $p < 0.01$) [8] and with better AVG secondary patency (RR = 0.70) [5].

However, aspirin was also associated with increased risk for myocardial infarction (RR = 1.21; $p = 0.001$) and cardiac events (RR = 1.08; $p < 0.01$). This association with negative outcomes is most likely due to the confounding effect of a prescription by indication bias, since aspirin is commonly prescribed for patients at elevated risk for cardiovascular events. Interestingly, no increase in gastrointestinal bleeding was described for patients receiving aspirin (RR = 1.01; $p = 0.4$).

Gastro-Protective Agents

Bailie et al. [9] reported wide variability in the prescription of gastro-protective agents and type of drug prescribed in DOPPS I. For instance, prescription of proton pump inhibitors) ranged from 0.8% in Japan to 27.3% in the UK; that of H_2 receptor antagonist (HA) from 3.4% in France to 36.9% in Italy. Prescription patterns also varied substantially across dialysis facilities, ranging from 0 to 94% of patients. Between 1996 and 2001, the proportion of DOPPS participants receiving gastro-protective drugs remained relatively constant (36–38%). However, significant changes were observed in the type of drug prescribed, with a decline in HA prescription and increase in proton pump inhibitor use. Prescription of gastro-protective drugs was more frequent in Italy, Spain and the UK compared to the USA and associated with several comorbidities (including gastrointestinal bleeding and coronary artery disease), low serum albumin, and with prescription of other medications, including corticosteroids, anti-inflammatory drugs, narcotics and antidepressant.

Analgesic

An analysis of DOPPS participants in the USA demonstrated that the prescription of analgesic declined over time (from 30.2% in 1996 to 24.3% in 2001) [10]. Analgesic prescription varies across facilities, ranging from 0 to 89.3% of patients. Overall, three quarters of patients reporting moderate to very severe pain did not have a prescription for analgesic. Factors associated with analgesic prescription included age, female gender, cardiovascular disease and malignancies. Interestingly, no association was found between analgesic prescription and loss of residual renal function or hospitalizations due to gastrointestinal bleeding.

Multivitamin

In an analysis of DOPPS I participants, prescription of water-soluble vitamins varied widely across DOPPS countries, ranging from 3.7% of patients in the UK to 71.9% in the USA. 6.4% of Italian patients in DOPPS I had a prescription for multivitamins [11]. Similar prescription rates were found in DOPPS II (fig. 1). Overall, multivitamin prescription was more frequent for younger patients with less comorbid conditions. However, use of vitamin was associated with improved clinical outcomes not only in patient-level models but also in practice-based models that may be able to better account for bias in multivitamin prescription [12]. Specifically, a 16% decreased mortality risk was observed in patient-level models (p = 0.001). The practice of prescribing more multivitamins was also associated with a significant survival benefit (RR = 0.98 per 10% more patients prescribed vitamins; p = 0.05).

Conclusions

This work summarizes the most relevant DOPPS findings concerning medication prescription and associated outcomes among a cohort of 'real-life' HD patients across the world. While randomized control trials are still needed to test potential clinical benefits of several agents, these data may contribute to inform the practice of medication prescription in dialysis units.

References

1   Young EW, Goodkin DA, Mapes DL, et al: The Dialysis Outomes and Practice Patterns Study (DOPPS): an international hemodialysis study. Kidney Int 2000;57:S74–S81.

2   Pisoni RL, Gillespie BW, Dickinson DM, et al: The Dialysis Outcomes and Practice Patterns Study (DOPPS): design, data elements, and methodology. Am J Kidney Dis 2004;44:7–15.
3   Port FK, Wolfe RA, Held PJ, et al: Random sample (DOPPS) versus census-based (registry) approaches to kidney disease research. Blood Purif 2003;21:85–88.
4   Bragg-Gresham JL, Fissell RB, Mason NA, et al: Diuretic use, residual renal function, and mortality among hemodialysis patients in the Dialysis Outcomes and Practice Pattern Study (DOPPS). Am J Kidney Dis 2007;49:426–431.
5   Saran R, Dykstra DM, Wolfe RA, et al: Association between vascular access failure and the use of specific drugs: the Dialysis Outcomes and Practice Patterns Study (DOPPS). Am J Kidney Dis 2002;40:1255–1263.
6   Bailie GR, Elder SJ, Mason NA, et al: Sexual dysfunction in dialysis patients treated with antihypertensive or antidepressive medications: results from the DOPPS. Nephrol Dial Transplant 2007;22:1163–1170.
7   Mason NA, Bailie GR, Satayathum S, et al: HMG-coenzyme a reductase inhibitor use is associated with mortality reduction in hemodialysis patients. Am J Kidney Dis 2005;45:119–126.
8   Ethier J, Bragg-Gresham JL, Piera L, et al: Aspirin prescription and outcomes in hemodialysis patients: the Dialysis Outcomes and Practice Patterns Study (DOPPS). Am J Kidney Dis 2007; 50:602–611.
9   Bailie GR, Mason NA, Elder SJ, et al: Large variations in prescriptions of gastrointestinal medications in hemodialysis patients on three continents: the Dialysis Outcomes and Practice Patterns Study (DOPPS). Hemodial Int 2006;10:180–188.
10 Bailie GR, Mason NA, Bragg-Gresham JL, et al: Analgesic prescription patterns among hemodialysis patients in the DOPPS: potential for underprescription. Kidney Int 2004;65:2419–2425.
11 Fissell RB, Bragg-Gresham JL, Gillespie BW, et al: International variation in vitamin prescription and association with mortality in the Dialysis Outcomes and Practice Patterns Study (DOPPS). Am J Kidney Dis 2004;44:293–299.
12 Johnston SC: Combining ecological and individual variables to reduce confounding by indication: case study–subarachnoid hemorrhage treatment. J Clin Epidemiol 2000;53:1236–1241.

Dr. Francesca Tentori
Arbor Research Collaborative for Health
315 W. Muron Street, Suite 360, Ann Arbor, MI 48103 (USA)
Tel. +1 734 665 4108, Fax +1 734 665 2103
E-Mail francesca.tentori@ArborResearch.org

Ronco C, Cruz DN (eds): Hemodialysis – From Basic Research to Clinical Trials.
Contrib Nephrol. Basel, Karger, 2008, vol 161, pp 55–62

....

Epigenetics and the Uremic Phenotype: A Matter of Balance

Peter Stenvinkel[a], *Tomas J. Ekström*[b]

[a]Division of Renal Medicine, Department of Clinical Science, Intervention and Technology, and [b]Department of Clinical Neuroscience, Karolinska Institutet, Stockholm, Sweden

Abstract

Epigenetics, which is the study of changes in gene expression that occur without changes in DNA sequence, is a novel discipline that has languished in the shadow of its genomic big brother. So far, studies of the epigenome have attracted little interest in nephrology. Chronic kidney disease is an example of complex disease in which the phenotype arises from a combination of environmental and heritable factors. Evidence suggests that the contribution made by the environment may be mediated via modifications of the epigenome. In the uremic milieu, several features such as inflammation, dyslipidemia, hyperhomocysteinema, oxidative stress as well as vitamin and nutritional deficiencies may affect aberrant global DNA methylation. However, as hyperhomocysteinemia seems to promote global DNA hypomethylation and persistent inflammation DNA hypermethylation, the effects of the uremic milieu on aberrant global DNA methylation may be complex and context-sensitive. It should be emphasized that in analogy to the unspecific nature of fever, aberrant global DNA methylation is only a sign of a generalized epigenetic dysregulation. Thus, to provide better understanding of the effects of aberrant DNA methylation on the uremic phenotype, further studies evaluating site-specific information on methylation in various candidate genes are needed. The science of epigenetics may not only uncover etiologic and pathogenic mechanisms in uremia, but may also be of help to develop novel treatment strategies targeting the unacceptable high death risk in cardiovascular complications in this patient population.

Copyright © 2008 S. Karger AG, Basel

An Introduction to Epigenetics

Epigenetics represent a novel approach in cardiovascular research that has started to attract interest in nephrology [1, 2]. As epigenetic mechanisms due to environmental factors have an impact on the normal function of the genome [3], more knowledge of the associations between the uremic milieu and epigenetic modifications are likely to add important understanding of the complex patho-physiological relationships that exist in this condition. Epigenetic analyses may turn out to be invaluable tools to explain how environment and lifestyle can impose on aberrant gene expression patterns in uremia. In principle, the epigenome denote properties of the genome that are not explained by the primary DNA sequence, but rather the results of modifications of DNA and DNA-associated proteins. These include dynamic changes in (a) cytosine methylation, (b) modifications of histones (such as methylation, acetylation and phophorylation), (c) energy-dependent chromatin remodeling or (d) RNA-based silencing. Among these epigenetic modifications, DNA methylation has attracted most interest as it regulates fundamental biological phenomena, such as genome stability, gene expression, X-chromosome inactivation and genomic imprinting. Studies of various species have shown that epigenetic control is critical for the normal function of the genome and if they occur improperly they may promote cancer [4]. It could be speculated that the loss of a normal epigenetic pattern over time could explain the late onset of common human diseases associated with age. Indeed, several CKD-related disease processes, such as hypertension [5], dyslipidemia [6], diabetes mellitus [7], ageing [8] and vascular disease [9], may be associated with epigenetic abnormalities.

Recent studies have demonstrated that epigenetic modifications due to environmental impact can be inherited for generations. Thus, alterations in the epigenotype may be one mechanism by which embryonic/fetal nutritional exposure in utero can influence gene expression and phenotype in the adult life. Indeed, a sex-specific transgenerational response to nutritional exposure has been reported in humans [10]. Of interest, one study showed that the diabetes mortality increased if the paternal grandfather was exposed to a surfeit of food during his slow growth prepubertal period [11]. The current literature, thus, suggests that we do not only inherit our gene sequence but also the effects of our ancestor's lifestyle in a partly Lamarckian way.

Methods to Study the Epigenotype

In contrast to genetic studies, the assessment of epigenetic modifications requires access to the tissue/cell type of interest. Unfortunately, this makes many epigenetic investigations in human studies very hard to conduct, and surrogate tissues and/or autopsy material have to be used in most cases. Several methods for global and gene-specific methylation analysis have been described in the literature [12]. The assessment of DNA methylation can be performed on most biological materials, fresh as well as frozen, at the genome-wide global scale, or gene-specific. Depending on the questions asked, both global and gene-specific DNA methylation analyses might be useful when assessing various pathological conditions. Global DNA methylation can be assessed in large patient materials using the luminometric assay (LUMA), which can be used as a quantitative rather than qualitative method [13]. Even though global analysis is a blunt tool, it should be emphasized that (in analogy to the unspecific nature of fever in various diseases) aberrant global DNA methylation is a sign of an epigenetic dysregulation that may provide important information of general disease states. Indeed, aberrant global DNA methylation has been demonstrated in various complex clinical conditions associated with ageing, atherosclerosis, inflammation, viral infections and carcinogenesis [14].

The Uremic Milieu – How Does It Affect the Epigenotype?

Considering the fact that hyperhomocysteinemia [15], inflammation [16], dyslipidemia [6] and oxidative stress [17] all may be associated with unbalanced DNA methylation and persistent change in chromatin organization, the effect of the uremic milieu on the epigenotype have been surprisingly little studied (fig. 1). In patients with vascular disease, increased homocysteine and S-adenosylhomocysteine (SAH) concentrations have been associated with DNA hypomethylation [18]. Thus, as plasma SAH levels are positively associated with lymphocyte DNA hypomethylation [19], elevation of homocysteine seems to have a negative effect on methylation reaction, mediated via an increase in intracellular SAH. In accordance, signs of global DNA hypomethylation were demonstrated in mononuclear cells in a small group of hyperhomocysteinemic HD patients [15]. However, as recent in vitro studies showed that homocysteine elevated inducible nitric oxide synthase (iNOS; a key enzyme in the regulation of vascular disease) promoter hypermethylation [20], and caused methylation of the ApoE (an important gene for anti-atherosclerosis) promoter [21] and the estrogen receptor (ER)-α gene [22], the effect of homocysteine on DNA methylation on a global and gene-specific level seems complex and could be context-sensitive. Indeed, Jiang et al. [23] demonstrated that different concentrations of homocysteine might have different effects on the epigenotype in rats. Whereas mild and moderate hyperhomocysteinemia might primarily influence the epigenetic regulation of gene expression through the interference of transferring methyl-group metabolism, the impact by high circulating homocysteine concentrations might be more injurious through oxidative stress, apoptosis and inflammation [23]. Thus, longitudinal studies are needed to investigate the effects of decreasing renal function on the epigenotype, and future interventions directed towards hyperhomocysteinemia in CKD should take into account the fact that homocysteine may have different effects on critical genes involved in atherogenesis dependent on the circulating levels [20].

In this context, persistent inflammation seems to be an important factor to take into account as it plays a part in the counterintuitive association between high homocysteine levels and better outcome in CKD [24]. Mediators of the inflammatory response, such as cytokines, free radicals, prostaglandins and growth factors, can induce epigenetic changes including DNA methylation and post-translational modifications. As this could cause alterations in critical pathways responsible for maintaining the normal cellular homeostasis, the impact of persistent inflammation on the uremic epigenotype needs further consideration. Whereas one study showed that the inflammatory cytokine IL-6 supports tumor suppressor gene promoter methylation [25], another study by the same group showed that IL-6 might exert an impact on epigenetic changes in cells via regulation of a DNA methyltransferase gene [26]. In another experiment in which embryonic stem cells were exposed to bacterial products (i.e. LPS), increased DNA methylation was found in the toll-like receptor (TLR)-4 gene upstream region [27]. In a recent clinical study of CKD patients we demonstrated that global DNA hypermethylation (assessed by LUMA) was associated with inflammation and poor outcome [16]. In an additional in vitro experiment we found that IL-6 promoted global DNA hypermethylation [16]. As a study of dialysis patients with renal neoplasm also showed evidence of DNA hypermethylation of various genes compared to renal neoplasm cases with normal renal function, current evidence suggests that uremia and/or the dialysis procedure per se promotes DNA hypermethylation [28]. One possible mechanism that may link inflammation to DNA hypermethylation in uremia is abnormal lipoprotein metabolism. Since Lund et al. [6] have shown that lipoproteins induce DNA hypermethylation in cultured cells, the effects of fatty acids and lipoproteins on the uremic epigenotype need further attention.

Folic acid is another factor that affects global DNA-methylation status in the genome and the regulation of imprinted genes [15], and represses the effects on DNA methylation induced by homocysteine [21]. Thus, vitamin status should be taken into account when studying the complex and context-sensitive interactions between unbalanced DNA methylation, vascular disease and outcome in CKD. As methylation status correlates with the transcriptional activity of a promoter, and methylation is associated with gene silencing [29], the effects of DNA hypermethylation on the expression of different genes in the uremic milieu should be further explored. In fact, one study showed that DNA hypermethylation causes silencing of erythropoietin expression [30]. Such studies may thus lead to a better understanding how the uremic milieu contributes to premature vascular disease and vascular ageing via up- or down-regulation of critical genes participating in atherosclerosis and smooth muscle cell proliferation (fig. 1).

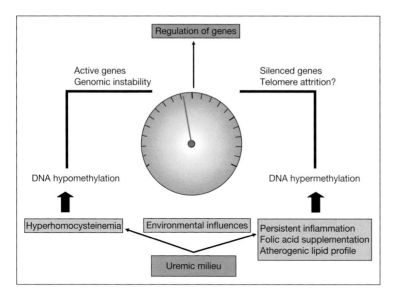

Fig. 1. Epigenetic mechanisms govern transcriptional regulation like a dynamic rheo-stat. In the unphysiological uremic milieu, several factors, such as hyperhomocysteinemia, vitamin B and folate status, dyslipidemia and persistent inflammation, affect the epigenome and gene function. Because of the effects on DNA methylation status by opposing factors, such as hyperhomocysteinemia and persistent inflammation, the balance of these factors will affect the epigenome, which via gene activation, silencing, or telomere attrition will ulti-mately regulate gene function.

Indeed, it has previously been shown that age-related inactivation due to methy-lation of the ER-α gene in vascular tissue might play a role in atherogenesis and ageing of the vascular system [31].

Can the Epigenotype Be Manipulated?

Epigenetics may not only uncover etiologic and pathogenic mechanisms, but also be a novel concept that may help to develop future treatment strategies targeting the primary epigenetic alterations. Currently, a number of epigenetic drugs, such as histone deacetylase inhibitors and DNA methylation inhibitors, exist at various stages of development [32]. As procainamide specifically inhibits DNA methyltransferase it has been suggested that this drug may be use-ful in the prevention of cancer [33]. Although promising results have been reported with epigenetic drugs, major concerns include their lack of target speci-ficity as well as their transient effects [32]. As interventions with folate in man

[15], and genistein in mice [34], may reverse epigenetic DNA unbalance, nutritional interventions may be another way of modifying the epigenome in CKD.

Conclusion

Our understanding of the role played by epigenetics in CKD remains in its infancy. Thus, further studies are needed to better understand the associations of aberrant DNA methylation in relation to homocysteine, dyslipidemia, vitamin deficiencies, oxidative stress and inflammation, as well as its presumably very complex interactions in the development of premature uremic vascular disease. Further research is also needed to study the association between aberrant global DNA methylation, gene level methylation status and silencing (or activation) of key genes associated with atherosclerosis (such as ApoE, ER-α and iNOS) in the context of uremia. As it is possible to modify the epigenome, the effects of various nutritional and pharmacological epigenetic interventions on unbalanced DNA methylation, gene expression, vascular health and outcome should be further explored in uremia.

Acknowledgements

The Swedish Medical Research Council (P.S.) and the Swedish Cancer Foundation (T.J.E.) supported the present work.

References

1   Stenvinkel P, Carrero JJ, Axelsson J, Lindholm B, Heimburger O, Massy Z: Emerging biomarkers for evaluating cardiovascular risk in the chronic kidney disease patient: How do new pieces fit into the uremic puzzle? Clin J Am Soc Nephrol 2008;3:505–521.
2   Stenvinkel P, Ekström T: Epigenetics – a helpful tool to better understand processes in clinical nephrology? Nephrol Dial Transpl 2008 (in press).
3   Richards EJ: Inherited epigenetic variation – revisiting soft inheritance. Nat Rev 2006;7:395–400.
4   Jones PA, Baylin SB: The epigenomics of cancer. Cell 2007;128:683–692.
5   Bogdarina I, Welham S, King PJ, Burns SP, Clark AJ: Epigenetic modifications of the renin-angiotensin system in the fetal programming of hypertension. Circ Res 2007;100:520–526.
6   Lund G, Andersson L, Lauria M, Lindholm M, Fraga MF, Villar-Garea A, et al: DNA methylation polymorphisms precede any histological sign of atherosclerosis in mice lacking apolipoprotein E. J Biol Chem 2004;279:29147–29154.
7   Gray S, De Meyts P: Role of histone and transcription factor acetylation in diabetes pathogenesis. Diabetes Metab Res Rev 2005;21:416–433.
8   Fraga MF, Esteller M: Epigenetics and aging: the targets and the marks. Trends Genet 2007; 23:413–418.
9   Dong C, Yoon W, Goldsmith-Clermont PJ: DNA methylation and atherosclerosis. J Nutr 2002; 132:2406S–2409S.

10   Pembrey ME, Bygren LO, Kaati G, Edvinsson S, Northstone K, Sjöström M, et al: Sex-specific, male-line transgenerational responses in humans. Eur J Hum Genet 2006;14:159–166.

11   Kaati G, Bygren LO, Edvinsson S: Cardiovascular and diabetes mortality determined by nutrition during parents' and grandparents' slow growth period. Eur J Hum Genet 2002;10:682–688.

12   Shen L, Waterland RA: Methods of DNA methylation analysis. Curr Opin Clin Nutr Metab Care 2007;10:576–581.

13   Karimi M, Johansson S, Ekström TJ: Using LUMA, a luminometric based assay for global DNA methylation. Epigenetics 2006;1:45–48.

14   Maekawa M, Watanabe Y: Epigenetics: relations to disease and laboratory findings. Curr Med Chem 2007;14:2642–2653.

15   Ingrosso D, Cimmino A, Perna AF, Masella L, de Santo NG, De Bonis ML, et al: Folate treatment and unbalanced methylation and changes of allelic expression induced by hyperhomocysteinemia in patients with uremia. Lancet 2003;361:1693–1699.

16   Stenvinkel P, Karimi M, Johansson S, Axelsson J, Suliman M, Lindholm B, et al: Impact of inflammation on epigenetic DNA methylation – a novel risk factor for cardiovascular disease? J Intern Med 2007;261:488–499.

17   Valinluck V, Tsai HH, Rogstad DK, Burdzy A, Bird A, Sowers LC: Oxidative damage to methyl-CpG sequences inhibits the binding of the methyl-CpG binding domain (MBD) of methyl-CpG binding protein 2 (MeCP2). Nucleic Acids Res 2004;32:4100–4108.

18   Castro R, Rivera I, Struys EA, Jansen EEW, Ravasco P, Camilo ME, et al: Increased homocysteine and S-adenosylhomocysteine concentrations and DNA hypomethylation in vascular disease. Clin Chem 2003;49:1292–1296.

19   Yi P, Melnyk S, Pogribna M, Pogribny IP, Hine RJ, James SJ: Increase in plasma homocysteine associated with parallel increases in plasma S-adenosylhomocysteine and lymphocyte DNA hypomethylation. J Biol Chem 2000;275:29318–29323.

20   Jiang Y, Zhang J, Xiong J, Cao J, Li G, Wang S: Ligands of peroxisome proliferator-activated receptor inhibit homocysteine-induced DNA methylation of inducible nitric oxide synthase gene. Acta Biochim Biophys Sin 2007;39:366–376.

21   Yi-Deng J, Tao S, Hui-Ping Z, Jian-Tuan X, Jun C, Gui-Zhong L, et al: Folate and ApoE DNA methylation induced by homocysteine in human monocytes. DNA Cell Biol 2007;26:737–744.

22   Huang Y, Peng K, Su J, Huang Y, Xu Y, Wang S: Different effects of homocysteine and oxidized low density lipoprotein on methylation status in the promoter region of the estrogen receptor α gene. Acta Biochim Biophys Sin 2007;39:19–26.

23   Jiang Y, Sun T, Xiong J, Cao J, Li G, Wang S: Hyperhomocysteinemia-mediated DNA hypomethylation and its potential role in rats. Acta Biochim Biophys Sin 2007;39:657–667.

24   Suliman ME, Barany P, Kalantar-Zadeh K, Lindholm B, Stenvinkel P: Homocysteine in uraemia – a puzzling and conflicting story. Nephrol Dial Transpl 2005;20:16–21.

25   Hodge DR, Peng B, Cherry JC, Hurt EM, Fox SD, Kelley JA, et al: Interleukin-6 supports the maintenance of p53 tumor suppressor gene promoter methylation. Cancer Res 2005;65:4673–4682.

26   Hodge DR, Xiao W, Clausen PA, Heidecker G, Szyf M, Farrar WL: Interleukin-6 regulation of the human DNA metyltransferase (HDNMT) gene in human erythroleukemia cells. J Biol Chem 2001;276:39508–39511.

27   Zampetaki A, Xiao Q, Zeng L, Hy Y, Xu Q: TLR4 expression in mouse embryonic stem cells and in stem cell-derived vascular cells is regulated by epigenetic modifications. Biochem Biophys Res Commun 2006;347:89–99.

28   Hori Y, Oda Y, Kiyoshima K, Yamada Y, Nakashima Y, Naito S, et al: Oxidative stress and DNA hypermethylation status in renal cell carcinoma arising in patients on dialysis. J Pathol 2007;212:218–226.

29   Meehan R, Lewis J, Cross S, Nan X, Jeppesen P, Bird A: Transscriptional regression by methylation of CpG. J Cell Sci 1992;16(suppl):9–14.

30   Yin H, Blanchard KL: DNA methylation represses the expression of the human erythropoietin gene by two different mechanisms. Blood 2000;95:111–119.

31   Post WS, Goldschmidt-Clermont PJ, Wilhide CC, Heldman AW, Sussman MS, Ouyang P, et al: Methylation of the estrogen receptor gene is associated with aging and atherosclerosis in the cardiovascular system. Cardiovasc Res 1999;43:985–991.

32   Ptak C, Petronis A: Epigenetics and complex disease: from etiology to new therapeutics. Annu Rev Pharmacol Toxicol 2008;48:257–276.
33   Lee BH, Yegnasubramanian S, Lin X, Nelson WG: Procainamide is a specific inhibitor of DNA methyltransferase-1. J Biol Chem 2005;280:40749–40756.
34   Day JK, Bauer AM, desBordes C, Zhuang Y, Kim B-E, Newton LG, et al: Genistein alters methylation patterns in mice. J Nutr 2002;132:2419S–2423S.

Peter Stenvinkel, MD, PhD
Department of Renal Medicine, K56
Karolinska University Hospital at Huddinge
SE–141 86 Stockholm (Sweden)
Tel. +46 8 5858 2532, Fax +46 8 711 4742, E-Mail peter.stenvinkel@ki.se

Ronco C, Cruz DN (eds): Hemodialysis – From Basic Research to Clinical Trials.
Contrib Nephrol. Basel, Karger, 2008, vol 161, pp 63–67

....

The Burden of Cardiovascular Disease in Patients with Chronic Kidney Disease and in End-Stage Renal Disease

Carmine Zoccali

Nephrology, Hypertension and Renal Transplantation, CNR-IBIM Clinical Epidemiology of Renal Diseases and Hypertension, Ospedali Riuniti, Reggio Calabria, Italy

Abstract

Patients who reach the end-stage phase of renal disease (ESRD) display an exceedingly high risk for cardiovascular (CV) complications. However it is still unclear whether in patients with chronic kidney disease (CKD) a critical glomerular filtration rate (GFR) threshold exists below which CV risk starts to rise. Analyses based on a medical database indicate that starting from the lower limit of the normal range (60 ml/min) a 30-ml/min GFR loss entails a doubling in the CV risk. In contrast, in population-based studies like the Atherosclerosis Risk in the Community (ARIC), the risk excess of stage 3 CKD is much lower, being about 30%. This discrepancy indicates that analyses based on medical databases provide an inflated estimate of the population risk for CV events associated with CKD. However, given the high prevalence of CKD at population level (about 8%–10%), a 30% increase in the risk of CV events would still have enormous public health implications. A considerable proportion of patients with CKD and occult or overt CV disease still remain largely undertreated. Multiple interventions on the multiple, modifiable risk factors of CKD at population and hospital level should be deployed if we are to curb the burden of CV sequelae of the CKD epidemics.

Chronic Kidney Disease as a Public Health Priority

Chronic kidney disease (CKD) is now considered as an established risk factor for death and cardiovascular disease (CVD) [1]. In particular, patients who reach the end-stage phase of renal disease (ESRD) display an exceedingly high risk. The proportion of patients dying because of cardiovascular complications in this population is remarkably similar to that in the general population,

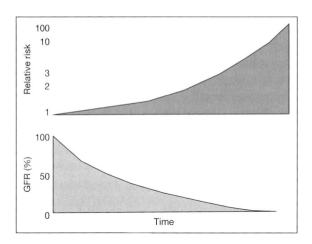

Fig. 1. Relationship between the GFR and the risk for CHD death. The graph was modeled according to data reported in references 2 and 3.

being about 50%. However, the absolute risk for overall and cardiovascular mortality in ESRD patients is so high that the probability of cardiovascular mortality in these patients is 5 (older cohorts) to 500 (younger cohorts) times higher than that in coeval individuals in the general population [2] with an average estimate of about 100 [3]. This exceedingly high risk is viewed as the terminal stage of a progressive disease that initiates in the early phase of renal disease (fig. 1). However, it is still unclear whether a glomerular filtration rate (GFR) threshold exists wherefrom individuals start to be exposed to a higher risk for cardiovascular complications. In general terms this is not a trivial question. Indeed it is relevant knowing at what CKD stage the excess risk takes an exponential shape. Mild and moderate degrees of renal impairment are much frequent (about 8–10%) and an early rise in the risk of cardiovascular events associated with renal function loss would entail a huge burden of cardiovascular complications at population level. In contrast, in a public health perspective, the cardiovascular sequelae of renal insufficiency would be much less concerning if the risk excess is confined to patients with severe GFR loss.

Is Chronic Kidney Disease a Real Cardiovascular Risk Equivalent to Diabetes?

Analyses by Go et al. [4] in the Francisco Bay area Kaiser Permanente enrollees demonstrated that, starting from the lower limit of the GFR range (conventionally, 60 ml/min per $1.73 \, m^2$ in this study) a 30 ml/min per $1.73 \, m^2$ decrease in the GFR (i.e. the lower limit of stage 3 CKD) entails a doubling in the risk of cardiovascular death. It was noted that such risk excess is similar to that of patients who had had a myocardial infarction and that therefore CKD should be considered as a 'risk equivalent' [5], i.e. a condition similar to diabetes mellitus which current guidelines, like the Adult Treatment Panel III guidelines (ATPIII), equate to a coronary event [6]. The concept of 'risk equivalent' is a pragmatic solution to directly identify high-risk individuals who deserve close surveillance and intensive treatment without resorting to the use of risk tables or risk calculators, i.e. two approaches that are difficult to implement in the busy clinical practice by the majority of physicians. It is expected that the application of the 'risk equivalent' concept improves the treatment of high-risk individuals and that it may eventually produce better clinical outcomes in CKD patients. To exemplify in the lipidology area, ATPIII guidelines assign a lower LDL cholesterol treatment goal to patients with diabetes or with peripheral atherosclerosis [6]. Because the relationship between LDL cholesterol and coronary heart disease (CHD) is linear across a wide range of LDL cholesterol values, setting a lower treatment goal in high-risk patients like diabetics would translate in a decrease in CHD event rates. The decision of considering CKD as a risk equivalent is not an economically neutral decision in that it would impose important costs to health systems. For example it can be estimated that in Italy about 300,000 additional patients would be prescribed a statin if the concept of 'risk equivalent' is applied to CKD.

Are We Overestimating the Cardiovascular Risk of CKD?

The number of studies associating CKD with cardiovascular risk is now very large. The association has been consistently found in patients with CVDs, particularly in patients in myocardial infarction or heart failure, and in community-level studies as well [1]. There is no question that this association is of clinical importance but eminent nephrologists believe that the public health implications of CKD are now overemphasized [7]. As mentioned before, the indication that CKD can be considered as a risk equivalent is based on the study of Go et al. [4], i.e. on detailed analyses in over 1 million persons enrolled with the Kaiser Permanente Center [4]. It is important to underline that these individuals were abstracted from a medical database and that therefore they were not representative of the general population. In other words, for creatinine to be ordered by a doctor there must be an underlying suspicion of a medical condition associated with or aggravated by renal insufficiency. To estimate the population risk of CVD attributable to CKD, studies performed at population level are needed.

Until now only one such study has been published. In this study [8], the Atherosclerosis Risk in Communities (ARIC), which enrolled middle-aged persons (45–64 years), stage 3 CKD signaled an increased risk for CHD. However, the relative risk estimate which materialized in this study was less than that in the study of Go et al. [4]. Indeed the incident risk for CHD or first non-fatal myocardial infarction in stage 3 CKD patients was almost halved in comparison to that in patients with past myocardial infarction and no CKD.

The Core Problem: Facing the Burden of the CKD Epidemics

Thus, sensu strictu, stage 3 CKD does not represent a CHD risk equivalent to diabetes mellitus and therefore stage 3 CKD patients should not automatically receive intensive treatment with lipid-lowering drugs. Yet it should be clearly recognized that the problem cannot be considered as having been definitively resolved. Disentangling the relative role of diabetes and CKD, and the high risk presented by patients having both diseases, is not a simple matter. CKD and diabetes frequently coexist and the resulting risk is higher than that of the two conditions considered separately. Past studies identifying diabetes or myocardial infarction as CHD risk equivalents more often than not failed to consider the interaction between these two conditions and CKD, and therefore did not exclude people with CKD or proteinuria. Thus the possibility remains that the excess risk of diabetes and myocardial infarction in part depends on coexistent CKD. However, it seems unlikely that, at community level, stage 3 CKD per se entails an independent risk sufficiently high to qualify this condition as a CHD equivalent. Yet, even though it cannot be considered as a risk equivalent, CKD (from stage 3 on) remains a main public health priority. Indeed, given the high prevalence of CKD at population level (about 8–10%), a 10–30% increase in the risk of cardiovascular events would still have enormous public health implications. Furthermore, it should not be forgotten that GFR levels <45 ml/min/1.73 m² (stage 3b), particularly in the presence of proteinuria, most likely entail a more than double risk excess for coronary events. At this phase of knowledge it appears fundamental not to lose the momentum in the fight against CKD, because CKD and proteinuria are often not properly taken into account in the clinical decision process by internists, cardiologists and general practitioners. In the real world of everyday clinical practice, a considerable proportion of patients with CKD and occult or overt CVD still remain largely undertreated [9]. Multiple interventions on the multiple, modifiable risk factors of CKD at population and hospital level should be deployed if we are to curb the burden of cardiovascular sequelae of the CKD epidemics.

References

1   Zoccali C: Traditional and emerging cardiovascular and renal risk factors: an epidemiologic per-
    spective. Kidney Int 2006;70:26–33.
2   Foley RN, Parfrey PS, Sarnak MJ: Clinical epidemiology of cardiovascular disease in chronic
    renal disease. Am J Kidney Dis 1998;32:S112–S119.
3   Baigent C, Burbury K, Wheeler D: Premature cardiovascular disease in chronic renal failure.
    Lancet 2000;356:147–52.
4   Go AS, Chertow GM, Fan D, McCulloch CE, Hsu CY: Chronic kidney disease and the risks of
    death, cardiovascular events, and hospitalization. N Engl J Med 2004 23;351:1296–1305.
5   Levey AS, Beto JA, Coronado BE, Eknoyan G, Foley RN, Kasiske BL, et al: Controlling the epi-
    demic of cardiovascular disease in chronic renal disease: What do we know? What do we need to
    learn? Where do we go from here? National Kidney Foundation Task Force on Cardiovascular
    Disease. Am J Kidney Dis 1998;32:853–906.
6   Executive Summary of the Third Report of the National Cholesterol Education Program (NCEP)
    Expert Panel on Detection, Evaluation, and Treatment of High Blood Cholesterol in Adults (Adult
    Treatment Panel III). JAMA 2001;285:2486–2497.
7   Couser WG: Chronic kidney disease the promise and the perils. J Am Soc Nephrol 2007;18:
    2803–2805.
8   Wattanakit K, Coresh J, Muntner P, Marsh J, Folsom AR: Cardiovascular risk among adults with
    chronic kidney disease, with or without prior myocardial infarction. J Am Coll Cardiol 2006;
    48:1183–1189.
9   Locatelli F, Zoccali C: Clinical policies on the management of chronic kidney disease patients in
    Italy. Nephrol Dial Transplant 2008;23:621–626.

Prof. Carmine Zoccali
CNR Laboratorio di Epidemiologia Clinica e Fisiopatologia
delle Malattie Renali e dell Ipertensione Arteriosa
Ospedale Riuniti, Via Vallone Petrara, IT–89124 Reggio Calabria (Italy)
Tel. +39 0965 397010, Fax +39 0965 56005, E-Mail carmine.zoccali@tin.it

Inflammation

Ronco C, Cruz DN (eds): Hemodialysis – From Basic Research to Clinical Trials.
Contrib Nephrol. Basel, Karger, 2008, vol 161, pp 68–75

·······················

BNP and a Renal Patient: Emphasis on the Unique Characteristics of B-Type Natriuretic Peptide in End-Stage Kidney Disease

Mikko Haapio[a], *Claudio Ronco*[b]

[a]Division of Nephrology, HUCH Meilahti Hospital, Helsinki, Finland, and
[b]Department of Nephrology, St. Bortolo Hospital, Vicenza, Italy

Abstract

Background: The widespread use of brain natriuretic peptide testing among patients with end-stage kidney disease (ESKD) has brought new insight to prognostic cardiovascular factors in this population, but has also raised questions regarding the diagnostic potential of B-type natriuretic peptide (BNP) and NT-proBNP in subjects with renal impairment. **Methods:** Highlighting the most important recent observations in the field, this review discusses the unique characteristics of BNP testing and interpretation in chronic kidney disease. **Results:** We review in detail the physiology and effects of BNP along with providing a thoughtful analysis of the limitations of BNP testing in patients with impaired kidney function. Additionally, the practicability of BNP in the management of renal patients with some rational suggestions for the use of BNP are presented. **Conclusion:** Although at present the use and interpretation of BNP testing in ESKD patients is complicated by altered renal clearance and frequent cardiac co-morbidity and, moreover, the complex and in many parts unknown interplay between the heart and the kidneys (cardiorenal syndrome), the prognostic value of elevated BNP is validated in the ESKD population. The importance of improving our understanding of the mechanisms of biomarkers in heart-kidney interdependence is emphasized.

Physiology of B-Type Natriuretic Peptide

B-type natriuretic peptide (BNP) belongs to a family of natriuretic peptides (NPs) which are vasodilatory neurohormones having an important role in controlling blood pressure and fluid homeostasis. Other members of the family are A-type natriuretic peptide (ANP), C-type natriuretic peptide (CNP), *Dendroaspis* or D-type natriuretic peptide (DNP) and urodilatin. ANP was the one first discovered and identified; a substance secreted mainly from cardiac atria, causing diuresis, natriuresis and vasodilation. It has a short half-life of 2–3 min, which with its rather complicated assay technique make it less useful in clinical practice. BNP was originally found in porcine brain by Sudoh and colleagues, but has since been recognized to be secreted mostly from cardiac ventricles. CNP secretion takes place in vascular endothelial cells and it causes vascular smooth muscle relaxation and possesses antimitogenic effects. DNP's actions are similar to ANP and BNP, but its function in humans is not fully understood. Urodilatin is a product of alternative ANP precursor processing in the kidney, is secreted into luminal part of distal nephron and causes diuresis, natriuresis and smooth muscle relaxation [1].

The secretion of BNP occurs mainly from myocytes in cardiac ventricles in response to excessive cardiac ventricular wall distension, shear stress, various pathological states (for instance, myocardial ischemia or cardiomyopathies) and increased release of catecholamines, renin, angiotensin II and endothelin [1, 2]. The precursor pro-BNP (108 amino acids) is first secreted, then cleaved to amino or N-terminal fragment (NT-proBNP, 76 amino acids) and BNP (32 amino acids). NT-proBNP is biologically almost inactive, with an 8.5-kDa molecular weight, and a serum half-life of 60–120 min. Its clearance is thought to occur principally by renal excretion. The biologically active BNP (MW 3.4 kDa, T½ 15–20 min) binds to and activates natriuretic peptide receptor A (NPR-A), causing production of cyclic guanosyl monophosphate (cGMP), followed by the biological effects of BNP. BNP is metabolized by natriuretic peptide receptor C, which is widespread in the human body (liver, lungs, kidney and vascular endothelium). BNP, unlike NT-proBNP, is further degraded by neutral endopeptidases (mainly renal tubular NEP) [1, 2].

Normal Physiological Effects of BNP

In the kidneys, BNP causes afferent arteriolar dilation and efferent arteriolar constriction, leading to an elevation in intraglomerular pressure and filtration. Mesangial cell relaxation allows the effective membrane surface and the fraction of filtered sodium to increase resulting in enhanced natriuresis and diuresis. BNP counteracts the overactivity of renin-angiotensin-aldosterone system commonly seen in heart failure, and antagonizes effects of vasopressin [1]. Cardiovascular effects of BNP include peripheral vasodilation of both arterial and venous circulatory beds, thereby decreasing systemic vascular resistance, blood pressure and central venous pressure. These are followed by a slight decline in cardiac output and blood volume. In the coronary arteries, with their vasodilation, improved perfusion of myocardium without an increase in

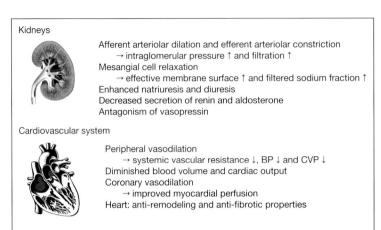

Kidneys

Afferent arteriolar dilation and efferent arteriolar constriction
    → intraglomerular pressure ↑ and filtration ↑
Mesangial cell relaxation
    → effective membrane surface ↑ and filtered sodium fraction ↑
Enhanced natriuresis and diuresis
Decreased secretion of renin and aldosterone
Antagonism of vasopressin

Cardiovascular system

Peripheral vasodilation
    → systemic vascular resistance ↓, BP ↓ and CVP ↓
Diminished blood volume and cardiac output
Coronary vasodilation
    → improved myocardial perfusion
Heart: anti-remodeling and anti-fibrotic properties

Central nervous system

Suppression of salt appetite and water intake
Decreased central sympathetic tone

Other

Lipolytic and lipid-mobilization effects?

Fig. 1. Physiological effects of BNP in healthy subjects. BP = Blood pressure; CVP = central venous pressure.

myocardial O_2 consumption takes place. BNP also possesses anti-remodeling and anti-fibrotic properties. In the central nervous system, central sympathetic tone decreases and suppression of salt appetite and water intake lessen systemic fluid overload [1]. There is some evidence that BNP also has lipolytic and lipid-mobilization effects (fig. 1). With all of these factors taken into account, BNP defends against the tendency for salt and water retention and reduces cardiac preload and filling pressures to counteract the vasoconstriction characteristic of such states as congestive heart failure.

BNP and Unique Characteristics of Renal Patients

With the above-described physiology of BNP and NT-proBNP in mind, it seems logical that renal insufficiency has an effect on the metabolism of BNP and NT-proBNP in particular. Owing to this fact and the frequent cardiac co-morbidity of renal patients, the clinical use of BNP and NT-proBNP has been complicated in patients with reduced glomerular filtration rate (GFR) under $60\,\text{ml/min}/1.73\,\text{m}^2$. The level of both BNP and NT-proBNP are negatively correlated to GFR in a graded fashion, yet both show a parallel behavior in elevation with NT-proBNP proportionally rising more than BNP as GFR approaches $15\,\text{ml/min}/1.73\,\text{m}^2$. In predialysis patients with left ventricular (LV) hypertrophy the reduction of estimated GFR of every $10\,\text{ml/min}/1.73\,\text{m}^2$ is associated with an increase of BNP about 20% and NT-proBNP about 38% [3]. In patients with chronic kidney disease, an abnormal circadian rhythmic oscillation of BNP has been recognized in which the frequency of pulsation is the same as in healthy subjects, but the secretion is abnormally high [4]. Furthermore, there is also a high intraindividual variation of NPs in end-stage kidney disease (ESKD) patients. NPs have a positive correlation to age and female gender and a negative correlation to body mass index.

In ESKD the risk of cardiovascular morbidity and mortality are grossly elevated and cardiovascular events are the leading cause for death in this population [5]. The prevalence of LV disorders is very common as only about 16% of ESKD patients present with a normal left ventricle assessed by echocardiography [6]. The pathological findings of the heart in uremia together with the commonly encountered anemia among these patients are associated with such cardiac derangements as cardiomegaly, diminished LV end systolic and diastolic volume (systolic and diastolic dysfunction), increased LV mass index and worsened LV ejection fraction, which in turn are associated with poor survival [6, 7]. LV hypertrophy is present in about 75%, congestive heart failure in approximately 40% and ischemic heart disease in 40% of ESKD patients [5].

With the commonness of cardiac pathology in ESKD, it is understandable that BNP values are above normal cut-off levels for heart failure in the majority of these patients; BNP in 94% and NT-proBNP in 100% of hemodialysis patients in one study [2]. This fact has aroused suspicion on the clinical utility of NPs, especially NT-proBNP, being affected more by the reduced renal clearance. Nonetheless, using above-normal cut-off values for ESKD patients, it has been shown in many studies that both BNP and NT-proBNP have independent predictive value for cardiovascular events and mortality. In the CREED study (Cardiovascular Risk Extended Evaluation in Dialysis patients), baseline BNP levels were higher in those patients who subsequently suffered a cardiovascular event than in event-free patients and in patients who died during follow-up ($p < 0.0001$ for both). A remarkable finding was that plasma BNP concentrations were only slightly elevated in patients with a normal LV mass index and LV geometry [8]. BNP concentrations are also higher in hemodialysis patients with coronary artery disease compared with those without [1].

About 60–80% of ESKD patients present with LV hypertrophy [6] which is often accompanied with congestive heart failure (CHF) and thereby a state in which serum BNP concentration is particularly elevated. Due to the closely

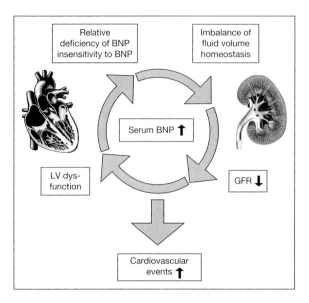

Fig. 2. A pathological cycle causing elevation of serum BNP. Cardiorenal and reno-cardiac connections with BNP. The heart and the kidneys are linked with neurohumoral signaling by BNP. Increased concentration of serum BNP is an independent predictor of cardiovascular morbidity and mortality in ESKD patients. BNP = B-type natriuretic peptide; LV = left ventricular, GFR = glomerular filtration rate.

linked and bidirectional control of fluid homeostasis between heart and kidneys, the issue of BNP elevation in this patient population has as yet not been clearly evaluated as far as the primary contributing factor elevating BNP is concerned. CHF (cardiac overload with fluid retention) in the presence of normal renal function raises BNP levels, and on the other hand a primary renal disease (without pre- or coexisting cardiac pathology) with reduced urine output also causes elevation of intravascular fluid volume with overload to heart chambers followed by a rise in BNP. Furthermore, altered clearance of NPs, specifically NT-proBNP, will add to the complex clinical consideration of the importance of NP elevation in these patients. The correct interpretation is further confounded by the recent findings that CHF in chronic kidney disease may well be a state of relative deficiency of BNP [9] as well as insensitivity to increased level of BNP [10], which could help to explain the controversy of high concentration of BNP without obviously seen clinical benefits of that elevation. It would be tempting to suggest that NP elevation is multifactorial, reflecting the elaborate mechanisms of cardiorenal and renocardiac syndromes in advanced heart and kidney diseases (fig. 2) [11].

Practicability of BNP in the Management of Renal Patients

Bearing in mind the close correlation between elevated NP levels and cardiac pathology, with inferior outcomes demonstrated in the ESKD population with elevated levels, choosing an appropriate way to utilize these biomarkers should prompt thorough investigation in this patient subpopulation. A high level of BNP could act as an alarm especially in ESKD patients without known preexisting cardiac pathology, to facilitate timely diagnostic and therapeutic interventions to prevent cardiovascular events. The awareness of a renal patient's NP level could also assist in hemodynamic assessment and subsequent treatment titration in heart failure.

There have been numerous trials aiming at establishing means for proper management of ESKD patient volume status with the aid of BNP level [12, 13]. Nevertheless, no clear correlation between hydration status, ultrafiltration volume and BNP has been found. Typically, the BNP level decreases during a HD session and either stays rather stable or increases somewhat before the next session. However, pre-HD session BNP can be used to distinguish patients with volume overload [12], and for patients with intradialytic BNP elevation the mortality risk is amplified [14].

The usefulness of BNP is further muddled by the conflicting evidence for BNP clearance by hemodialysis process. As it has not been proven whether the intradialytic drop in BNP level reflects lessened volume load on the heart (diminished production of BNP) or clearance by hemodialysis filter (in particular when high-flux dialyzer is applied), drawing conclusions based solely on BNP levels is not possible. It seems that at least partially the fall in BNP and NT-proBNP is caused by hemodialysis clearance [15].

Discussion

The readily available testing of brain NP has made it increasingly popular and broadly used, and both BNP and NT-proBNP have established a very sound and solid role in managing cardiac patients. Unfortunately the same has still not been possible for renal patients. To create plausible cut-off values for BNP and NT-proBNP in renal impairment has been troublesome, caused by the interdependence of the heart and the kidneys with simultaneous altered renal clearance and cardiac morbidity together with plural confounding factors (serum albumin, hemoglobin, β-blockade, age). A reliable biomarker should have a reference range wherein the changes of the parameter value are mirrored with a sufficient degree of precision in clinical status. Moreover, the reference range should take into account the level of renal dysfunction. Studies aiming at clarifying the possible usefulness of BNP with combined biomarker information are ongoing. At this point, all that can be summarized based on present knowledge of use of BNP and NT-proBNP in ESKD is that both parameters have an excellent negative predictive value in excluding myocardial distress. However, all that being said, BNP can to some extent provide us valuable and independent prognostic information in the day-to-day management of our complex ESKD patients. To make the most of BNP, there clearly is a pressing need for more research activity especially to find out the true role of BNP in the context of cardiorenal syndrome.

References

1 Suresh M, Farrington K: Natriuretic peptides and the dialysis patient. Semin Dial 2005;18: 409–419.
2 Racek J, Kralova H, Trefil L, Rajdl D, Eiselt J: Brain natriuretic peptide and N-terminal proBNP in chronic haemodialysis patients. Nephron Clin Pract 2006;103:c162–c172.
3 Austin WJ, Bhalla V, Hernandez-Arce I, Isakson SR, Beede J, Clopton P, Maisel AS, Fitzgerald RL: Correlation and prognostic utility of B-type natriuretic peptide and its amino-terminal fragment in patients with chronic kidney disease. Am J Clin Pathol 2006;126:506–512.
4 Pedersen EB, Bacevicius E, Bech JN, Solling K, Pedersen HB: Abnormal rhythmic oscillations of atrial natriuretic peptide and brain natriuretic peptide in chronic renal failure. Clin Sci (Lond) 2006;110:491–501.
5 Sarnak MJ, Levey AS, Schoolwerth AC, Coresh J, Culleton B, Hamm LL, McCullough PA, Kasiske BL, Kelepouris E, Klag MJ, Parfrey P, Pfeffer M, Raij L, Spinosa DJ, Wilson PW: Kidney disease as a risk factor for development of cardiovascular disease: a statement from the American Heart Association Councils on Kidney in Cardiovascular Disease, High Blood Pressure Research, Clinical Cardiology, and Epidemiology and Prevention. Hypertension 2003;42:1050–1065.
6 Foley RN, Parfrey PS, Harnett JD, Kent GM, Murray DC, Barre PE: The prognostic importance of left ventricular geometry in uremic cardiomyopathy. J Am Soc Nephrol 1995;5:2024–2031.
7 Silverberg DS, Wexler D, Iaina A, Steinbruch S, Wollman Y, Schwartz D: Anemia, chronic renal disease and congestive heart failure–the cardio renal anemia syndrome: the need for cooperation between cardiologists and nephrologists. Int Urol Nephrol 2006;38:295–310.
8 Zoccali C, Mallamaci F, Benedetto FA, Tripepi G, Parlongo S, Cataliotti A, Cutrupi S, Giacone G, Bellanuova I, Cottini E, Malatino LS: Cardiac natriuretic peptides are related to left ventricular mass and function and predict mortality in dialysis patients. J Am Soc Nephrol 2001;12: 1508–1515.
9 Liang F, O'Rear J, Schellenberger U, Tai L, Lasecki M, Schreiner GF, Apple FS, Maisel AS, Pollitt NS, Protter AA: Evidence for functional heterogeneity of circulating B-type natriuretic peptide. J Am Coll Cardiol 2007;49:1071–1078.
10 Forfia PR, Lee M, Tunin RS, Mahmud M, Champion HC, Kass DA: Acute phosphodiesterase-5 inhibition mimics hemodynamic effects of B-type natriuretic peptide and potentiates B-type natriuretic peptide effects in failing but not normal canine heart. J Am Coll Cardiol 2007;49: 1079–1088.
11 Ronco C, House AA, Haapio M: Cardiorenal syndrome: refining the definition of a complex symbiosis gone wrong. Intensive Care Med 2008 (in press).
12 Lee SW, Song JH, Kim GA, Lim HJ, Kim MJ: Plasma brain natriuretic peptide concentration on assessment of hydration status in hemodialysis patient. Am J Kidney Dis 2003;41:1257–1266.
13 Sheen V, Bhalla V, Tulua-Tata A, Bhalla MA, Weiss D, Chiu A, Abdeen O, Mullaney S, Maisel A: The use of B-type natriuretic peptide to assess volume status in patients with end-stage renal disease. Am Heart J 2007;153:244.e1–244.e5.

14   Biasioli S, Zamperetti M, Borin D, Guidi G, De Fanti E, Schiavon R: Significance of plasma
      B-type natriuretic peptide in hemodialysis patients: blood sample timing and comorbidity burden.
      ASAIO J 2007;53:587–591.
15   Wahl HG, Graf S, Renz H, Fassbinder W: Elimination of the cardiac natriuretic peptides B-type
      natriuretic peptide (BNP) and N-terminal proBNP by hemodialysis. Clin Chem 2004;50:
      1071–1074.

Dr. Mikko Haapio
HUCH Meilahti Hospital
Haartmaninkatu 4, FI–00029 Helsinki (Finland)
Tel. +358 9 4711, Fax +358 9 47177246, E-Mail mikko.haapio@helsinki.fi

Ronco C, Cruz DN (eds): Hemodialysis – From Basic Research to Clinical Trials.
Contrib Nephrol. Basel, Karger, 2008, vol 161, pp 76–82

....

Potential Interplay between Nutrition and Inflammation in Dialysis Patients

Martin K. Kuhlmann[a], *Nathan W. Levin*[b]

[a]Vivantes Klinikum im Friedrichshain, Berlin, and [b]Renal Research Institute,
New York, N.Y., USA

Abstract

Chronic inflammation, which is widely seen in long-term dialysis patients, is associated with malnutrition, atherosclerosis and an increased mortality risk. The relationship between inflammation and nutrition is certainly bidirectional with inflammation affecting nutritional status and dietary factors influencing the state of inflammation. Cytokines, such as IL-6 and TNF-α, interfere with the satiety center inducing loss of appetite, delayed gastric emptying and catabolism of skeletal muscle protein. High adipokine levels may also contribute to the development of malnutrition. On the other hand, dietary factors may interfere directly or indirectly with inflammatory activity. For example, dietary AGEs intake may aggravate inflammation while natural antioxidants, such as polyphenolic flavones or vitamin C from fruits and vegetables may even decrease inflammatory activity. Although there is a lack of good prospective nutritional studies in CKD patients, the individual patient should be advised to follow a more Mediterranean-style diet, restrain from broiling meats in order to avoid dietary AGEs, and take multivitamins regularly.

Patients undergoing maintenance hemodialysis have a high prevalence of protein-energy malnutrition and inflammation in association with atherosclerosis. This ferocious triad is strongly associated with outcome and it has been hypothesized that inflammation is the cause of both malnutrition and atherosclerosis. A definite link between inflammation and atherosclerosis has been established in recent years. On the other hand, the interrelationship between chronic inflammation and malnutrition is certainly bidirectional, with inflammation affecting nutritional status and dietary factors influencing the state of inflammation. We have previously discussed this topic at the Vicenza Course on Hemodialysis in 2005 [1] and are now updating the information in this article.

Pathogenesis of Inflammation

Chronic inflammation is characterized by increased plasma levels of pro-inflammatory (IL-1, IL-6, TNF-α, etc.) and decreased plasma levels of anti-inflammatory cytokines (IL-10). Pro-inflammatory cytokines are released from activated monocytes and macrophages, whereas IL-10 is a product of mainly monocytes and lymphocytes. An activated inflammatory response is a common feature of ESRD patients and predicts outcome. Pro-inflammatory mediators induce the hepatic synthesis of acute phase proteins (CRP) and inhibit the hepatic generation of negative acute phase reactants, such as albumin. In ESRD patients the balance between pro- and anti-inflammatory cytokines is disturbed, thus, that not only high levels of pro-inflammatory cytokine are correlated with severity and progression of carotid atherosclerosis [2], but that also low levels of anti-inflammatory cytokines are associated with increased morbidity and mortality.

There are multiple potential causes for inflammation in CKD patients, both dialysis-related and non-dialysis-related. The most frequent dialysis-related causes are suboptimal water quality in conjunction with dialysate back-filtration, and, as it is more and more recognized, the long-term placement of central venous dialysis catheters and the use of grafts for vascular access. Non-dialysis-related causes include decreased renal cytokine clearance, metabolic syndrome, insulin resistance, increased body fat mass, chronic heart failure, and accumulation of advanced glycation end products (AGEs). Much attention has been given recently to the effects of certain pro-inflammatory adipokines, which in renal failure are retained and not adequately eliminated [3].

Effect of Inflammation on Nutritional State

Besides their pronounced effects on atherosclerosis, pro-inflammatory cytokines also have profound effects on nutritional state. Initial findings from animal studies showing that cytokines interfere with the satiety center inducing loss of appetite, delayed gastric emptying (IL-6) and contribute to catabolism of skeletal muscle protein [4] have recently been confirmed in dialysis patients. Kalantar-Zadeh et al. [5] were able to demonstrate a strong and consistent association between poor appetite and high levels of inflammatory markers IL-6 and TNF-α, also known as cachectin. In this study the mortality risk in anorexic HD patients was 4–5 times that in those with normal appetite. Data from the DOPPS study recently pointed out that lack of appetite is also associated with depression and a higher risk of hospitalization [6]. Leptin and its receptors share structural and functional similarities with members of the cytokine family and an inverse relationship between leptin levels and spontaneous dietary energy intake has been reported. In uremic children, high leptin levels are associated with decreasing lean body mass [7]. In contrast, a recent study in 71 adult hemodialysis patients described low leptin levels as an independent predictor of mortality, adding to the discussion of the role of body composition and fat mass to outcome in ESR patients [8]. Taken together, there are many data indicating a direct link between chronic inflammation and the development of malnutrition in ESRD patients.

Effects of Dietary Factors on Inflammation

At least in the general population the saying 'we are what we eat' more and more turns out to hold some truth. Similarly, an increasing number of studies in the ESRD population also suggest that the inflammatory status can either be further triggered or even attenuated by diet modification. While up to 2004 most studies demonstrated some relation between dietary compounds and levels of selected cytokines, clinical studies in recent years put their focus on the biological effects of chronic inflammation, such as endothelial dysfunction.

Pro-oxidant and pro-inflammatory effects of advanced AGEs are well established [9]. These compounds are commonly elevated in patients with advanced CKD. While it had initially been assumed that AGEs are mainly produced endogenously, it is now accepted that an increased dietary AGE load can also contribute to elevated plasma AGE levels in dialysis patients [10]. Dietary AGEs are formed during heating of common foods due to spontaneous reactions between reducing sugars and proteins or lipids. These so-called dietary glycotoxins are generated in high amounts during roasting, broiling and oven frying, and considerably less during boiling, poaching, stewing and steaming of foods. The amount of AGEs ingested with a conventional diet is much higher than the total amount of AGEs in plasma and tissue. Roughly 10% of the dietary AGE amount ingested is absorbed and out of this fraction two thirds are retained in tissues in a bioactive form [9]. As a proof of concept it was demonstrated that circulating AGE levels can be decreased in dialysis patients by consumption of modified diets with low AGE content [11]. Lower serum AGE levels were accompanied by parallel changes in serum CRP levels. Recent data further support the relevance of the dietary AGE concept, as administration of a single oral load of AGEs to diabetics as well as healthy subjects led to an increase in circulating PAI-1 levels and an acute impairment of arterial flow-mediated dilation, an early indicator of endothelial dysfunction [12].

In HD patients, plasma isoprostanes, markers of oxidative lipid peroxidation, are significantly higher compared to healthy controls and are directly correlated with serum CRP levels, indicating a link between oxidative stress and inflammation [13]. A disruption of the natural balance between the generation of oxidants and the activity of antioxidant systems has been documented and plasma antioxidant capacity has been reported to be impaired in dialysis patients. Various vitamins, endogenous antioxidants (e.g. glutathione) and natural antioxidants mainly derived from fruits, such as polyphenolic flavones and catechins are acting as the main antioxidants in humans and need to be replenished regularly. In dialysis patients, however, the consumption of fresh fruits is restricted and absolute or functional vitamin deficit has been documented. Low vitamin C levels, even within the scorbutic range, can be found in a large percentage of dialysis patients [14]. Since vitamin C constitutes one of the most important water-soluble antioxidants in plasma and serves as the primary intracellular antioxidant in concert with glutathione, a severe depletion of this compound may well contribute to reduced antioxidant status and chronic inflammation.

A deficit in vitamins B_{12}, B_6 and folic acid in association with hyperhomocysteinemia is frequently found in dialysis patients. Besides being considered a non-traditional risk factor for cardiovascular disease, homocysteine (Hcy) it is also viewed as an oxidant and as an indicator of oxidative stress in dialysis patients. Although normalization of Hcy levels can be achieved in over 90% of HD patients by administering folic acid, vitamin B_6 and vitamin B_{12} intravenously during dialysis [15], several randomized, prospective folic acid intervention trials were not able to demonstrate significant effects on outcome in CKD and non-CKD patients [16]. Therefore, current recommendations do not support folic acid treatment to lower or normalize Hcy levels in dialysis patients.

Prescription of multivitamins is generally recommended for dialysis patients, but in practice this is not consistently the case. Among 308 representative dialysis facilities throughout Europe, Japan and the USA, the percentage of patients administered water-soluble vitamins varied largely, being highest in the USA (71.9%) and lowest in Japan (5.6%) with Europe in between, where it ranged from 3.7% in the UK to 37.9% in Spain [17]. Use of water-soluble vitamins was independently associated with a 16% reduction of relative risk for mortality. Still, no information is available from this study on the effects of multivitamins on inflammatory markers. In general, research is mainly focusing on supplementation of vitamin D analogues and not of multivitamins.

In 2004 data from the cross-sectional ATTICA study involving more than 3,000 healthy subjects from Greece reported significant associations between coffee consumption and inflammatory markers, blood pressure and hypercholesterolemia in healthy persons [18]. However, it was not sure whether the observed effect could be solely explained by caffeine intake, or whether other factors were involved. Meanwhile these data have been challenged by two new epidemiological studies reporting contrary, even anti-inflammatory effects of coffee consumption [19, 20]. Coffee may even serve as a relevant source of antioxidants, such as caffeine, polyphenols, pyrroles, furans, imidazoles and pyrazines. Many of these compounds are efficiently absorbed and plasma antioxidants increase after coffee intake [21]. The Iowa Women's Health Study concluded that coffee may inhibit inflammation and thereby reduce the risk of cardiovascular and other inflammatory diseases in postmenopausal women [19]. In a cross-sectional study on 730 healthy women with type 2 diabetes from the Nurses' Health Study I cohort, higher caffeinated coffee intake was associated with lower plasma concentrations of E-selectin, a marker of endothelial function, and lower CRP levels [20]. Further, more detailed studies on potential pro- or anti-inflammatory effects of coffee will be necessary before Starbucks will view dialysis units as a new promising market for their business.

Mediterranean diet, which is characterized by high intakes of vegetables, legumes, fruits and nuts, cereals, fish, and olive oil and relatively low intakes of dairy products and meat, is associated with a significantly lower mortality risk [22]. In the ATTICA study, adherence to a Mediterranean diet was associated with lower levels of inflammatory markers, such as CRP and IL-6. These data are now corroborated by a randomized, single-blinded, trial in 180 patients with metabolic syndrome, where the intervention group (n = 90) followed a Mediterranean-style diet and the control group a 'prudent diet' (50–60% carbohydrates, 15–20% proteins and <30% fat) for a period of 2 years. The main outcome measures were endothelial function assessed as blood pressure and platelet aggregation response to L-arginine, the natural precursor of nitric oxide, in addition to measuring circulating levels of the pro-inflammatory cytokines CRP, IL-6, IL-7 and IL-18. After 2 years, patients in the intervention group had significant decreases in body weight, body mass index, waist circumference, HOMA score and blood pressure compared to the control group. In addition, serum concentrations of the inflammatory markers were significantly reduced and endothelial function score improved in the intervention group but remained stable in the control group. There was an inverse relation between changes in endothelial function score and changes in CRP levels and HOMA score [23]. Taken together, Mediterranean diet appears to be a promising tool to reduce cardiovascular mortality among CKD 3–4 patients. For dialysis patients the complex Mediterranean diet will be associated with an increase in dietary phosphate intake, which needs to be compensated for by more intensive dialysis or higher phosphate binder dose.

Soy protein diets have received increasing attention because of their nutritional properties and their high content of isoflavones, natural antioxidants with anti-inflammatory potency. Blood levels of the isoflavone genistein are commonly used as markers of dietary soy intake and have been shown to accumulate in ESRD patients as a function of dietary soy intake. Small studies of short term soy protein diet in ESRD patients had reported an inverse correlation between plasma-isoflavone concentration and serum CRP levels. In a recent study in transplant patients, flow-mediated dilation of the brachial artery, an indicator of endothelial dysfunction, was improved after 5 weeks of soy diet [24]. This effect, which disappeared after soy withdrawal, was independent of changes in oxidative stress or isoflavone levels.

Taken together, data published between 2004 and 2008 further strengthen the interrelation between inflammation and nutrition and vice versa. Although no general recommendations can be made from these studies, the individual CKD or dialysis patient should be advised to follow a more Mediterranean-style diet, restrain from broiling meats in order to avoid dietary AGEs, and take his vitamins regularly.

References

1   Kuhlmann MK, Levin NW: Interaction between nutrition and inflammation in hemodialysis patients. Contrib Nephrol. Basel, Karger, 2005, vol 149, pp 200–207.
2   Pecoits-Filho R, Lindholm B, Stenvinkel P: The malnutrition, inflammation, and atherosclerosis syndrome – the heart of the matter. Nephrol Dial Transplant 2002;17:28–31.
3   Axelsson J, Heimbürger O, Stenvinkel P: Adipose tissue and inflammation in chronic kidney disease. Contrib Nephrol. Basel, Karger, 2006, vol 151, pp 165–174.
4   Ikizler TA: Role of nutrition for cardiovascular risk reduction in chronic kidney disease patients. Adv Chronic Kidney Dis 2004;11:162–171.
5   Kalantar-Zadeh K, Block G, McAllister CJ, Humphreys MH, Kopple JD: Appetite and inflammation, nutrition, anemia, and clinical outcome in hemodialysis patients. Am J Clin Nutr 2004;80: 299–307.
6   Lopes AA, Elder SJ, Ginsberg N, Andreucci VE, et al: Lack of appetite in haemodialysis patients associations with patient characteristics, indicators of nutritional status and outcomes in the international DOPPS. Nephrol Dial Transplant 2007;22:3538–3546.
7   Stenvinkel P, Pecoits-Filho R, Lindholm B: Leptin, ghrelin, and proinflammatory cytokines: compounds with nutritional impact in chronic kidney disease? Adv Ren Replace Ther 2003;10:155–169.
8   Scholze A, Rattensperger D, Zidek W, Tepel M Low serum leptin predicts mortality in patients with chronic kidney disease stage 5. Obesity 2007;15:1617–1622.
9   Vlassara H, Cai W, Crandall J, et al: Inflammatory mediators are induced by dietary glycotoxins, a major risk factor for diabetic angiopathy. Proc Natl Acad Sci USA 2002;99:15596–15601.
10 Uribarri J, Peppa M, Cai W, et al: Dietary glycotoxins correlate with circulating advanced glycation end product levels in renal failure patients. Am J Kidney Dis 2003;42:532–538.
11 Uribarri J, Peppa M, Cai W, et al: Restriction of dietary glycotoxins reduces excessive advanced glycation end products in renal failure patients. J Am Soc Nephrol 2003;14:728–731.
12 Uribarri J, Stirban A, Sander D, Cai W, et al: Single oral challenge by advanced glycation end products acutely impairs endothelial function in diabetic and nondiabetic subjects. Diab Care 2007;30:2579–2582.
13 Spittle MA, Hoenich NA, Handelman GJ, et al: Oxidative stress and inflammation in hemodialysis patients. Am J Kidney Dis 2001;38:1408–1413.
14 Richter A, Kuhlmann MK, Seibert E, Kotanko P, et al: Vitamin C deficiency and secondary hyperparathyroidism in chronic hemodialysis patients. Nephrol Dial Transplant 2008 (in press).

15   Obeid R, Kuhlmann MK, Kohler H, Herrmann W: Response of homocysteine, cystathionine, and methylmalonic acid to vitamin treatment in dialysis patients. Clin Chem 2005;51:196–201.

16   Suliman ME, Lindholm B, Bárány P, Qureshi AR, Stenvinkel P: Homocysteine-lowering is not a primary target for cardiovascular disease prevention in chronic kidney disease patients. Semin Dial 2007;20:523–529.

17   Fissell RB, Bragg-Gresham JL, Gillespie BW, et al: International variation in vitamin prescription and association with mortality in the Dialysis Outcomes and Practice Patterns Study (DOPPS). Am J Kidney Dis 2004;44:293–299.

18   Zampelas A, Panagiotakos DB, Pitsavos, et al: Associations between coffee consumption and inflammatory markers in healthy persons: the ATTICA study. Am J Clin Nutr 2004;80:862–867.

19   Andersen LF, Jacobs DR Jr, Carlsen MH, Blomhoff R: Consumption of coffee is associated with reduced risk of death attributed to inflammatory and cardiovascular diseases in the Iowa Women's Health Study. Am J Clin Nutr 2006;83:1039–1046.

20   Lopez-Garcia E, van Dam RM, Qi L, Hu FB: Coffee consumption and markers of inflammation and endothelial dysfunction in healthy and diabetic women. Am J Clin Nutr 2006;84:888–893.

21   Illy E: The complexity of coffee. Sci Am 2002;50:5480–5484.

22   Chrysohoou C, Panagiotakos DB, Pitsavos C, et al: Adherence to the Mediterranean diet attenuates inflammation and coagulation process in healthy adults: the ATTICA Study. J Am Coll Cardiol 2004;44:152–158.

23   Esposito K, Marfella R, Ciotola M, Di Paolo C, et al: Effect of a Mediterranean-style diet on endothelial dysfunction and markers of vascular inflammation in the metabolic syndrome. JAMA 2004;292:1440–1446.

24   Cupisti A, Ghiadoni L, D'Alessandro C, Kardasz I, et al: Soy protein diet improves endothelial dysfunction in renal transplant patients. Nephrol Dial Transplant 2007;22:229–234.

Martin K. Kuhlmann, MD
Klinik für Innere Medizin, Nephrologie
Vivantes Klinikum im Friedrichshain, Landsberger Allee 49
DE–10249 Berlin (Germany)
Tel. +49 30 13023 1322, Fax +49 30 13023 2046, E-Mail martin.kuhlmann@vivantes.de

Ronco C, Cruz DN (eds): Hemodialysis – From Basic Research to Clinical Trials.
Contrib Nephrol. Basel, Karger, 2008, vol 161, pp 83–88

....

Microinflammation and Endothelial Damage in Hemodialysis

Ana Merino, Sonia Nogueras, Paula Buendía, Raquel Ojeda,
Julia Carracedo, Rafael Ramirez-Chamond, Alejandro Martin-Malo,
Pedro Aljama

Department of Nephroplogy and Research Unit, University Hospital Reina Sofia,
Cordoba, Spain

Abstract

Background: Chronic kidney disease (CKD) stage 4-5 patients have increased cardiovascular morbidity and mortality rates compared with the general population. Chronic inflammation has been proposed as a cardiovascular risk factor. We have previously demonstrated that the majority of CKD patients show a microinflammatory state with an increased percentage of CD14+/CD16+ monocytes in peripheral blood, even in patients who do not show clinical evidence of inflammatory disease. However, the role played by these microinflammatory cells on the endothelial damage that precede the development of cardiovascular disease has not been investigated. **Methods:** To study the effect of microinflammation on endothelial cell injury we have developed an experimental co-culture model in which isolated CD14+/CD16+ cells were seeded in 24-well tissue-culture plates. Human umbilical vein endothelial cells were placed on the top of the culture well in a insert that permitted intercellular soluble network communication. To stimulate the release of proinflammatory products, monocytes were activated with substimulating doses of bacterial DNA. Endothelial injury was characterized measuring intracellular reactive oxygen species activity and cell apoptosis. **Results:** Only CD14+/CD16+ cells released proinflammatory cytokines when they were stimulated by bacterial DNA. In the culture wells in which inflammatory cytokines were detected, endothelial cells showed an increased reactive oxygen species activity and features of apoptosis. **Conclusions:** Our results support the hypothesis that independently of uremia, in CKD stage 4–5 patients microinflammation mediated by CD14+/CD16+ cells induces endothelial damage and thus may contribute to the increased risk of atherosclerosis and cardiovascular disease that has been reported in this population.

Patients with chronic kidney disease (CKD) stage 4-5 have a greater risk of developing cardiovascular disease, which is associated with higher rates of morbidity and mortality. Several studies have reported that the microinflammatory status chronically present in CKD patients is associated with endothelial dysfunction, an early event in atherosclerotic disease that precedes the appearance of cardiovascular diseases [1].

The inflammatory response plays an important role in protecting against tissue injury. The function of this immune response is to destroy and remove agents that can injure cells and tissues. However, this response is non-specific, and inflammatory mediators may produce unwanted damage. For this reason, the inflammatory process should cease after tissue structures have been repaired and their normal functions have been restored [2]. However, in chronic inflammatory diseases, when inflammation occurs in an uncontrolled manner, the excessive cellular damage may result in the destruction of normal tissue. Reactive oxygen species (ROS), such as the superoxide anion liberated by phagocytes recruited to sites of inflammation, have been suggested as a major cause of the cell and tissue damage, including apoptosis that is associated with many chronic inflammatory diseases. Excessive production of ROS, usually considered a signal of oxidative stress, results from an imbalance between pro- and antioxidant mechanisms in the cell. In vascular tissue, endothelial cells are susceptible to the injurious effects of oxidants. Although endothelial cells possess antioxidant enzymatic and non-enzymatic systems, which act in concert to detoxify ROS, a number of proatherogenic stimuli induce high rates of production of ROS that may induce endothelial cell damage and subsequently endothelial dysfunction and atherosclerosis [3].

A relationship between inflammation, oxidative stress and endothelial damage in CKD patients [4] is supported by numerous studies that correlate levels of inflammatory mediators, oxidative stress and markers of endothelial damage. However, the biological pathway by which inflammation of CKD patients induces endothelial damage is poorly understood. This is probably due to the lack of experimental models that assess the relationship between inflammatory activity induced by immunocompetent cells and endothelial cells.

In previous studies, we have reported that most CKD patients present a microinflammatory state with a raised percentage of CD14+/CD16+ monocytes in peripheral blood, even when there is no clinical evidence of inflammatory disease, such as elevated CRP or proinflammatory serum cytokine levels [5]. CD14+/CD16+ monocytes have been described as a subset of cells that show a shorter telomere than normal CD14++/CD16− monocytes, and which accumulate in the peripheral blood as a result of their enhanced resistance to proapoptotic stimuli [6–8]. Unlike CD14++/CD16− monocytes, CD14+/CD16+ cells contain intracytoplasmic preformed cytokines that are released to the extracellular

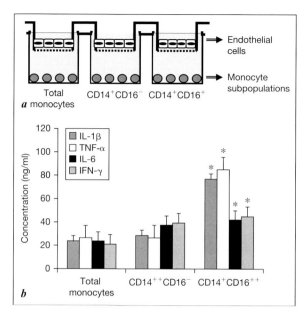

Fig. 1. a Schematic diagram of co-culture model. HUVEC cells were seeded into 0.45-μm pore-size cell culture inserts placed on culture plates. On another culture plate, peripheral blood monocytes, isolated CD14++/CD16− monocytes or CD14+/CD16+ monocytes were seeded into culture medium at a density of 1×10^5/cells. For the co-culture experiment, inserts containing HUVEC were washed and deposited on the top of the wells containing monocytes. ***b*** Cytokine levels were measured in the culture supernatant by flow cytometry, using a CBA assay kit. *p < 0.05 vs. total monocytes and vs. CD14++/CD16−.

medium, even when these monocytes are activated by stimuli, such as bacterial DNA, that are insufficient to induce an inflammatory response in normal CD14++/CD16− monocytes [9].

Suitable models of human 'pathological endothelium in CKD' could greatly expand our knowledge of the mechanisms responsible for initiation and progression of endothelial damage. The role of microinflammation-mediated CD14+/CD16+ monocytes in endothelial damage in CKD patients is still unknown. In order to study the effect of inflammatory products released by activated CD14+/CD16+ cells on endothelial cells, we have developed an experimental co-culture model in which isolated CD14+/CD16+ cells were seeded in 24-well tissue-culture plates. Human umbilical vein endothelial cells (HUVEC) were placed on the top of the culture well in a insert that permitted intercellular soluble network communication (fig. 1a). This experimental set-up conserves network signaling between inflammatory and endothelial cells.

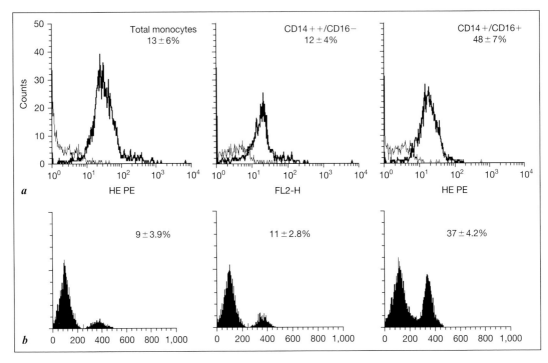

Fig. 2. Percentage of cells and representative graphs of cytofluorometry analysis of ROS activity and apoptosis in HUVEC co-cultured with (1) a total monocyte population, (2) isolated CD14++/CD16− monocytes, and (3) isolated CD14+/CD16+ monocytes. The percentage of endothelial cells showing ROS activity (**a**) or features of apoptosis (**b**) was greater in endothelial cells co-cultured with CD14+/CD16+ monocytes than in endothelial cells co-cultured with CD14++/CD16− monocytes or total monocytes ($p < 0.01$).

Thus, inflammatory products released by activated mononuclear cells may act on endothelial cells, and soluble mediators released by endothelial cells in response to these signaling can also interact with mononuclear cells. In order to stimulate the release of inflammatory cytokines, cells were cultured for 24 h in the presence of bacterial DNA (1.8 µg/ml), to evaluate endothelial damage, ROS activity and apoptosis were measured by flow cytometry in HUVEC As figure 1b shows, only CD14+/CD16+ cells released proinflammatory cytokines when they were stimulated by bacterial DNA, supporting our hypothesis that this subset of monocytes consists of activated monocytes with proinflammatory activity that play an important role in maintaining microinflammatory disease in hemodialysis patients.

Increased ROS activity in endothelial cells is believed to be an important factor in the endothelial damage associated with CKD. We have measured ROS activity in HUVEC co-cultured with non-isolated monocytes (total monocytes), CD14++/CD16– monocytes or CD14+/CD16+ monocytes. Only HUVEC cultures in the presence of CD14+/CD16+ monocytes showed ROS activity (fig. 2a). Furthermore, features of apoptosis were only observed in HUVEC cultures in the presence of CD14+/CD16+ monocytes, supporting the idea that oxidative stress induced by microinflammation in endothelial cells is sufficient to induce endothelial injury.

In conclusion, our results support the hypothesis that independently of uremia, in CKD stage 4-5 patients microinflammation mediated by CD14+/CD16+ cells induces endothelial damage and thus may contribute to the increased risk of atherosclerosis and cardiovascular disease that has been reported in this population.

Acknowledgments

This work was supported by grants from ISCIII-Fondo de Investigaciones Científicas de la Seguridad Social (FIS PI05/0896, PI06/0724, PI06/0747, PI07/0204, RETICs Red Renal RD06/0016/0007), Junta de Andalucía (207/05, TCRM 0006/2006), and Fundación Nefrológica. We are grateful M.J. Jiménez for technical assistance. J. Carracedo was supported by contract ISCIII-Fundación Progreso y Salud (Programa de Estabilización e Incentivación de la Investigación 2006).

References

1   Methe H, Weis M: Atherogenesis and inflammation – was Virchow right? Nephrol Dial Transplant 2007;22:1823–1827.
2   Barton GM: A calculated response: control of inflammation by the innate immune system. J Clin Invest 2008;118:413–420.
3   Zhang DX, Gutterman DD: Mitochondrial reactive oxygen species-mediated signaling in endothelial cells. Am J Physiol 2007;292:H2023–2031.
4   Morena M, Delbosc S, Dupuy AM, Canaud B, Cristol JP: Overproduction of reactive oxygen species in end-stage renal disease patients: a potential component of hemodialysis-associated inflammation. Hemodial Int 2005;9:37–46.
5   Ramirez R, Carracedo J, Merino A, Nogueras S, Alvarez-Lara MA, Rodríguez M, Martin-Malo A, Tetta C, Aljama P: Microinflammation induces endothelial damage in hemodialysis patients: the role of convective transport. Kidney Int 2007;72:108–113.
6   Carracedo J, Ramirez R, Soriano S, Alvarez de Lara MA, Rodriguez M, Martin-Malo A, Aljama P: Monocytes from dialysis patients exhibit characteristics of senescent cells: does it really mean inflammation? Contrib Nephrol. Basel, Karger, 2005, vol 149, pp 208–218.
7   Skinner NA, MacIsaac CM, Hamilton JA, Visvanathan K: Regulation of Toll-like receptors 2 and 4 on CD14dimCD16+ monocytes in response to sepsis-related antigens. Clin Exp Immunol 2005;141:270–278.

8   Belge KU, Dayyani F, Horelt A, et al: The proinflammatory CD14+CD16+DR++ monocytes are a major source of TNF. J Immunol 2002;168:3536–3542
9   Navarro MD, Carracedo J, Ramírez R, Madueño JA, Merino A, Rodríguez M, Martín-Malo A, Aljama P: Bacterial DNA prolongs the survival of inflamed mononuclear cells in haemodialysis patients. Nephrol Dial Transplant 2007;22:3580–3585.

Prof. Pedro Aljama
Department of Nephrology
University Hospital Reina Sofia
ES–14004 Cordoba (Spain)
Tel. +34 957 010 440, Fax +34 957 010 307, E-Mail pedro.aljama.sspa@juntadeandalucia.es

Ronco C, Cruz DN (eds): Hemodialysis – From Basic Research to Clinical Trials.
Contrib Nephrol. Basel, Karger, 2008, vol 161, pp 89–98

....

Oxidative Stress and Anemia in Chronic Hemodialysis: The Promise of Bioreactive Membranes

Dinna N. Cruz, Massimo de Cal, Claudio Ronco

Department of Nephrology, Ospedale San Bortolo and the International
Renal Research Institute Vicenza (IRRIV), Vicenza, Italy

Abstract

Patients with advanced chronic kidney disease are characterized by an imbalance
between pro- and antioxidant factors, and increased oxidative stress has been associated with
complications of end-stage renal disease such as atherosclerosis, β_2-microglobulin amyloidosis and anemia. Antioxidants such as vitamin E work by inhibiting LDL oxidation by oxidants and by limiting cellular response to oxidized LDL, and are potentially useful adjuncts
to the usual medical therapy provided to such patients. In chronic hemodialysis (HD)
patients, vitamin E therapy may be administered in the form of dietary supplementation, or
as an integral part of the HD procedure in the form of bioreactive dialysis membranes, in
which the blood surface has been modified with α-tocopherol. Since blood membrane interaction plays a key role in generating oxidative stress, direct free radical scavenging at the
membrane site is a logical approach. Dialysis with vitamin E-coated membranes (VECM) is
associated with an improvement in circulating biomarkers of lipid peroxidation. Other than
antioxidant activity, the modified surface appears to render these dialyzers more biocompatible, in that cellulose-based membranes behave similar to synthetic dialyzers in terms of
cytokine induction. In small studies in chromic HD patients, both dietary vitamin E supplementation as well as use of VECM have been associated with reduced RBC fragility, prolonged RBC lifespan, and improvements in hemoglobin and rHuEpo requirements. Newer
VECM based on polysulfone bring us further down the road towards complete biocompatibility, and represent a promising therapy against oxidative stress in chronic HD patients.

Chronic kidney disease (CKD) is characterized by an imbalance between
pro- and antioxidant elements. Among patients on chronic hemodialysis (HD),
the interaction of blood with cellulose membranes leads to a rapid and massive
complement activation with leukopenia, and to the release of cytokines. At the

same time, the activation of neutrophil and monocyte oxygen metabolism induces a series of cytotoxic effects commonly described as 'oxidative stress'. The administration of intravenous iron for anemia therapy is also believed to result in production of free radicals, further contributing to the level of oxidative stress in the uremic milieu [1]. There is accumulation of short-chain fatty aldehydes, such as malonyldialdehyde (MDA), because of reduced renal excretion (and insufficient removal through HD), and uremia-induced alterations in pentose-phosphate shunt activity. Moreover, several deficiencies in antioxidant defense mechanisms have been demonstrated in CKD patients, such as reduced levels of vitamins C and E and selenium, as well as deficiency in the glutathione scavenging system. This is in part due to the increased consumption of vitamin E as an antioxidant agent, resulting in lower vitamin E content in the plasma and, ultimately, cellular membranes. All these factors contribute to increased oxidative stress in chronic HD patients, and this has been implicated in the pathogenesis of typical clinical complications, including atherosclerosis and anemia.

Antioxidant therapy works by inhibiting low-density lipoprotein (LDL) oxidation by oxidants and by limiting cellular response to oxidized LDL. Auto-oxidation inhibitors can be divided into primary antioxidants, which reduce the rate at which new free radicals are formed, and secondary antioxidants, which break the chain by trapping the highly reactive chain-propagating peroxyl free radicals. Vitamin E is the most effective chain-breaking lipid-soluble antioxidant in biological membranes. It contributes to the stability of the cell membrane and protects the cell structures from damage caused by oxygen free radicals and the products of lipoperoxidation. Vitamin E also modulates the metabolism of the cascade of arachidonic acid initiated by lipoxygenase and/or cyclo-oxygenase. In addition to its antioxidant function, vitamin E affects cell response to oxidative stress through modulation of signal-transduction pathways [2]. Antioxidant therapy in the form of vitamin E can be 'administered' as a dietary supplement, or as an integral part of the HD process with the use of dialyzers with a modified surface. Vitamin E-coated membranes (VECM) consist of a multilayer membrane bearing a hydrophilic polymer on the blood surface that strongly binds liposoluble α-tocopherol (fig. 1) [3].

Vitamin E Therapy in Chronic Hemodialysis: Per Orem or 'Per Membrane'?

Dietary supplementation with vitamin E is an attractively simple solution to the problem of oxidative stress in uremic patients. Several small short-term studies have reported favorable changes in the levels of various markers of oxidative stress, including MDA, thiobarbituric acid-reactive substance, erythrocyte

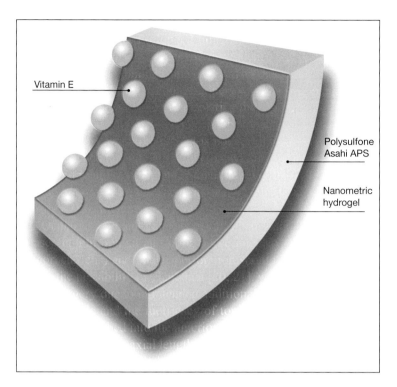

Vitamin E

Polysulfone
Asahi APS

Nanometric
hydrogel

Fig. 1. Schematic representation of the VECM. On the blood side, α-tocopherol (circles) is linked to the membrane surface via hydrophobic interaction, rendering it biologically active. APS = Asahi polysulfone.

superoxide dismutase, catalase, when oral vitamin E was given to patients [4–7]. However, the balance of oxidant/antioxidant systems appears to be more complex in patients on chronic HD. A recent randomized clinical trial in 27 chronic HD patients failed to demonstrate a significant long-term decrease in levels of lipid peroxidation products despite a twofold increase in circulating α-tocopherol level after oral vitamin E supplementation [8]. The increase was accompanied by a halving of γ-tocopherol levels. Presumably, supplementation with α-tocopherol competitively inhibits α-tocopherol transfer protein of dietary γ-tocopherol. γ-tocopherol and its metabolites, but not α-tocopherol, inhibit cyclooxygenase activity and thus have strong anti-inflammatory properties. In comparison, α-tocopherol may be less potent in modulating inflammatory pathways. Furthermore, γ-tocopherol may have unique specificity for protection against reactive nitrogen species. Although the study suffered from insufficient statistical power, the authors suggested that the decrease in γ-tocopherol levels might paradoxically result in an increase in inflammation with dietary vitamin E supplementation. Another possible pro-oxidant effect of α-tocopherol supplementation is the production of tocopheryl quinone from oxidation of α-tocopherol, resulting in a concomitant decrease in transition metal ions. These ions then mediate reductive cleavage of hydroperoxides to alkoxy radicals. Thus, vitamin E can in theory promote the generation of alkoxy radicals from lipid hydroperoxides.

In contrast to dietary supplementation, direct free radical scavenging at the membrane site is an attractive approach to the problem, given that blood membrane interaction plays a key role in generating oxidative stress. Dialysis with VECM decreases the peroxidation of red blood cell (RBC) and plasma lipids, decreases the level of advanced glycation end products, and appears to normalize immune function [9–11]. In a recent meta-analysis of 14 studies, Pereira and colleagues [12] concluded that the conversion of dialysis patients to a vitamin E-coated dialyzer is associated with an improvement in circulating biomarkers of lipid peroxidation, such as MDA and thiobarbituric acid-reactive substances. Vitamin E in the dialyzer acts as an antioxidant, which effectively inhibits oxidation of free radicals by donating electrons [3]. The bond between vitamin E and oleyl alcohol on the membrane surface on the blood side also tends to reduce the oxidative stress, thereby reducing the activation of the polymorphonuclear cells and the consequent generation of free radicals.

These divergent results point to a fundamental difference between vitamin E localized to the HD membrane versus dietary supplementation. Not only would gastrointestinal absorption of oral supplements be affected by several factors, but also any generation of oxidative products related to α-tocopherol can be readily cleared by the dialysis process when α-tocopherol is localized to the membrane [8]. In contrast, they would remain in situ in tissue and in the circulation in the presence of high systemic levels of α-tocopherol, as occurs with systemic administration.

Vitamin E-Coated Membranes: Is It Only Antioxidant Activity?

Although generated cellulose membranes have clearance and mechanical properties which make them extremely suitable as dialyzers, these membranes lead to strong complement activation through their reactive hydroxyl groups. Therefore much effort has been made to render dialyzer membranes more biocompatible to reduce cellular activation during HD. Two common approaches to this issue are the modification of the hydroxyl groups (substituted cellulose membranes) or the use of fully synthetic membranes. A novel concept in the effort to improve membrane biocompatibility is the covering of reactive groups on the surface of membranes by vitamin E (fig. 1) [3].

To evaluate this effectiveness of this innovation, Perterosa et al. [13] compared a vitamin E-modified cellulose membrane to a non-modified cellulose acetate membrane with equivalent dialysis performance in terms of mononuclear cell activation and complement alternative pathway activation. The vitamin E-modified cellulose membrane showed significantly lower C5b-9 levels and abrogated the increase in levels of cytoplasmic tyrosine phosphorylated proteins that was seen with the non-modified cellulose membrane. Similarly, Girndt et al. [14] compared the biocompatibility of a polyamide membrane with a vitamin E-modified cellulose membrane in a crossover study. Being cellulose-based, the vitamin E-coated dialyzers demonstrated, as expected, higher complement activation compared to the synthetic membrane. Despite this, the two membranes were similar with respect to cytokine induction and acute cellular effects, such as T-cell activation and sequestration of activated cells from circulation. The coating of HD membranes with vitamin E lead to an improvement of biocompatibility that makes a dialyzer membrane based on cuprophane behave similar to a synthetic polyamide dialyzer in terms of cytokine induction. Improvement in passive biocompatibility as shown by these criteria seems not to be only the effect of the vitamin E coating as it does not explain the contradiction between high complement and low cytokine activation. Vitamin E seems to exert active effects in that it suppresses directly the production of proinflammatory cytokines in monocytes, an effect which reached its maximum only after 4 weeks of treatment [14]. These experiments demonstrate the VECM was superior in inhibiting complement activation and transient decreases in leukocytes while maintaining the membrane performance.

Oxidative Stress and Anemia: Does Vitamin E Help?

Other than erythropoeitin and iron deficiency, there is increased hemolysis and reduced RBC lifespan in patients on chronic HD. This is related to several factors, including RBC sodium pump inhibition by uremic factors in the plasma, microangiopathy, RBC rigidity due to hypophosphatemia, and oxidative stress. RBCs of HD patients demonstrate a disorder in glucose metabolism, in which there is inefficient phosphoglyceromutase activity. This then decreases pentose-phosphate shunt activity, leading to decreased production of NADPH, and ultimately resulting in an increased production of NAD [15]. These then lead to the formation of hydroxyl radicals, responsible for RBC membrane lipid peroxidation. RBC peroxidation affects the mechanical behavior of the actual membrane, and has been associated with decreased cell deformability. This then increases the RBC's sensitivity to hemolysis and shortens RBC lifespan.

The toxic effects of the oxidizing radicals may be offset by the membrane antioxidant systems, of which the most important is vitamin E.

The basic function of vitamin E in biological membranes is to protect membrane phospholipids from oxidative damage. In fact, vitamin E deficit related to intestinal malabsorption increases hemolysis due to an increase in the fragility of the RBC membrane. In certain genetic hematologic diseases such as sickle cell anemia and β-thalassemia, there is a high potential for oxidative damage due to chronic redox imbalance in red cells which manifest clinically as hemolysis in these patients [16]. An increase in superoxide dismutase, a decrease in catalase activity, and change in erythrocyte membrane protein pattern are seen in thalassemia patients, and these changes are ameliorated with oral vitamin E [16]. Supplementation with α-tocopherol in this instance, as well as in glutathione synthase deficiency and G6PD deficiency, may increase the average RBC lifespan and decrease the number of reticulocytes.

With regard to anemia in end-stage renal disease, there have been conflicting results concerning the effect of systemic administration of vitamin E (table 1). Two studies reported a post-treatment decrease in erythrocyte osmotic fragility with oral administration of vitamin E for periods ranging from 30 days to 20 weeks [4, 17]. Their results would suggest that oral vitamin E would be a useful adjunct in anemia management in HD patients. One study reported a statistically significant improvement in Hct levels, while in two studies, patients were able to maintain Hct levels with a lower rHuEpo dose when oral vitamin E was added to the treatment regimen [5, 17, 18]. In contrast, other authors found no significant effect on Hb or Hct levels or transfusion needs [4, 19, 20]. All these studies are limited by uncontrolled study design, small sample size and short follow-up.

A number of studies have also looked at the effect of VECM on hematologic parameters (table 1) [1–9]. Usberti et al. [21, 22] were able to maintain Hb levels while patients were dialyzed with VECM on half the previous rHuEpo dose. This effect was even more pronounced when the use of VECM was combined with glutathione [21]. However, the results may have been confounded by the use of less biocompatible membranes in some patients at baseline. Similarly, other authors have noted an ability to maintain the patients' Hb on comparatively lower rHuEpo doses [23–25] or even with complete suspension of rHuEpo [26] while dialyzing on VECM. Nakatan et al. [27] saw a statistically significant increase in Hb from 9.5 to 10.7 g/dl after switching patients to VECM, with no significant change in rHuEpo dose. There was no change in reticulocyte count, suggesting that the improvement in Hb was not due to increased hematopoeisis. They speculated that this was due to better RBC survival, as supported by prolonged RBC lifespan demonstrated in their own, as well as other, studies [21, 22, 27]. When patients switched back to their previous polysulfone dialyzer, Hb and Hct trended down, necessitating an increase in

Table 1. Effect of vitamin E therapy on various anemia parameters of chronic HD patients

Reference	Vitamin E therapy	Duration of vitamin E therapy	Population studied	n	RBC survival/ lifespan	RBC fragility	Hb g/dl	Hct %	rHuEpo dose
4	Oral	20 w	HD, PD	56		↓			
19	Oral	20 w	HD	35				↔	
17	Oral	30 d	HD	30		↓	↑	↑	
5	Oral	3 m	HD	46			↔		↓
20	Oral	3 m	HD	24			↔	↔	
7	Oral	2 w	HD (pediatric)	10			↔	↔	
18	Oral	6 m	HD	12			↔		↓
21	VECM	7 m	HD	38	↑		↑	↑	↓
23	VECM	6 m	HD	16			↔		↓
24	VECM	12 m	HD	17				↔	↓
27	VECM	12 m	HD	18	↑		↑	↑	↔
29	VECM	13 w	HD	12	↑ but returned to baseline		↔	↔	↔
31	VECM	4 w	HD	75			↔		
22	VECM	4–6 m	HD	9	↑		↔		↓
28	VECM	12 m	HD	10			↔	↔	↔
26	VECM	12 m	HD	10			↔	↔	↓

Hb = Hemoglobin; Hct = hematocrit; HD = hemodialysis; PD = peritoneal dialysis; RBC = red blood cell; VECM = vitamin E-coated membranes; d = days; w = weeks; m = months;

rHuEpo doses [27]. The superior RBC survival may be consequent to a decrease in dysmorphic erythrocytes, improved RBC rheology and viscosity seen with the use of VECM [24], resulting in less hemolysis [25]. However, the exact mechanism for better blood counts remains unclear, as other studies noted an increase in reticulocyte count [21, 26]. It is likely that multiple mechanisms are involved. In the majority of cases, these favorable hematologic changes were associated with augmented levels of plasma or erythrocyte vitamin E, as well as lower levels of oxidative stress, as represented by oxidized LDL, asymmetric dimethylarginine, MDA and MDA-LDL [21–23, 25]. In contrast, Triolo et al. [28] failed to see significant changes in Hb, Hct, or rHuEpo doses on VECM despite lower MDA levels. Another small study noted a greater degree of unsaturation of fatty acids in the RBC membrane after patients were shifted to VECM compatible with reduced oxidative stress [29]. Erythrocytes also demonstrated enhanced resistance to hemolysis after 6 weeks of dialysis with VECM, but this reverted back to baseline levels by 13 weeks.

Towards a More Biocompatible Membrane: What Next?

Earlier studies have shown that coating of HD membranes with vitamin E makes a dialyzer membrane based on cuprophane behave similar to a synthetic polyamide dialyzer in terms of cytokine induction [13, 14]. It would be logical to move forward on this continuum, and presume that a vitamin E-modified synthetic membrane would be even more biocompatible. A vitamin E-modified polysulfone membrane dialyzer has been realized (fig. 1) [30]. The membrane is said to simulate the structure of a living cell membrane, with a hydrophobic inner layer sandwiched between two hydrophilic outer layers. On the blood side, α-tocopherol is linked to the membrane surface via hydrophobic interaction, rendering it biologically active. In vitro studies demonstrated the antioxidative activity of the modified membrane [29]. A cross-over study confirmed that use of the polysulfone VECM reduced the level of oxidative stress markers as compared to a standard polysulfone membrane. Downstream effects on clinical complications such as anemia, β_2-microglobulin amyloidosis and cardiovascular events remain to be evaluated in properly designed trials.

Conclusion

Oxidative stress plays a key role in long-term complications of CKD, particularly in chronic HD, including cardiovascular and infectious diseases, cancer, dialysis-related amyloidosis, and anemia. Significant research efforts have been directed towards investigating new strategies for antioxidant therapy and improvement of dialysis biocompatibility. Going beyond the notion of standard methods of supplementation of antioxidants such as vitamin E is the novel concept of bioreactivity, in which dialyzers become biological surfaces interacting with chemical and biological properties of the blood flowing in contact with them. A growing body of evidence demonstrates the superiority of VECM in terms of oxidative stress markers and intermediate clinical endpoints such as anemia. Newer VECM bring us further down the road towards complete biocompatibility, and represent a promising therapy against the specter of oxidative stress.

Acknowledgments

Figure 1 was provided by courtesy of Asahi Kasei Medical Europe GmbH Italy Branch. This work has been made possible by the International Society of Nephrology-funded fellowship of Dr. Dinna Cruz.

References

1 Locatelli F, Canaud B, Eckardt KU, Stenvinkel P, Wanner C, Zoccali C: Oxidative stress in end-stage renal disease: an emerging threat to patient outcome. Nephrol Dial Transplant 2003;18: 1272–1280.

2 Taccone-Gallucci M, Lubrano R, Meloni C: Vitamin E as an antioxidant agent. Contrib Nephrol. Basel, Karger, 1999, vol 127, pp 32–43.

3 Sasaki M, Hosoya N, Saruhashi M: Development of vitamin E-modified membrane. Contrib Nephrol. Basel, Karger, 1999, vol 127, pp 49–70.

4 Uzum A, Toprak O, Gumustas MK, Ciftci S, Sen S: Effect of vitamin E therapy on oxidative stress and erythrocyte osmotic fragility in patients on peritoneal dialysis and hemodialysis. J Nephrol 2006;19:739–745.

5 Inal M, Kanbak G, Sen S, Akyuz F, Sunal E: Antioxidant status and lipid peroxidation in hemodialysis patients undergoing erythropoietin and erythropoietin-vitamin E combined therapy. Free Radic Res 1999;31:211–216.

6 Giardini O, Taccone-Gallucci M, Lubrano R, Ricciardi-Tenore G, Bandino D, Silvi I, Paradisi C, Mannarino O, Citti G, Elli M: Effects of α-tocopherol administration on red blood cell membrane lipid peroxidation in hemodialysis patients. Clin Nephrol 1984;21:174–177.

7 Németh I, Túri S, Haszon I, Bereczki C: Vitamin E alleviates the oxidative stress of erythropoietin in uremic children on hemodialysis. Pediatr Nephrol 2000;14:13–17.

8 Lu L, Erhard P, Salomon RG, Weiss MF: Serum vitamin E and oxidative protein modification in hemodialysis: a randomized clinical trial. Am J Kidney Dis 2007;50:305–313.

9 Wanner C, Bahner U, Mattern R, Lang D, Passlick-Deetjen J: Effect of dialysis flux and membrane material on dyslipidaemia and inflammation in haemodialysis patients. Nephrol Dial Transplant 2004;19:2570–2575.

10 Baragetti I, Furiani S, Vettoretti S, et al: Role of vitamin E-coated membrane in reducing advanced glycation end products in hemodialysis patients: a pilot study. Blood Purif 2006;24: 369–376.

11 Girndt M, Lengler S, Kaul H, Sester U, Sester M, Kohler H: Prospective crossover trial of the influence of vitamin-E coated dialyzer membranes on T-cell activation and cytokine induction. Am J Kidney Dis 2000;35:95–104

12 Sosa MA, Balk EM, Lau J, Liangos O, Balakrishnan VS, Madias NE, Pereira BJ, Jaber BL: A systematic review of the effect of the Excebrane dialyser on biomarkers of lipid peroxidation. Nephrol Dial Transplant 2006;21:2825–2833.

13 Pertosa G, Grandaliano G, Valente M, Montinaro V, Soccio M, Gesualdo L, Schena FP: In vivo evaluation of biocompatibility of a new dialyzer employing the vitamin E-modified cellulose membrane 'Excebrane E': study of mechanisms involved in mononuclear cell activation. Contrib Nephrol. Basel, Karger, 1999, vol 127, pp 200–207.

14 Girndt M, Kaul H, Lengler S, Sester U, Sester M, Köhler H: Immunological biocompatibility characterization of a vitamin E-bonded membrane. Contrib Nephrol. Basel, Karger, 1999, vol 127, pp 226–242.

15 Yawata Y, Jacobs HS: Abnormal red cell metabolism in patients with chronic uremia: nature of the defect and its persistence despite adequate hemodialysis. Blood 1975;45:231–239.

16 Das N, Das Chowdhury T, Chattopadhyay A, Datta AG: Attenuation of oxidative stress-induced changes in thalassemic erythrocytes by vitamin E. Pol J Pharmacol 2004;56:85–96.

17 Ono K: Effects of large dose vitamin E supplementation on anemia in hemodialysis patients. Nephron 1985;40:440–445.

18 Cristol JP, Bosc JY, Badiou S, Leblanc M, Lorrho R, Descomps B, Canaud B: Erythropoietin and oxidative stress in haemodialysis: beneficial effects of vitamin E supplementation. Nephrol Dial Transplant 1997;12:2312–2317.

19 Sinsakul V, Drake JR, Leavitt JN Jr, Harrison BR, Fitch CD: Lack of effect of vitamin E therapy on the anemia of patients receiving hemodialysis. Am J Clin Nutr 1984;39:223–226.

20 Aguilera A, Teruel JL, Villatruela JJ, Rivera M, Ortuño J: Effect of vitamin E administration on erythropoietin values and anaemia in hemodialysis patients. Nephrol Dial Transplant 1993;8:379.

21 Usberti M, Gerardi G, Micheli A, Tira P, Bufano G, Gaggia P, Movilli E, Cancarini GC, De Marinis S, D'Avolio G, Broccoli R, Manganoni A, Albertin A, Di Lorenzo D: Effects of a vitamin E-bonded membrane and of glutathione on anemia and erythropoietin requirements in hemodialysis patients. J Nephrol 2002;15:558–564.

22 Usberti M, Gerardi G, Bufano G, Tira P, Micheli A, Albertini A, Floridi A, Di Lorenzo D, Galli F: Effects of erythropoietin and vitamin E-modified membrane on plasma oxidative stress markers and anemia of hemodialyzed patients. Am J Kidney Dis 2002;40:590–599.

23 Morimoto H, Nakao K, Fukuoka K, Sarai A, Yano A, Kihara T, Fukuda S, Wada J, Makino H: Long-term use of vitamin E-coated polysulfone membrane reduces oxidative stress markers in haemodialysis patients. Nephrol Dial Transplant 2005;20:2775–2782.

24 Kobayashi S, Moriya H, Aso K, Ohtake T: Vitamin E-bonded hemodialyzer improves atherosclerosis associated with a rheological improvement of circulating red blood cells. Kidney Int 2003;63:1881–1887.

25 Usberti M, Bufano G, Lima G, Gazzotti RM, Tira P, Gerardi G, Di Lorenzo D: Increased red blood cell survival reduces the need of erythropoietin in hemodialyzed patients treated with exogenous glutathione and vitamin E-modified membrane. Contrib Nephrol. Basel, Karger, 1999, vol 127, pp 208–214.

26 Taccone-Gallucci M, Meloni C, Lubrano R, Morosetti M, Palombo G, Cianciulli P, Scoppi P, Castello MA, Casciani CU: Chronic haemolysis and erythrocyte survival in haemodialysis patients treated with vitamin E-modified dialysis filters. Contrib Nephrol. Basel, Karger, 1999, vol 127, pp 44–48.

27 Nakatan T, Takemoto Y, Tsuchida AK: The effect of vitamin E-bonded dialyzer membrane on red blood cell survival in hemodialyzed patients. Artif Organs 2003;27:214–217.

28 Triolo L, Malaguti M, Ansali F, Comunian MC, Arcangeloni O, Coppolino F, Marrocco F, Sicoli R, Biagini M: Vitamin E-bonded cellulose membrane, lipoperoxidation, and anemia in hemodialysis patients. Artif Cells Blood Substit Immobil Biotechnol 2003;31:185–191.

29 Westhuyzen J, Saltissi D, Stanbury V: Oxidative stress and erythrocyte integrity in end-stage renal failure patients hemodialysed using a vitamin E-modified membrane. Ann Clin Lab Sci 2003; 33:3–10.

30 Sasaki M: Development of vitamin E-modified polysulfone membrane dialyzers. J Artif Organs 2006;9:50–60.

31 Al-Jondeby MS, Cabaguing IT, Pajarillo AA, Hawas FA, Mousa DH, Al-Sulaiman MH, Shaheen FA, Al-Khader AA: Comparative crossover controlled study using polysulphone and vitamin E-coated dialyzers. Saudi Med J 2003;24:265–268.

Dinna N. Cruz, MD, MPH
Department of Nephrology, San Bortolo Hospital
Viale Rodolfi 37, IT–36100 Vicenza (Italy)
Tel +39 0444 753 650, Fax +39 0444 753 973, E-Mail dinnacruzmd@yahoo.com

Ronco C, Cruz DN (eds): Hemodialysis – From Basic Research to Clinical Trials.
Contrib Nephrol. Basel, Karger, 2008, vol 161, pp 99–107

·······················

Consequences of Overhydration and the Need for Dry Weight Assessment

J. Raimann, L. Liu, D. Ulloa, P. Kotanko, N.W. Levin

Renal Research Institute, New York City, N.Y., USA

Abstract

Despite significant progress in the fields of dialysis technology and medical therapy, mortality of hemodialysis (HD) patients remains high. Chronic overhydration is a major contributor to the high cardiovascular morbidity and mortality observed in HD patients. The difficulty of measuring excess fluid accurately and the determination of 'dry weight' are reflected in the abundant literature on overhydration. Data indicate that a significant proportion of HD patients are not at 'dry weight'. Considering its impact on cardiovascular diseases, the relation between excess fluid, sodium, interdialytic weight gain, hypertension and cardiac diseases needs more attention. Clearly the reduction of sodium intake is of prime importance. This can be achieved by a reduction of dietary sodium intake, individualized dialysate sodium concentration, avoidance of sodium profiling and use of hypertonic saline during dialysis. These measures are expected to result in less thirst and consecutive water intake, thereby facilitating achieving dry weight (DW). In concert, the application of new tools for DW assessment such as continuous intradialytic bioimpedance spectroscopy measurement, means to prevent intradialytic symptoms (e.g. glucose bolus instead of hypertonic saline; improved hemodynamic stability by reduced dialysate temperature) may be operative in reducing morbidity and mortality in HD patients.

Copyright © 2008 S. Karger AG, Basel

Despite technical and pharmacological progress, morbidity and mortality of chronic hemodialysis (HD) patients has not improved substantially [1]. The leading cause of mortality is cardiovascular disease with overhydration being a major contributing factor.

The prevalence of overhydration in dialysis patients differs among populations. These differences are due to the lack of a generally accepted definition of overhydration and dialysis modalities, particularly length of dialysis. Overhydration was diagnosed in 30–37% based on increased inferior vena caval diameter [2, 3]. Using extracellular volume (ECV) measured by bioimpedance spectroscopy (BIS), 24% of HD patients at 'clinical dry weight' were fluid over-loaded [4]. Unfortunately, all these studies suffer from low patient numbers (19–50 patients). Therefore, sufficiently powered studies in chronic kidney disease (CKD), HD and peritoneal dialysis patients are needed to more clearly delineate the prevalence of overhydration.

Since there is no easy way to measure the ECV in a larger number of end-stage renal disease patients, surrogate estimates of dry weight (DW) have been used to calculate required ultrafiltration volume. In the 1960s, Thomson introduced the term 'dry weight', defining it as the reduction of blood pressure to hypotensive levels during ultrafiltration. This definition was of limited value when hypotension was due to antihypertensive drugs and more importantly due to the presence of cardiovascular disease. In 1996, Charra suggested 'the post-dialysis weight at which the patient is and remains normotensive until the next dialysis in spite of the interdialytic fluid retention without anti-hypertensive medication' as a definition of 'dry weight'. Daugirdas' defines DW as 'the post-dialysis weight at which all or most excess body fluid has been removed, below which the patient, more often than not, will develop symptoms of hypotension'. Physiologically DW may be defined as the weight at which the ECV is in the normal range of the individual patient.

Assessment of Dry Weight

Multiple methods have been proposed for DW assessment (table 1). The measurement of ECV by tracer dilution techniques is adequate for small-scale epidemiological studies but cannot be considered as a gold standard for DW assessment. Due to technical problems, its invasive nature and costs, dilution methods are not used clinically for this purpose.

In everyday practice in most dialysis units worldwide, DW is assessed using one of the clinical definitions described above. Symptoms related to ECV excess (dyspnea, headache and hypertension) and ECV depletion (postural dizziness, fatigue and cramps) are neither sufficiently specific nor sensitive and show a large inter- and intra-individual variability.

In adults, clinical examination fails to determine ECV expansion of up to 2–3 liters of ECV. The earliest physical sign of fluid overload is an increase in the jugular venous pressure (JVP). An elevated JVP is the classic sign of right-sided heart failure. Unfortunately, JVP is rarely examined in most dialysis units.

Cardiothoracic ratio measured by chest X-ray lacks sensitivity as a measure of DW; the same notion holds true for the findings of pulmonary congestion.

Table 1. Available techniques for DW assessment

Modality	What is measured	Pros	Cons
Inferior vena cava	Intravascular volume	Noninvasive Strong correlation with right heart failure	Cost Best time after HD not defined Inter-operator error Difficult to use in heart failure patients
Biochemical markers	Intravascular volume	Noninvasive Ease of use High sensitivity for overhydration	Wide variability Poor correlation with normo- and underhydration Not available in most laboratories Difficult to assess in patients with CKD, CHF, tricuspid/mitral disease
Blood volume monitoring	Intravascular volume	Ease of use Ease of interpretion Real-time monitoring Decreases intradialytic hypotensive events	Cost Individual variability Requires active interventions by HD nurses Reflects the shifts from intravascular space and its refilling rate: may be reduced in presence of excess ECV Measures relative volume change only
Bioimpedance	ECV ICV TBW Resistance and resistivity of the calf	Ease of use Reproducibility Assessment of body composition Estimates fluid shifts between compartments	Best time after HD not defined Underestimates volume shifts from trunk Accurate measurement of ECV or ICV confounded by body position, body composition and skin thickness May be uncomfortable because of restriction of leg movement during intradialytic measurement Variability in normal range confounds volume estimate except when the patient is his/her own control

DW = Dry weight; HD = hemodialysis, ECV = extracellular volume, ICV = intracellular volume, TBW = total body water, CHF = chronic heart failure, CKD = chronic kidney disease.

Inferior vena caval diameter and collapsibility on deep inspiration correlate well with right atrial central venous pressure. It is noninvasive and enables the rapid evaluation of intravascular volume status. However, the clinical application is limited by cost, need for staff training, inter-observer variability, and the waiting time needed for reaching the stabilization after dialysis.

Atrial natriuretic peptide, brain natriuretic peptide (BNP), their second messenger cyclic guanosine monophosphate, and more recently NT-pro-BNP (a precursor of biologically active BNP) have been used to identify patients with increased plasma volume in renal failure. These molecules are essentially produced by stretched atrial and ventricular cardiomyocytes. Neither atrial natriuretic peptide nor cyclic guanosine monophosphate have proved practically useful. NT-pro-BNP did not correlate with ECV/total body water ratio in a study with 66 patients [5].

Continuous measurements of relative blood volume (BV) changes are frequently performed in HD patients. This is achieved by online monitoring changes in hematocrit or blood protein concentration. This technique measures the relative BV changes which depend on ultrafiltration rate (UFR) and plasma refilling rate. BV monitoring is easy to use and interpret. Unfortunately, no practically useful normal ranges have been established and relative BV changes. Intradialytic BV dynamics depend heavily on the plasma refilling rate, which is only weakly related to ECV status. Plasma refilling may be reduced in overhydrated patients, particularly diabetics, with autonomic dysfunction.

Bioimpedance analysis (BIA) techniques have been broadly used to detect changes in both extracellular and, to a lesser extent, intracellular fluid volumes. BIA is a safe, noninvasive, simple and shows a high level of intra-individual reproducibility. Due to high variability of physiological ECV ranges, whole-body BIA is of limited use in DW evaluation. DW assessment by whole-body BIA and by the relation of reactance to resistance is confounded by differences in body composition. To overcome these limitations, intradialytic online measurement of calf resistance employing a combination of criteria (plateauing of resistance and calf resistivity approaching the normal range) is currently under intensive investigation [6].

Consequences of Sodium Excess and Overhydration

The multiple consequences of overhydration are summarized in figure 1. Hypertension is a major manifestation of inadequate ECV removal in the overhydrated patient. Scribner stated 40 years ago clearly that the volume of the extracellular space influences the blood pressure and merely the combination of ultrafiltration and dietary sodium restriction would permit regulation of the ECV [7]. Guyton showed that the retention of water and sodium increases venous preload and cardiac output. When all other mechanisms to eliminate hypervolemia are not effective, the vessels react with vasoconstriction in order to prevent hyperperfusion. This autoregulatory mechanism normalizes tissue perfusion but also results in elevated arterial pressure [7]. Longstanding mechanical strain alters gene expression resulting in increased production of growth factors in endothelial cells, changes the anatomical and morphologic structure of vessels, increasing their stiffness [8].

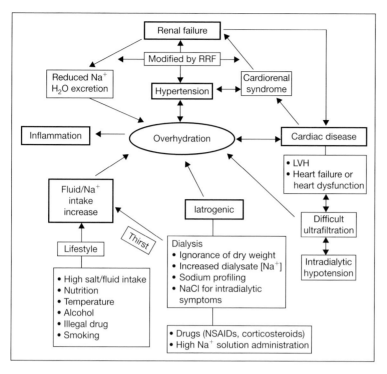

Fig. 1. Pathophysiology of overhydration in CKD. RRF = Residual renal function; LVH = left ventricular hypertrophy; NSAID = non-steroidal anti-inflammatory drug.

Large interdialytic weight gains (IDWG) associated with high sodium intake and hypertension frequently results in eccentric and concentric left ventricular hypertrophy due to chronic volume preload and increased arterial stiffness.

A further consequence of permanent hypervolemia and an activated renin-angiotensin system is hyperactivity of the sympathetic nerve system. In addition, factors such as renal ischemia, chronic inflammation, obesity, nocturnal hypoxia and elevated levels of asymmetric dimethylarginine contribute to this increased sympathetic activity [9].

The sequelae are elevated arterial pressure, cardiac arrhythmias, increased myocardial oxygen demand and in concert with arterial hypertension a reduced compliance of large arteries [9]. In addition to its volume effects, sodium exerts direct profibrotic effects with the potential of aggravating kidney and cardio-vascular diseases. Salt directly increases oxidative stress [10] and is associated with the secretion of an endogenous ouabain-like substance from the adrenal gland. This digitalis-like compound induces myocardial cell hypertrophy in vitro and correlates with left ventricular mass in HD patients, independent of arterial pressure and delivered dialysis dose [11].

In renal patients, residual renal function (RRF) contributes significantly to the excretion and the catabolism of uremic toxins, but another major RRF effect relates to sodium and fluid removal. Therefore, strategies to preserve RRF are of prime importance [12].

Sodium intake is associated with increase of urinary albumin excretion in microalbuminuric subjects [13]. Retrospective data analysis suggests that the progression of kidney disease is less in patients adhering to a low salt diet. Sodium-related progression of kidney failure may be due to the vascular effects of angiotensin II and aldosterone [14].

Several recent studies have shown an association of overhydration with inflammatory markers in CKD. One explanation is bowel wall edema with consecutive barrier breakdown and endotoxin translocation from the gut [15, 16].

Noteworthy, in patients with congestive heart failure, therapy with loop diuretics resulted in lower levels of circulating endotoxins, presumably due to less intestinal translocation. Bowel edema may also result in protein losing enteropathy and fat malabsorption [17, 18]. In addition, levels of intestinal hormones such as ghrelin (which may be explained by hyperactivity of the sympathetic nerve system [19]) and leptin are elevated in HD patients and the presumed resistance to them may contribute to malnutrition [20].

Overhydration may also cause an apparent decrease in predialytic hematocrit levels. Controlled and strict ECV reduction resulted in an increase of hematocrit from 23.4 to 29.1% [21]. Otherwise, unexplained anemia in HD patients may occasionally be caused by hemodilution [16].

Modulation of Overhydration

Overhydration can be modulated by various interventions (table 2). The aim is to gradually reduce excess fluid in order to achieve DW and then subsequently maintain this DW by an ultrafiltration volume equal to IDWG. Data acquired in Tassin showed that drug-free blood pressure control by controlled ECV reduction was possible in 712 patients on routine dialysis. This required both long dialysis times and a low salt diet [22]. This may not apply globally as genetic background, lifestyle and nutritional habits differ. However, effective DW assessment and maintenance with a continuing reduction of ECV leads to normalization of blood pressure and the withdrawal of all antihypertensive drugs.

Salt intake changes the serum osmolarity and triggers thirst, thus education about salt intake will be more efficient than about fluid intake alone [23]. Restriction of salt intake to <5 g sodium chloride per day, which equals

Table 2. Factors modulating overhydration

Modulation	Aim and challenges
Precise dry weight assessment	A major challenge in dialysis
Re-assessment of DW	Regular repetition of assessment, aiming to recognize weight loss and for avoidance of excess fluid
Preservation of RRF	Sodium and fluid removal, numerous advantages in terms of kidney function
Ultrafiltration	Tool to remove excess fluid, which equals the IDWG at dry weight
Salt-restricted diet	Prevention of thirst and high IDWG, lowers occurrence of cardiovascular
KDOQI: salt intake <5 g/day	disease and mortality, reduces oxidative stress, helps preservation of RRF
Dialysate [Na$^+$] = patient's serum [Na$^+$]	
Avoidance of Na$^+$ profiling	
Prevention of intradialytic symptoms	Intravenous hyperosmolar glucose (20 ml of 50% glucose = 10 g glucose) instead of i.v. administration of saline causing thirst and excess fluid gain
Reduced core temperature	Improves hemodynamic stability
Increase of treatment time	Safe removal of excess fluid, most effective prevention of intradialytic symptoms, particularly in patients with diastolic dysfunction
Low UFR/prolonged treatment time	<10 ml/h/kg body weight, associated with lower mortality

85 mmol sodium (KDOQI recommendation), will lower the direct effects of sodium as well as the IDWG. Salt restriction also helps to achieve normotension and represents another way to preserve RRF [24].

An important source of sodium is the dialysate and a positive correlation of sodium gradient and IDWG and blood pressure has been reported. Patients may have an individual Na$^+$-setpoint, triggering thirst when the plasma sodium level exceeds that threshold. This underlines the importance of individualization of dialysate Na$^+$ [25].

While sodium profiling might prevent intradialytic symptoms, it may result in intradialytic sodium loading and interdialytic thirst, thereby increasing IDWG.

In the event of intradialytic cramps or hypotension the injection of hyperosmolar glucose instead of isotonic or hypertonic saline may be a preferred intervention, because it avoids additional sodium loading and is followed by positive impacts on BV, stroke volume and also induces an increase in total peripheral resistance [26].

Reduction of core temperature during dialysis increases the total peripheral resistance and myocardial contractility in association with higher levels of plasma epinephrine [27].

UFR and treatment time directly relates to IDWG, which determines the fluid to be removed. Keeping the UFR as low as possible is beneficial in terms of intradialytic symptoms. These findings have been confirmed in the DOPPS study, which retrospectively analyzed survival in 22,000 HD patients. Longer treatment time and a UFR <10 ml/h/kg was associated with lower mortality [28]. Prolonged treatment time and low UFR is particularly necessary in patients with diastolic dysfunction to achieve DW, since reduction in filling pressure can markedly reduce cardiac output. In conclusion, a low UFR can be achieved by low IDWG and prolonged treatment times, but in practice neither of these is frequently present.

References

1   Foley RN, Collins AJ: End-stage renal disease in the United States: an update from the United States Renal Data System. J Am Soc Nephrol 2007;18:2644–2648.
2   Yashiro M, Kamata T, Yamadori N, Tomita M, Muso E: Evaluation of markers to estimate volume status in hemodialysis patients: atrial natriuretic peptide, inferior vena cava diameter, blood volume changes and filtration coefficients of microvasculature. Ther Apher Dial 2007;11:131–137.
3   Oe B, de Fijter CW, Geers TB, Vos PF, Donker AJ, de Vries PM: Diameter of inferior caval vein and impedance analysis for assessment of hydration status in peritoneal dialysis. Artif Organs 2000;24:575–577.
4   Kouw PM, Kooman JP, Cheriex EC, Olthof CG, de Vries PM, Leunissen KM: Assessment of post-dialysis dry weight: a comparison of techniques. J Am Soc Nephrol 1993;4:98–104.
5   Van de Pol AC, Frenken LA, Moret K, Baumgarten R, van der Sande FM, Beerenhout CM, et al: An evaluation of blood volume changes during ultrafiltration pulses and natriuretic peptides in the assessment of dry weight in hemodialysis patients. Hemodial Int 2007;11:51–61.
6   Zhu F, Leonard EF, Carter M, Levin NW: Continuous measurement of calf resistivity in hemodialysis patients using bioimpedance analysis. Conf Proc IEEE Eng Med Biol Soc 2006;1:5126–5128.
7   Ritz E, Passlick-Deetjen J, Zeier M, Amann K: Blood pressure on dialysis: an ongoing controversy. Saudi J Kidney Dis Transpl 2002;13:1–13.
8   Chien S, Li S, Shyy YJ: Effects of mechanical forces on signal transduction and gene expression in endothelial cells. Hypertension 1998;31:162–169.
9   Koomans HA, Blankestijn PJ, Joles JA: Sympathetic hyperactivity in chronic renal failure: a wake-up call. J Am Soc Nephrol 2004;15:524–537.
10 Kitiyakara C, Chabrashvili T, Chen Y, Blau J, Karber A, Aslam S, et al: Salt intake, oxidative stress, and renal expression of NADPH oxidase and superoxide dismutase. J Am Soc Nephrol 2003;14:2775–2782.
11 Stella P, Manunta P, Mallamaci F, Melandri M, Spotti D, Tripepi G, et al: Endogenous ouabain and cardiomyopathy in dialysis patients. J Intern Med 2007.
12 Wang AY, Lai KN: The importance of residual renal function in dialysis patients. Kidney Int 2006;69:1726–1732.
13 Verhave JC, Hillege HL, Burgerhof JG, Janssen WM, Gansevoort RT, Navis GJ, et al: Sodium intake affects urinary albumin excretion especially in overweight subjects. J Intern Med 2004;256:324–330.
14 Joffe HV, Adler GK: Effect of aldosterone and mineralocorticoid receptor blockade on vascular inflammation. Heart Fail Rev 2005;10:31–37.
15 Avila-Diaz M, Ventura MD, Valle D, Vicente-Martinez M, Garcia-Gonzalez Z, Cisneros A, et al: Inflammation and extracellular volume expansion are related to sodium and water removal in patients on peritoneal dialysis. Perit Dial Int 2006;26:574–580.

16   Ortega Marcos O, Rodriguez I, Gallar P, Oliet A, Vigil A: Importance of dry-weight assessment in well-being, appetite, nutritional status, and anaemia correction in haemodialysis patients. Nephrol Dial Transplant 1998;13:2424.

17   King D, Smith ML, Chapman TJ, Stockdale HR, Lye M: Fat malabsorption in elderly patients with cardiac cachexia. Age Ageing 1996;25:144–149.

18   King D, Smith ML, Lye M: Gastrointestinal protein loss in elderly patients with cardiac cachexia. Age Ageing 1996;25:221–223.

19   Mundinger TO, Cummings DE, Taborsky GJ Jr: Direct stimulation of ghrelin secretion by sympathetic nerves. Endocrinology 2006;147:2893–2901.

20   Bossola M, Tazza L, Giungi S, Luciani G: Anorexia in hemodialysis patients: an update. Kidney Int 2006;70:417–422.

21   Ozkahya M, Ok E, Cirit M, Aydin S, Akcicek F, Basci A, et al: Regression of left ventricular hypertrophy in haemodialysis patients by ultrafiltration and reduced salt intake without antihypertensive drugs. Nephrol Dial Transplant 1998;13:1489–1493.

22   Charra B, Bergstrom J, Scribner BH: Blood pressure control in dialysis patients: importance of the lag phenomenon. Am J Kidney Dis 1998;32:720–724.

23   Cook NR, Cutler JA, Obarzanek E, Buring JE, Rexrode KM, Kumanyika SK, et al: Long-term effects of dietary sodium reduction on cardiovascular disease outcomes: observational follow-up of the trials of hypertension prevention. BMJ 2007;334:885.

24   Ritz E, Dikow R, Morath C, Schwenger V: Salt – a potential 'uremic toxin'? Blood Purif 2006;24: 63–66.

25   Keen ML, Gotch FA: The association of the sodium 'setpoint' to interdialytic weight gain and blood pressure in hemodialysis patients. Int J Artif Organs 2007;30:971–979.

26   Nette RW, Krepel HP, van den Meiracker AH, Weimar W, Zietse R: Specific effect of the infusion of glucose on blood volume during haemodialysis. Nephrol Dial Transplant 2002;17:1275–1280.

27   Maggiore Q, Pizzarelli F, Santoro A, Panzetta G, Bonforte G, Hannedouche T, et al: The effects of control of thermal balance on vascular stability in hemodialysis patients: results of the European randomized clinical trial. Am J Kidney Dis 2002;40:280–290.

28   Saran R, Bragg-Gresham JL, Levin NW, Twardowski ZJ, Wizemann V, Saito A, et al: Longer treatment time and slower ultrafiltration in hemodialysis: associations with reduced mortality in the DOPPS. Kidney Int 2006;69:1222–1228.

Dr. Nathan W. Levin
207 East 94th Street, Suite 303
New York, NY 10128 (USA)
Tel. +1 212 360 4900, Fax +1 212 996 5905, E-Mail nlevin@rriny.com

Ronco C, Cruz DN (eds): Hemodialysis – From Basic Research to Clinical Trials.
Contrib Nephrol. Basel, Karger, 2008, vol 161, pp 108–114

....

Body Composition and Outcomes in Chronic Hemodialysis Patients

Padam Hirachan, Stephan Thijssen, Nathan W. Levin, Peter Kotanko

Renal Research Institute, New York, N.Y., USA

Abstract

In contrast to epidemiological data from the general population, maintenance hemodialysis (MHD) patients with a naturally small body size experience an increased mortality rate compared to their larger fellow patients. Since body mass index is a poor surrogate of body composition, attempts were made to delineate muscle, fat and visceral organ mass in MHD patients. Several lines of evidence indicate that (a) increased fat and muscle mass exerts protective effects, (b) some markers of inflammation may be increased with fat mass, and (c) a high visceral mass per body weight is associated with a reduced survival time. The reasons for the positive effects of fat and muscle mass on survival are not clear. A novel hypothesis predicts lower uremic toxin concentrations in larger subjects. This is based on the observation that both in healthy subjects and in dialysis patients, visceral organ mass is inversely related to body mass. Since visceral organs are the most prominent source of uremic toxins, large patients may have a lower toxin production rate per unit of body mass. Moreover, large patients have a greater volume of distribution (total body water, fat mass) resulting in lower toxin concentrations. Future studies should aim to tackle the Janus-like duality of obesity by a system biology approach.

Copyright © 2008 S. Karger AG, Basel

In contrast to epidemiological data from the general population, in maintenance hemodialysis (MHD) patients small body size (defined by low body mass index (BMI)) is correlated with poorer outcomes compared to larger patients. A similar relationship between BMI and survival has been reported in chronic kidney disease patients not yet on dialysis [1]. A decrease in mortality risk with higher BMI was reported for the first time in a population of mostly young, non-diabetic patients treated with MHD in France during the 1970s [2]. Subsequently, several investigators have found a significant inverse relationship between mortality risk and body size, unaffected by adjustments for comorbidities, in prevalent and incident hemodialysis patients [3–5].

The 'obesity paradox' is not limited to patients with renal disease. In a large population with hypertension and coronary heart disease, overweight and obese patients had decreased risk of major cardiovascular events, particularly mortality, compared with 'normal' weight patients [6]. These data are in agreement with a recent meta-analysis that demonstrated better cardiovascular outcomes in overweight and mildly obese coronary heart disease patients compared with those with ideal weight and especially compared with underweight patients [7]. In this meta-analysis the better outcomes for cardiovascular and total mortality seen in the overweight and mildly obese groups could not be explained by adjustment for confounding factors. In addition, it also supports the results of a recent study from nearly 7,000 male non-heart failure veterans referred for stress testing that demonstrated a similar obesity paradox [8].

Correlations of Body Composition

BMI is a poor surrogate of body composition and subjects with the same BMI may have a quite different body composition. More sophisticated techniques are needed to assess body composition in detail in terms of muscle, fat (total adipose tissue, visceral adipose tissue, subcutaneous adipose tissue), bone (table 1A). Body composition can also be estimated by indirect techniques, utilizing validated regression models (table 1B, C). Importantly, all these regression models are based on adequate reference techniques such as MRI and dilution methods. Bioimpedance measurements provide additional means to assess body composition, whereby multiple frequency methods enable simultaneous determination of extra- and intracellular volume. Bioimpedance models can also be employed for estimating fat free mass and total body muscle mass. Some of those models are summarized in table 1D.

Body composition as determined by various techniques has been associated with an array of epidemiological and functional findings in dialysis patients (table 2). Beyond the well-known fact that higher BMI associates with better survival, the broad overall picture suggests that adipose tissue is associated with increased inflammation, reflected in higher levels of C-reactive protein and interleukin-6. Despite this, in African-Americans, EPO dose and EPO resistance are reduced with higher fat mass. In females unlike males a higher muscle mass confers less EPO resistance [9]. So we are confronted with the puzzling phenomenon that some indicators of inflammation are increased in parallel with fat mass, but despite this, overall survival is improved. Multiple explanations for this surprising observation have been proposed [10], such as reverse causation, competing risks for the adverse events that are associated

Table 1. A Assessment of body composition by tracer and imaging techniques

	TBW	ECF	ICF	PV	LBM	BM	MM	TAT	VAT	SAT	VM	BCM
DEXA					X	X		X		X		
Bioimpedance analysis	X	X	X		X		X	X				X
Magnetic resonance imaging					X	X	X	X	X	X	X	
Computer tomography					X	X	X	X	X	X	X	
^{40}K whole body counting												X
D$_2$O distribution volume	X											
H$_3$O distribution volume	X											
NaBr distribution volume		X										
Urea distribution volume	X											
Infrared					X			X		X		
Ultrasound						X			X	X		
^{125}I-albumin distribution volume				X								
^{51}Cr-labeled red blood cells distribution volume				X								
Underwater weighing								X				

DEXA = Dual-energy x-ray absorptiometry; TBW = total body water; ECF = extracellular fluid volume; ICF = intracellular fluid volume; PV = plasma volume; LBM = lean body mass; BM = bone mass; MM = muscle mass; TAT = total adipose tissue; VAT = visceral adipose tissue; SAT = subcutaneous adipose tissue; VM = visceral mass; BCM = body cell mass; D$_2$O = deuterium dilution method; H$_3$O = tritium dilution method; NaBr = sodium bromide.

Table 1. B Anthropometric models to estimate extracellular (ECV) and intracellular (ICV) volume (in liters)

Gender	Parameter	ECV	ICV
Male	height, m	9.78	7.92
Male	weight, kg	0.245	0.198
Male	BSA, m^2	9.22	7.45
Male	LBM, kg LBM	0.303	0.244
Female	height, m	8.44	7.04
Female	weight, kg	0.220	0.186
Female	BSA, m^2	8.18	6.84
Female	LBM, kg	0.302	0.248
Both	LBM, kg	0.3027	0.2456

Table 1. C Anthropometric models to estimate total body water (TBW), lean body mass (LBM), and visceral organ mass

Domain	Model
TBW (males >16 years), liters [Hume & Weyers]	$(0.194786 \cdot (\text{height, cm})) + (0.296785 \cdot \text{weight, kg})) - 14.012934$
TBW (females >16 years), liters [Hume & Weyers]	$(0.344547 \cdot (\text{height, cm})) + (0.183809 \cdot (\text{weight, kg})) - 35.270121$
TBW (males), liters [Watson]	$(-0.09516 \cdot (\text{age, years})) + (0.1074 \cdot (\text{height, cm})) + (0.3362 \cdot (\text{weight, kg})) + 2.447$
TBW (females), liters [Watson]	$(0.1069 \cdot (\text{height, cm})) + (0.2466 \cdot (\text{weight, kg})) - 2.097$
LBM (males >16 years), kg [Hume & Weyers]	$(0.32810 \cdot (\text{body weight, kg})) + (0.33929 \cdot (\text{height, cm})) - 29.5336$
LBM (adult males), kg [Boer]	$(0.407 \cdot (\text{body weight, kg})) + (26.7 \cdot (\text{height, m})) - 19.2$
LBM (females >30 years), kg [Hume & Weyers]	$(0.29569 \cdot (\text{body weight, kg})) + (0.41813 \cdot (\text{height, cm})) - 43.2933$
LBM (adult females), kg [Boer]	$(0.252 \cdot (\text{body weight, kg})) + (47.3 \cdot (\text{height, m})) - 48.3$
Visceral organ mass, kg [(Gallagher et. al.]	$1.223 - 0.008 \cdot \text{age [years]} + 0.801 \cdot \text{height [m]} + 0.016 \cdot \text{BW [kg]} + 0.305 \cdot \text{Sex [0 if female; 1 if male]} - 0.251 \cdot \text{Race [0 if white; 1 if black]}$

Table 1. D Body composition analysis based on bioimpedance

Tissue	Model
FFM, kg [Deurenberg]	$(0.671 \cdot (10^4) \cdot ((\text{height, m})^2/(\text{resistance}, \Omega)) + (3.1 \cdot (\text{gender value})) + 3.9$ Gender value = 0 if female, 1 if male
TBW (hemodialysis patients), kg [Chertow]	$(-0.07493713 \cdot (\text{age})) - (1.01767992 \cdot (\text{points for gender})) + (0.12703384 \cdot (\text{height})) - (0.04012056 \cdot (\text{weight})) + (0.57894981 \cdot (\text{points for diabetes})) - (0.00067247 \cdot (\text{weight}) \cdot (\text{weight})) - (0.03486146 \cdot (\text{age}) \cdot (\text{points for gender})) + (0.11262857 \cdot (\text{points for gender}) \cdot (\text{weight})) + (0.00104135 \cdot (\text{age}) \cdot (\text{weight})) + (0.00186104 \cdot (\text{height}) \cdot (\text{weight}))$ *Height, cm; weight, kg; age, years; gender point = 0 if female, 1 if male; diabetes point = 1 if diabetic, 0 if not*
Total body muscle mass, kg [Kaysen]	$9.52 + 0.331 \cdot \text{ICV} \cdot (\text{by BIS, ml}) + 2.77 \cdot (\text{male; 0 if female}) + 0.180 \cdot \text{weight} \cdot (\text{kg}) - 0.133 \, \text{age} \cdot (\text{years})$
FFM (males), kg [Chumlea]	$-10.68 + 0.65 \cdot \text{height} \cdot (\text{cm})^2/\text{resistance} \, (\Omega) + 0.26 \cdot \text{weight} \, (\text{kg}) + 0.02 \, \text{resistance} \, (\Omega)$
FFM (females), kg [Chumlea]	$-9.53 + 0.69 \cdot \text{height} \, (\text{cm})^2/\text{resistance} \, (\Omega) + 0.17 \cdot \text{weight} \, (\text{kg}) + 0.02 \cdot \text{resistance} \, (\Omega)$

LBM = Lean body mass; ECF = extracellular fluid volume; ICF = intracellular fluid volume; FFM = fat free mass; TBW = total body water.

Table 2. Body composition and outcomes

	BMI	Weight	MM	VM	TAT	VAT	SAT	MAC	TBW
Survival	↑	↑	↑	↓	↑	↑	↑		↑
HGB	↑		±		±		±		
EPO dose	↓		↓ (F)		↓		↓		
ERI	↓		↓ (F)		↓		↓		
Lipids (TGS)	↑	↑			↑	↑	↑		
CRP	↑	↑			↑	↑			
IL-6						↑			
CVM	↓								
Leptin	↑				↑	↑	↑	↑	↓
Adiponectin					±	±	±		
Albumin	↓		±		±		±		
N/L ratio			±		±		±		

↑ = Positive association; ↓ = negative association; ± = no relation; F = female only; BMI = body mass index; MM = muscle mass; VM = visceral mass; TAT = total adipose tissue; SAT = subcutaneous adipose tissue; MAC = maximum abdominal circumference; TBW = total body water; ECF = extracellular fluid volume; HGB = hemoglobin; EPO dose = erythropoietin dose; ERI = erythropoietin resistance index; CRP = C-reactive protein; IL-6 = interleukin-6; CVM = cardiovascular mortality; N/L ratio = neutrophil/lymphocyte ratio.

with overnutrition and malnutrition, a more stable intradialytic hemodynamic situation, and beneficial neurohormonal constellations [for review, see 11].

The reduced survival in MHD patients with a low BMI has been recently explained by a novel hypothesis [Levin N, Gotch F: J Am Soc Nephrol 12:452A, 2001(abstract) and 12, 13]. Briefly, both in healthy and MHD subjects, visceral organ mass relative to whole body mass is inversely related to weight and urea distribution volume (V). V as determined by urea kinetic modeling is closely related to muscle mass [12], whereas fat mass contributes only marginally to V. Viscera are the most likely source of uremic toxins and their production rate may be related to visceral mass. According to that hypothesis the concentration of uremic toxins in V is higher in subjects with a naturally low V (and thus low muscle mass and low BMI), resulting in an underdialysis in low-BMI patients. Dialysis dose is currently prescribed based on V with the basic assumption that body composition variability is not relevant and the only differences between individuals having different values for V is quantitative and not qualitative. In addition to the dilution of uremic toxins in a larger volume in patients with naturally larger body mass (and thus larger V), uremic toxins may be metabolized and stored in adipose tissues and skeletal muscle. This may be particularly relevant for lipophilic uremic toxins such as *p*-cresol and pentosidine. It has recently been shown that the concentration of pentosidine, a protein-bound advanced glycation end product and uremic toxin, is indeed higher in MHD patients with lower BMI [14].

There are no easy means to measure visceral mass directly in dialysis patients. Recently, mathematical models were developed to estimate visceral mass in black and white dialysis subjects of both genders [15]. These regression models were applied to a cohort of 2,004 stable chronic hemodialysis patients [16]. Gender- and race-specific visceral mass relative to body weight was then related to survival. This study revealed an inverse relationship between the relative organ mass and survival, so that patients in the higher tertile of relative organ mass experienced a significantly shorter survival time when compared to the lowest tertile (1,031 vs. 876 days, $p < 0.0001$). This finding is in line with the hypothesis that the uremic toxin load is a function of organ mass, with muscle and fat tissue (the main components of body weight) serving as dilution compartment. This study also showed that the mass of visceral organs (in g) relative to urea distribution volume (expressed in liters) is higher both in black and white females when compared to males (white females by +3.6 g/l (95% CI 2.2–5.1); black females +2.9 g/l (95% CI 1.3–4.5)). This could result in a higher uremic toxin load per liter of V. When dialysis prescription is solely based on V, females could suffer from underdialysis because of their higher uremic toxin load per unit of V. This result may be of relevance in the light of the finding from the HEMO study that females were among those subgroups benefiting from higher dialysis dose.

Well-designed longitudinal studies are necessary to test this hypothesis, encompassing kinetics of uremic toxins and their tissue levels, pro- and anti-cytokines, lipids, and fetuin A, amongst others, in relationship to well-defined measures of body composition.

In summary, the finding that increased BMI translates into improved outcome in chronic dialysis patients is a robust one. Obesity exerts protective effects despite some pro-inflammatory properties of fat tissue. Future studies should aim to tackle the obvious Janus-like duality [10] of obesity by an integrative system biological approach.

References

1   Kovesdy CP, Anderson JE, Kalantar-Zadeh K: Paradoxical association between body mass index and mortality in men with CKD not yet on dialysis. Am J Kidney Dis 2007;49:581–591.
2   Degoulet P, Legrain M, Reach I, Aime F, Devries C, Rojas P, et al: Mortality risk factors in patients treated by chronic hemodialysis. Report of the Diaphane Collaborative Study. Nephron 1982;31:103–110.
3   Leavey SF, Strawderman RL, Jones CA, Port FK, Held PJ: Simple nutritional indicators as independent predictors of mortality in hemodialysis patients. Am J Kidney Dis 1998;31:997–1006.

4   Port FK, Ashby VB, Dhingra RK, Roys EC, Wolfe RA: Dialysis dose and body mass index are strongly associated with survival in hemodialysis patients. J Am Soc Nephrol 2002;13:1061–1066.

5   Kalantar-Zadeh K, Kopple JD: Obesity paradox in patients on maintenance dialysis. Contrib Nephrol. Basel, Karger, 2006, vol 151, pp 57–69.

6   Uretsky S, Messerli FH, Bangalore S, Champion A, Cooper-Dehoff RM, Zhou Q, et al: Obesity paradox in patients with hypertension and coronary artery disease. Am J Med 2007;120:863–870.

7   Romero-Corral A, Montori VM, Somers VK, Korinek J, Thomas RJ, Allison TG, et al: Association of body weight with total mortality and with cardiovascular events in coronary artery disease: a systematic review of cohort studies. Lancet 2006;368:666–678.

8   McAuley P, Myers J, Abella J, Froelicher V: Body mass, fitness and survival in veteran patients: another obesity paradox? Am J Med 2007;120:518–524.

9   Kotanko P, Thijssen S, Levin NW: Association between erythropoietin responsiveness and body composition in dialysis patients. Blood Purif 2008;26:82–89.

10 Ikizler TA: Resolved: being fat is good for dialysis patients: the Godzilla effect. J Am Soc Nephrol 2008.

11 Kalantar-Zadeh K, Block G, Humphreys MH, Kopple JD: Reverse epidemiology of cardiovascular risk factors in maintenance dialysis patients. Kidney Int 2003;63:793–808.

12 Sarkar SR, Kuhlmann MK, Kotanko P, Zhu F, Heymsfield SB, Wang J, et al: Metabolic consequences of body size and body composition in hemodialysis patients. Kidney Int 2006;70: 1832–1839.

13 Kotanko P, Thijssen S, Kitzler T, Wystrychowski G, Sarkar SR, Zhu F, et al: Size matters: body composition and outcomes in maintenance hemodialysis patients. Blood Purif 2007;25:27–30.

14 Slowick-Zylka D, Safranow K, Dziedziejko V, Dutkiewicz G, Ciechanowski K, Chlubek D: The influence of gender, weight, height and BMI on pentosidine concentrations in plasma of hemodialyzed patients. J Nephrol 2006;19:65–69.

15 Gallagher D, Albu J, He Q, Heshka S, Boxt L, Krasnow N, et al: Small organs with a high metabolic rate explain lower resting energy expenditure in African-American than in white adults. Am J Clin Nutr 2006;83:1062–1067.

16 Kotanko P, Levin NW: The impact of visceral mass on survival in chronic hemodialysis patients. Int J Artif Organs 2007;30:993–999.

Peter Kotanko, MD
Renal Research Institute, 207 East 94th Street, Suite 303
New York, NY 10128 (USA)
Tel. +1 646 672 4042, Fax +1 212 996 5905, E-Mail pkotanko@rriny.com

Ronco C, Cruz DN (eds): Hemodialysis – From Basic Research to Clinical Trials.
Contrib Nephrol. Basel, Karger, 2008, vol 161, pp 115–118

....

Whole-Body Spectroscopy (BCM) in the Assessment of Normovolemia in Hemodialysis Patients

Volker Wizemann[a], Christiane Rode[a], Peter Wabel[b]

[a]Georg Haas Dialysezentrum Giessen and [b]Fresenius Medical Care, Bad Homburg, Germany

Abstract

Whole-body impedance spectroscopy (BCM) has been validated by comparing isotope dilution methods for precisely measuring body volume compartments. Clinical assessment as well as comparison to other methods shows that BCM predicts a reliable individual dialysis target weight in kilograms, which corresponds to a physiological (normal) extracellular volume. BCM is helpful in the management of volume status and arterial hypertension in hemodialysis patients as well as in patients with chronic kidney disease. Quantified by BCM, overhydration is a powerful predictor of death in hemodialysis patients.

Description of the Model

The description is based on the assumption that overhydration in anuric dialysis patients is primarily expressed in an expanded extracellular volume (ECV). A normal ECV then represents the goal of ultrafiltration therapy, which is equivalent to a normal 'dry weight'. However, normal ECVs in healthy adults range from 10 to >20 liters depending on the body composition. Thus, by body composition analysis, an individual normal ECV can be defined in healthy persons in absolute terms such as liters or kilograms. In a dialysis patient with exactly an identical body composition as the measured healthy person, predicted normal ECV would be identical, which means that this individual ECV

This article is restricted to the description and clinical evaluation of a model which targets to define an individual dry weight (in kg) for HD patients by means of whole-body spectroscopy.

value is equivalent with a state achieved in an individual and normal 'dry weight' following ultrafiltration.

In contrast to all other methods of dry weight assessment such as clinical work-up, inferior vena cava diameter, blood volume changes, monofrequency bioimpedance as well as segmental impedance during dialysis, our model is the only one which predicts not relative changes but an absolute endpoint in kilograms.

Validation of the Model

Initially, bioimpedance (Hydra bioimpedance analyzer) was performed in 68 normal healthy volunteers, weight range 14.5–120 kg. In the mean time the healthy reference group was extended to over 1,000 persons of both sexes. A subgroup study was performed in healthy adult persons as well as hemodialysis patients with extreme body compositions and weights ranging up to 176 kg. In these patients there was a good accordance between total body water assessed by urea kinetics and studied by the bioimpedance method.

Isotope dilution methods are considered as gold standard for measuring intra- and extracellular volumes. Our model has been validated in multicenter simultaneous comparisons of isotope and bioimpedance spectroscopy measurements in healthy as well as in hemodialysis patients where a good correlation between both approaches was found (for ECW:BCM vs. Na Br –0.2 liter) [1]. It is safe to say that the bioimpedance spectroscopy method (marketed as Body Composition Monitor = BCM) is equivalent to isotope dilution methods in predicting ECV and ICV which per se are not suitable for clinical application.

Clinical Validation

Bioimpedance spectroscopy has been validated in 17 patients starting with hemodialysis therapy. As control method a thorough clinical assessment with scoring of symptoms and signs by an experienced clinician in combination with serial inferior vena cava diameter measurements and changes in relative blood volumes was chosen. The blinded BCM predictions of dialysis target weight corresponded well with the clinically achieved dry weight. A mean of 6 liters excess ECW water had to be removed per patient during the target weight-finding process and all patients achieved a normotensive state without antihypertensive medication [2].

Detection limits for volume changes during ultrafiltration were excellent for the BCM method in comparison to other established methods for volume state evaluation. The BCM method sensed a volume change of 0.89 ± 0.64 kg in contrast to the VCI method (1.74 ± 1.56 kg) and the relative blood volume method (2.3 ± 1.00 kg) [3].

In a single-center study involving 193 hemodialysis patients there was a close correlation between the routinely defined dry weight and the BCM method (applied for the first time), where the mean deviation from the routine target weight was –1.5 ± 2.2 kg [Wizemann et al., unpubl. data].

In 310 hemodialysis patients from two centers, according to BCM, 48% of all patients were normohydrated and within the 2 kg acceptable overweight before dialysis. 23% were classified as hypovolemic (less than –1.2 kg to BCM target weight before dialysis) and 29% as hypervolemic (>2 kg of the BCM target weight). Interesting to note is that only 15% of the whole group had hypervolemia and simultaneous arterial hypertension and 21% of patients were hypertensive and were classified as hypovolemic. It appears that arterial hypertension in dialysis patients is not necessarily a sequela of hypervolemia and that the proportion of true hypertonic patients is comparable to that of the general population. In this group, antihypertensives are rather indicated than volume loss. On the other hand there was a group of 14% of the whole population, which – according to BCM – was overhydrated and had arterial hypotension (defined as BP <100 predialysis). Closer inspection of those patients revealed underlying cardiac failure, where careful fluid loss and serial left ventricular function monitoring might be helpful. Thus, assessment by BCM appears to create a useful diagnostic basis for differential therapy [Wabel et al., to be published].

We applied BCM in more than 400 patients with chronic renal failure stage 1–5. Statistically, there was a reverse significant relationship between excretory renal function and volume expansion of ECV. Although there was a large interindividual variation probably partly due to different pretreatment regimens, BCM in individual follow-up was an important instrument to modify antihypertensive and diuretic therapy.

In a study including 254 hemodialysis patients from two centers, 76 deaths occurred in a 10-year time span. Cox proportional hazard analysis revealed that the volume state assessed by BCM before dialysis is an independent predictor of mortality.

Comments

Whole-body impedance with the model of BCM is an easily applicable method in hemodialysis as well as chronic renal failure patients to define an individual normal ECV and thereby dry weight. The BCM method is the only one which predicts a normal volume state not only in indicative relative changes of volume state but in endpoints (in kilograms extracellular water or dry weight). This renders the BCM method ideal for wide routine application in renal failure patients.

There are however limitations to the method: although BCM is equivalent to isotope dilution methods in assessing volume state, a predicted normal ECW for an individual patient must not necessarily be the optimum ECW for a multi-morbid hemodialysis patient. For example, in a hemodialysis patient with cardiac output failure, the magnitude of left ventricular systolic function is the most important parameter for the prognosis and quality of life for the patient. Volume state and thereby ventricular filling volume as well as ventricular pressure is one important determinate of ventricular systolic function and is highly modifiable by the magnitude of volume removal by dialysis. At present it is unclear whether a normal volume state as predicted by BCM for a completely healthy person is also the optimal endpoint for a patient with cardiac systolic failure. The optimum lies certainly within a narrow range of normal ECW but additional clinical assessment and echocardiographic follow-up is necessary to find that range. This example indicates that the BCM prediction of a 'normal' dry weight – although in itself quite accurate – is a *suggestion* for the treating nephrologists who should modify it according to the clinical situation. This statement is also true for application of BCM in diagnosing and treating volume state (and hypertension) in predialysis chronic renal failure patients.

Thus in a vast sea of endless water, BCM is not a kind of GPS for the 15th century ocean sailor, it is rather a very helpful landmark for otherwise difficult navigation.

References

1   Moissl U, Wabel P, Chamney P, et al: Body fluid volume determination via body composition spectroscopy in health and disease. Physiol Meas 2006;27:921–933.
2   Chamney PW, Krämer M, Rode C, Wizemann V: A new technique for establishing dry weight in hemodialysis patients via whole-body bioimpedance. Kidney Int 2002;61:2250–2258.
3   Krämer M, Rode C, Wizemann V: Detection limit of methods to assess fluid status changes in dialysis patients. Kidney Int 2006;69:1609–1620.

Prof. Volker Wizemann
Johann-Sebastian-Bachstrasse 40
DE–35392 Giessen (Germany)
Tel. +49 641 92207 15, Fax +49 641 29187, E-Mail wizemann.volker@phv-dialyse.de

Ronco C, Cruz DN (eds): Hemodialysis – From Basic Research to Clinical Trials.
Contrib Nephrol. Basel, Karger, 2008, vol 161, pp 119–124

··· · ···· · ···· · ····

Blood Volume Monitoring

Roland E. Winkler[a], Wolfgang Pätow[a], Peter Ahrenholz[b]

[a]PDA Rostock, Department of Internal Medicine, Nephrology and Dialysis, and
[b]BioArtProducts GmbH, Rostock, Germany

Abstract

Background: In CKD stage 5 diabetic patients (DM), only approximately half of the interdialytic weight gain was accounted for by sodium intake. The other half was due to pure water gain, probably caused by hyperglycemia. Dialysis treatment faces two major troubles: the removal of the extra amount of water and the therapy of the compromised compensatory mechanisms. The described situation is the reason why new technologies in hemodialysis were developed. Blood volume monitoring (BVM) with regulation of ultrafiltration and sodium (Hemocontrol, Hospal, Belgium; Hameomaster, Nikkiso Co. Ltd, Japan) was evaluated to describe the advantages for efficacy and compatibility in hemodialysis therapy. **Methods:** 18 cardiovascular instable patients (DM) were included into the study (age 56.4 ± 12.5, 7 female, 11 male). Begin of dialysis 39 ± 9.3 months before the study, dialysis time/session 258.3 ± 15.4 min, 3 sessions/week, blood flow 250 ml/min, dialysate flow 500 ml/min, prephase: standard bicarbonate dialysis (HD; HCO_3^- 35 mmol/l) 2 weeks, BVM: 48 weeks. Clinical parameters evaluated before BVM and 48 weeks after BVM: number of muscle cramps (MC) and hypotensive episodes (HypoEp) during dialysis, optimal weight (OptW), single pool Kt/V (sp Kt/V), equilibrated Kt/V (db Kt/V), systolic blood pressure (BP), antihypertensive drugs (AntiDr), cardiac ejection fraction (EF) and left ventricular mass index (LVMI). **Results:** In comparison with HD after 48 weeks with BVM, we can demonstrate a reduction of MC by 83.7%, HypoEp by 88.9%, OptW by 1.7%. The improved refilling and reduction of OptW led to an increase of sp Kt/V by 34.8% and db Kt/V by 33.3%. AntiDr were reduced to 56.6% compared to HD, BP lowered by 4.4%. Due to BVM, EF increases to 123.8% and LVMI decreases by 25.2%. **Conclusion:** BVM can improve clinical parameters for adequacy of hemodialysis. It offers a unique possibility to treat diabetic patients according to their special needs.

Background

The dialysis population has changed in the last decade to a majority of patients with severe cardiovascular morbidity, especially in diabetics, which has had a great impact on the complication rate during hemodialysis treatment. Several factors are involved in the pathogenesis of dialysis discomfort – the most important one is a decrease in blood volume caused by an imbalance between ultrafiltration (UF) and plasma interstitial refilling rate, which has been reported frequently. Augmenting conditions are the excessive interdialytic water intake, boosted by hyperglycemia, the disturbance of cardiovascular compensation mechanisms, such as baroreflex and vascular tonus, and the abundance of interacting medication. In addition, for the clinician the assessment of volume state is difficult, in spite of tools such as ultrasound-estimated vena cava tension and the presence or absence of edema in the clinical examination. Intradialytic hypotension and cramping are frequent complications of hemodialysis (up to 20%) following excessive rate or volume of fluid removal. On the other hand, less invasive but inadequate low volume removal may lead to chronic volume overload manifesting as arterial hypertension, left ventricular hypertrophy and consecutive systolic and diastolic heart failure. It therefore became a challenge for the dialysis staff and a landmark of dialysis quality to estimate the hydration state and manage a well-tolerated water removal. For this purpose, devices that continuously and non-invasively monitor the changes of relative blood volume during the treatment have been developed as a tool to maintain an adequate volume of the intravascular compartment. Such devices include sensors for the measurement of temperature and hematocrit as well as measurement of blood flow rate. Many manufacturers have incorporated a blood volume monitor in their dialysis monitors and some have developed biofeedback systems that control volume changes, answered by variations of UF rate and/or dialysate conductivity. Such biofeedback technologies seem to diminish the severity and frequency of dialysis hypotension, ensure the efficiency of the treatment and may, by improvement of physiological conditions, lead to an overall reduction in morbidity and mortality.

Material and Methods

Eighteen diabetic patients undergoing regular hemodialysis therapy with cardiovascular disease and complications like muscle cramps and hypotensive episodes during dialysis sessions were included into the clinical evaluation. The start of renal replacement therapy before the study was 39 ± 9.3 months. 7 female and 11 male patients with an age of 56.4 ± 12.5 years (range 34–71) took part in this study. The study was performed as descriptive clinical evaluation.

In the prephase we carried out standard bicarbonate dialysis with high-flux membranes (polyarylethersulfonate, polyamide; Gambro Hospal GmbH, Germany), bicarbonate in dialysate 35 mmol/l, blood flow (Q_b) 250 ml/min, dialysate flow (Q_d) 500 ml/min, ultrapure dialysis water. We started the regimen of blood volume monitoring (BVM) with UF and sodium regulation (Biofeedback System Hemocontrol, Hospal, Belgium) after 2 weeks with standard bicarbonate dialysis (prephase). To estimate the advantages of BVM, we measured parameters of efficacy and compatibility in the prephase and under the conditions of BVM at

Table 1. Changes in clinical parameters in prephase standard bicarbonate dialysis compared to BVM dialysis

Parameter	Prephase HD	BVM			Dimension	t test
		12 weeks	40 weeks	48 weeks		
sysBP	132.7 ± 3.9	136.9 ± 6.8		125.8 ± 3.6	mm Hg	n.s.
EF	42.9 ± 4.9	45.6 ± 5.1	49.9 ± 4.3	53.1 ± 5.9	%	n.s.
LVMI	163.4 ± 10.4*	165.1 ± 11.2	134.1 ± 8.9	121.9 ± 11.9*	g/m^2	p < 0.05
AntiDr	3 ± 1.2	3 ± 0.6		1.7 ± 0.5		n.s.
MC	6 ± 1.2*	3 ± 0.7	1*	1*		p < 0.01
HypoEp	9 ± 0.9*	1*	1*	1*		p < 0.01
OptW	0	0	−0.6 ± 0.3	−1.7 ± 0.4	Δ kg	n.s.
sp Kt/V	1.09 ± 0.09*	1.23 ± 0.12	1.28 ± 0.08	1.47 ± 0.15*		p < 0.05
db Kt/V	0.96 ± 0.07*	1.09 ± 0.09	1.18 ± 0.06	1.28 ± 0.11*		p < 0.05

sysBP = Systolic blood pressure before dialysis; EF = cardiac ejection fraction; LVMI = left ventricular mass index; AntiDr = antihypertensive drugs; MC = muscle cramps; HypoEp = hypotensive episodes; OptW = optimal weight; sp Kt/V = single pool Kt/V; db Kt/V = double pool Kt/V.
    * = Significance t-test.

the time t_0 (prephase), t_1 (12 weeks BVM), t_2 (40 weeks BVM) and t_3 (48 weeks BVM). Systolic blood pressure (sysBP) was measured by the dialysis monitor at the start of dialysis session and every hour. Table 1 compares the sysBP at the beginning of dialysis sessions. At time 0, 1, 2 and 3, we examined cardiac function such as cardiac ejection fraction (EF) and left ventricular mass index (LVMI) by echocardiography, the number of muscle cramps (MC) and hypotension episodes (HypoEp) during dialysis session, the optimal weight (OptW) after hemodialysis, the amount of antihypertensive drugs (AntiDr) and the single pool (sp) Kt/V and double pool (dp) Kt/V by the method of Daugirdas. Statistical analysis was performed descriptively by mean ± SD. Statistical significance was estimated by paired t test (p < 0.05).

Results

After BVM over 48 weeks we can state a benefit in all clinical parameters versus standard bicarbonate high-flux dialysis (fig. 1). Surprisingly, BVM seems to be able to correct the cardiac function with a reduction of the overload of additionally pure water caused by diabetes and intermittent hyperglycemia. Therefore, we can demonstrate the possibility to reduce the OptW (–1.7 ± 0.4 kg (n.s.)) in combination with lowering the AntiDr by –1.7 ± 0.5 (n.s.) medicaments. Although there is a reduction in drug therapy, the sysBP dropped from 132.7 ± 3.9 to

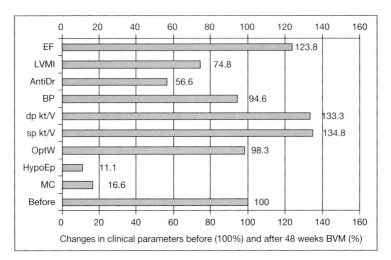

Fig. 1. Changes in clinical parameters in % (before: standard bicarbonate dialysis 100%). EF = Cardiac ejection fraction; LVMI = left ventricular mass index; AntiDr = antihypertensive drugs; BP = blood pressure; dp Kt/V = double pool Kt/V; sp Kt/V = single pool Kt/V; OptW = optimal weight; HypoEp = hypotensive episodes; MC = muscle cramps; Before = prephase standard bicarbonate dialysis.

125.8 ± 3.6 mm Hg (n.s.). The hypothesized better refilling into the intravascular compartment leads to an improvement of cardiac function with increasing EF (from 42.9 ± 4.9 to 53.1 ± 5.9% (n.s.)) and a near normalization of LVMI (from 163.4 ± 10.4 to 121.9 ± 11.9 g/m^2 (p < 0.05)). Due to a reduction of V and the improvement of cardiac function, sp Kt/v increased from 1.09 ± 0.09 to 1.47 ± 0.15 (p < 0.05), and db Kt/V from 0.96 ± 0.07 up to 1.28 ± 0.11 (p < 0.05), respectively. We observed a dramatic reduction of MC (6 ± 1.2 to 1 (p < 0.01) and HypoEP (9 ± –0.9 to 1 (p < 0.01)) (table 1).

Discussion

The worldwide dialysis population is growing between 3 and 7% annually [1]. In Germany the incidence and prevalence of diabetic patients in dialysis is approaching 40% and the development of CKD stage 5 in patients >70 years has increased by more than 10% in the last 3 years [2]. In diabetic patients a higher rate of intradialytic complications occurs due to cardiovascular disease and the lack of regulatory mechanisms (autonomic neuropathy).

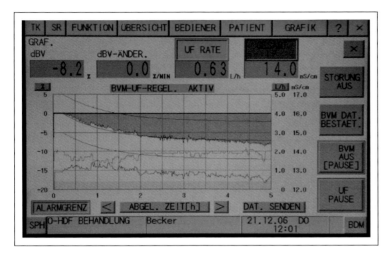

Fig. 2. Screenshot of BVM with UF and conductivity regulation with Haemomaster (Nikkiso Co. Ltd, Japan).

Increased extracellular fluid osmolarity resulting from hyperglycemia induces intracellular dehydration and central stimulation of thirst. Hyperglycemia-induced thirst stimulates increased fluid ingestion, resulting in excess interdialytic weight gain in dialyzed diabetic patients. There is a positive correlation between interdialytic weight gain and glycemic control [3]. Three BVM technologies can be used: (a) BVM with regulation of UF rate (Fresenius Medical Care, Germany); (b) Haemomaster with regulation of UF and conductivity (Nikkiso Co. Ltd, Japan, fig. 2), or (c) the biofeedback system Hemocontrol with regulation of UF and conductivity (Hospal, Gambro Renal Products, Belgium). The lack of conductivity regulation (BVM, Fresenius Medical Care, Germany) leads to a prolongation of dialysis time if the limits of blood volume changes are exceeded. The monitoring of blood volume changes during hemodialysis sessions in combination with a biofeedback system including the regulation of conductivity (sodium) and UF may be helpful to prevent intradialytic complications (Hemocontrol) [4]. In cardiovascular instable patients the continuous BVM enables the achievement of optimal weight and the removal of the extra amount of pure water [5]. Due to a mathematical model of sodium kinetics the sodium balance will be unchanged during BMV sessions (equivalent conductivity) [5]. The BVM treatment has to be individualized for each patient due to varying refilling capacities inter- and intraindividually [6]. The improvement of fluid balance with lower optimal weight after dialysis session and reduced antihypertensive drugs seems to be responsible for the efficacy (sp Kt/V, db Kt/V) and compatibility (EF, LVMI).

Conclusions

The fluid balance in diabetic patients with cardiovascular disease will be improved by blood volume-regulated hemodialysis. Due to a combination of fluid and sodium balance regulation, dialysis dosage/time (intradialytic refilling) might improve. Fluid balance and sodium kinetics are responsible for the reduction of optimal weight without well-known complications such as muscle cramps and hypotensive episodes. In BVM the mean systolic blood pressure can be normalized. It seems that the correction of fluid balance may influence the cardiac parameter EF positively. The improvement of the LVMI is a direct parameter for the prevention of cardiovascular death [7]. BVM is able to improve parameters for adequacy of hemodialysis. It offers a unique possibility to treat diabetic patients according to their special needs. The small number of patients and the descriptive kind of evaluation only allows the demonstration of trends. Randomized, multicentric, prospective clinical studies have established the advantages and benefits of BVM [8, 9]. The optimization of BVM, measuring and regulating dialysis technologies to validate this extracorporeal procedure, represents another important clinical problem [10].

References

1 Lysaght MJ: Maintenance dialysis population dynamics: current trends and long-term implications. J Am Soc Nephrol 2002;13(suppl 1):37–40.
2 Frei U, Schober-Halstenberg HJ: Nierenersatztherapie in Deutschland 2005–2006. Berlin, QuasiNiere, 2006.
3 Ifudu O, Dulin AL, Friedman EA: Interdialytic weight gain correlates with glycosylated hemoglobin in diabetic hemodialysis patients. Am J Kidney Dis 1994;23:686–691.
4 Locatelli F, Buoncristiani U, Canaud B, Kohler H, et al: Haemodialysis with on-line monitoring equipment: tools or toys? Nephrol Dial Transplant 2005;20:22–23.
5 Bonello M, House AA, Cruz Y, et al: Integration of blood volume, blood pressure, heart rate and bioimpedance monitoring for the achievement of optimal dry body weight during chronic hemodialysis. Int J Artif Org 2007;30:1098–1108.
6 Brummelhuis WJ, van Schelven LJ, Boer WH: Continuous, online measurement of the absolute plasma refill rate during hemodialysis using feedback regulated ultrafiltration: preliminary results. ASAIO J 2008;54:95–99.
7 Levin A, Singer J, Thompson CR, et al: Prevalent left ventricular hypertrophy in the predialysis population: identifying opportunities for intervention. Am J Kidney Dis 1996;27:347–354.
8 Santoro A, Mambelli E, Canova C, et al: Biofeedback in dialysis. J Nephrol 2003;16(suppl 7):48–56.
9 Santoro A, Mancini E, Basile C, et al: Blood volume controller hemodialysis in hypotension-prone patients: a randomized, multicenter controller trial. Kidney Int 2002;62:1034–1045.
10 Agarwal R, Kelley K, Light RP: Diagnostic utility of blood volume monitoring in hemodialysis patients. Am J Kidney Dis 2008;51:242–254.

Roland E. Winkler, MD, PhD, MBA
PDA Rostock, Department for Internal Medicine, Nephrology and Dialysis
St.-Petersburger-Strasse 18c, DE–18107 Rostock (Germany)
Tel. +49 381 776810, Fax +49 381 7768149, E-Mail roland.winkler@praxisverbund-rostock.de

Ronco C, Cruz DN (eds): Hemodialysis – From Basic Research to Clinical Trials.
Contrib Nephrol. Basel, Karger, 2008, vol 161, pp 125–131

· ·

From Uremic Toxin Retention to Removal by Convection: Do We Know Enough?

R. Vanholder, N. Meert, E. Schepers, G. Glorieux

Nephrology Section, University Hospital, Gent, Belgium

Abstract

The uremic syndrome is defined by a complex clinical picture, characterized by the dysfunction of most organs which are affected by the retention of multiple solutes. Recent research has helped to unravel the pathophysiology and to identify several as yet unknown responsible compounds. In this publication, we summarize which compounds play the most important pathophysiologic role, and which dialysis strategies can be considered to decrease their concentration and improve outcomes. The main pathophysiologic role is played by molecules which are so-called 'difficult to remove by dialysis'. Essentially observational studies have suggested that enhancement of removal of these molecules, by improving convection (hemodiafiltration), creates an improvement of survival. The knowledge of uremic toxicity is still far from complete however, and we need extra information about responsible compounds and mechanisms, eventually leading to a classification of the most important culprits, to allow the development of even more efficient or specific removal strategies.

Uremia and Uremic Toxicity

The term *uremia* defines the condition occurring when kidney function regresses during chronic kidney disease (CKD). During uremia, the function of almost every organ system fails; the totality of clinical problems registered during uremia is called the *uremic syndrome*. A host of compounds are no more or insufficiently removed by the kidneys and remain in the body. They are called *uremic retention solutes*. In as far as they exert biological and/or biochemical activities, they are named *uremic toxins*. In the latter case, they contribute to the uremic syndrome. Even if uremic retention solutes are biologically/biochemically inert, they may be useful markers for the retention or the removal of other, more toxic compounds; a current example is urea which is universally used as a marker but which is biologically relatively inert.

A variety of toxic effects have been attributed to several of the compounds retained during progressive renal failure [1, 2]. One of the major concerns is the increased cardiovascular morbidity and mortality in CKD so that outcome is affected to a similar extent as in diabetes mellitus [3]. Many of the other organic disturbances which are at play during uremia also indirectly contribute to cardiovascular morbidity and mortality (e.g. anemia, inflammation).

Whereas these deleterious effects in general are most preponderant at the final stage (stage 5) of CKD when renal replacement therapy is necessary, organ damage related to the uremic syndrome starts to occur already at much earlier stages. Cardiovascular mortality increases already from a glomerular filtration rate of $60\,ml/min \cdot 1.73\,m^2$ on (CKD stage 3, corresponding to a decrease of renal function by 50%), and according to some sources even earlier [3, 4].

Hence, CKD and the uremic syndrome are a major source of morbidity and mortality. Knowledge of the retained compounds and of their pathophysiologic role might help to develop strategies to remove these solutes or to counteract their deleterious effects.

The Complexity of Uremic Retention

During the last two decades, our knowledge of uremic retention has grown so rapidly, that in a review in 2003, 90 different uremic retention solutes were identified [5].

By applying gas chromatography-mass spectrometry, even more than 1,000 different peptidic compounds with MW $>800\,D$ were found in ultrafiltrate from patients on dialysis [6]. Several of these compounds have an important pathophysiologic impact, as depicted in several recent reviews which have just been published or are on the verge of being published [7, 8].

One such example of a newly detected group of toxins are the dinucleoside polyphosphates; they are characterized by a chemical structure of one nucleoside at each end, linked by a variable number of phosphates (usually 3–6). Dinucleoside polyphosphates are a group of substances involved in the regulation of vascular tone as well as in the proliferation of vascular smooth muscle cells [9] and mesangial cells [10]. Specific members of this group, the diadenosine polyphosphates, were detected in hepatocytes, human plasma and platelets. In addition, concentrations of diadenosine polyphosphates are increased in platelets from hemodialysis patients [11]. Recently, uridine adenosine tetraphosphate (Up4A) was isolated and identified as a novel endothelium-derived vasoconstrictive factor. Its vasoconstrictive effects, its plasma concentration and its release upon endothelial stimulation strongly suggest a functional vasoregulatory role [12].

Another newly detected compound with potential interest is *p*-cresylsulfate. Although most of the pioneering research on the phenolic compounds has been focused on the concentration and the toxicity of the mother compound *p*-cresol, later work revealed that genuine *p*-cresol was present at very low up to undetectable concentrations in patients with renal failure and that most of the *p*-cresol, generated by the intestinal flora, was conjugated to *p*-cresylsulfate in the intestinal wall and to *p*-cresylglucuronide in the liver [13, 14]. Both conjugates are characterized by a strong protein binding. The reason for the previous emphasis on *p*-cresol was due to the fact that most determination methods were based on deproteinization by acidification, causing disintegration of the conjugates by hydrolysis. Application of deproteinization methods without acidification revealed the presence of the conjugate *p*-cresylsulfate [13].

Further studies indicated that the biochemical impact of the mother compound *p*-cresol is not necessarily the same as that of the conjugate. Whereas *p*-cresol suppresses the activity of leukocytes, especially after their activation, *p*-cresylsulfate essentially appeared to be linked to baseline leukocyte activation [15]. Nevertheless, since there is very likely a correlation between former *p*-cresol estimations and current *p*-cresylsulfate measurements, previously held conclusions about protein binding and relationship with clinical outcome parameters of *p*-cresol [16–18] might still be valid.

In vitro Assessment of Uremic Toxicity

Many uremic compounds are first studied in an in vitro setting, prior to clinical or epidemiological evaluations. To define which compounds are at play in uremic cardiovascular disease, numerous in vitro studies have been undertaken, concentrating on the four major cell systems involved in this process: leukocyte (granulocyte and monocyte) activation; endothelial damage; thrombocyte activation, and smooth muscle cell proliferation [2]. From a survey in 2001, it appeared that essentially molecules that are 'difficult to remove by dialysis', such as larger 'middle' molecules and protein-bound uremic retention molecules, had been shown to play a role in these processes [2]. The current generally applied method to assess dialysis adequacy, which is based on the kinetics of the small water-soluble compound urea, conceivably is not representative for the behavior during dialysis of the latter compounds.

Newly collected information confirms the major pathophysiologic role of these 'difficult to remove' molecules and refers amongst others to middle molecules such as the diadenosine polyphosphates, structural variants of angiotensin II, fibrinogen fragments and newly detected cytokines, as well as to protein-bound molecules, such as the phenols, indoles and phenylacetic acid. In addition, several guanidino compounds, amongst which also asymmetric and symmetric dimethylarginine, are to be mentioned. Although guanidino compounds are small water-soluble compounds with supposed similar physicochemical characteristics as our current markers urea and creatinine, they display a kinetic behavior which is largely different so that even these molecules classify among 'the difficult to remove molecules' [19].

Results of in vitro studies about uremic toxins should always be considered with the necessary care. On the one hand, methodological approaches should be applied in a consistent way, preferably based on strict methodological rules or recommendations like those recently formulated [20]; on the other hand, application of incorrect concentrations is another potential bias of these in vitro approaches [21, 22].

A recent example of such a bias emanated from studies showing that AOPP concentrations measured with classical methods [23] are biased by a hard to fathom background noise created at least in part by triglycerides and coagulation factors [24, 25].

Additional information for the future assessment of uremic toxicity is expected from proteomic and genomic studies, which could be of help to identify as yet undetected substances with a potential impact in certain uremic disease processes. While starting from previously specified conditions or complications (e.g. comparing patients with and without cardiovascular disease or with and without malnutrition, and assessing plasma or RNA samples of both conditions with sophisticated analytical and biostatistical methods), such approaches might be of help to unveil as yet unknown pathophysiological mechanisms and responsible compounds [26].

Translation into Clinical Studies

Based on the experience gained from in vitro studies, the next step is to translate this knowledge into improvements of the therapeutic conditions for patients.

Our current knowledge that several of the known larger 'middle' molecules have the potential to induce mechanisms responsible for cardiovascular damage, emanated in a number of studies assessing dialyzers with a large pore size, comparing them to standard dialyzers with small pores and no or little removal capacity for these 'difficult to remove molecules'.

The first controlled study in this domain was the HEMO study showing no difference in overall outcome at primary analysis between high- and low-flux membranes [27]. Secondary analyses learned, however, that the frequency of the following conditions was lower with high-flux membranes: (1) for the entire population, the risk of cardiac death and of cardiac death plus hospitalization for cardiac reasons [27]; (2) overall mortality for those patients enrolled in the study after a time on dialysis above the median (3.7 years) [28]; (3) frequency of cerebrovascular accidents, especially in patients with baseline presence of cerebrovascular disease [29]. In addition, irrespective of membrane flux, an inverse correlation was observed between plasma concentration of β_2-microglobulin and survival, again pointing to a relationship between average concentration of large 'middle' molecules and outcome [30].

The HEMO study was a four-armed study (considering not only dialyzer flux but also dialysis adequacy as estimated by Kt/V_{urea}), targeting for a population of 900 patients, running over 1–5 years, evaluating incident patients, allowing dialyzer reuse and imposing a rather restrictive definition of high flux. In contrast, the more recent European MPO study was two-armed (only focusing on flux), targeting for a population of 660 patients (thus potentially more powered than the HEMO study in function of only two arms), running over 3–7.5 years, evaluating prevalent patients, not allowing dialyzer reuse and imposing a liberal definition of high flux [31]. The study was essentially focusing on a patient population with hypoalbuminemia, which is carrying a higher mortality risk than the normoalbuminemic dialysis population, since hypoalbuminemia is a reflection of poor nutritional status, inflammation and/or fluid overload. In the MPO study, outcome was superior for high-flux membranes in this hypo-albuminemic population, and also in the subgroup with diabetes mellitus [F. Locatelli, communication at the ERA-EDTA Meeting, Barcelona 2007].

The data collected by Cheung et al. [30] from the HEMO database and showing a direct correlation between β_2-microglobulin concentrations and mortality, suggest that further enhancing larger molecule removal, e.g. by increasing convection, could induce an additional benefit. Recent evolutions in hemodialysis have enabled to purify dialysate to such an extent that it can be used as substitution fluid in hemodiafiltration strategies, hence increasing possibilities for convective removal of large molecules. For the time being, the two available outcome studies on convective strategies were observational, but showed both a survival advantage if enough plasma water was ultrafiltered and substituted [32, 33].

Conclusions

The sequence of the steps depicted in the above example shows how knowledge collected from in vitro evaluations and observational or epidemiological clinical studies ultimately can lead to development of well-conceived clinical studies and funded therapeutic strategies to improve outcome and quality of life of patients with CKD. Our spectrum of basic pathophysiologic knowledge should further be extended if we want to design new therapeutic approaches to improve the condition of this population.

References

1   Vanholder R, De Smet R: Pathophysiologic effects of uremic retention solutes. J Am Soc Nephrol 1999;10:1815–1823.
2   Vanholder R, Argiles A, Baurmeister U, et al: Uremic toxicity: present state of the art. Int J Artif Organs 2001;24:695–725.
3   Vanholder R, Massy Z, Argiles A, et al: Chronic kidney disease as cause of cardiovascular morbidity and mortality. Nephrol Dial Transplant 2005;20:1048–1056.
4   Van Biesen W, De Bacquer D, Verbeke F, et al: The glomerular filtration rate in an apparently healthy population and its relation with cardiovascular mortality during 10 years. Eur Heart J 2007;28:478–483.
5   Vanholder R, De Smet R, Glorieux G, et al: Review on uremic toxins: classification, concentration, and interindividual variability. Kidney Int 2003;63:1934–1943.
6   Weissinger EM, Kaiser T, Meert N, et al: Proteomics: a novel tool to unravel the pathophysiology of uraemia. Nephrol Dial Transplant 2004;19:3068–3077.
7   Vanholder R, Van Laecke S, Glorieux G: What is new in uremic toxicity. Pediatr Nephrol 2008 (in press).
8   Vanholder R, Van Laecke S, Glorieux G: The middle molecule hypothesis thirty years after: lost and rediscovered in the universe of uremic toxicity? J Nephrol 2008 (in press).
9   Ogilvie A, Blasius R, Schulze-Lohoff E, Sterzel RB: Adenine dinucleotides: a novel class of signalling molecules. J Auton Pharmacol 1996;16:325–328.
10 Heidenreich S, Tepel M, Schluter H, Harrach B, Zidek W: Regulation of rat mesangial cell growth by diadenosine phosphates. J Clin Invest 1995;95:2862–2867.
11 Jankowski J, Hagemann J, Yoon MS, et al: Increased vascular growth in hemodialysis patients induced by platelet-derived diadenosine polyphosphates. Kidney Int 2001;59:1134–1141.
12 Jankowski V, Tolle M, Vanholder R, et al: Uridine adenosine tetraphosphate: a novel endothelium-derived vasoconstrictive factor. Nat Med 2005;11:223–227.
13 Martinez AW, Recht NS, Hostetter TH, Meyer TW: Removal of p-cresol sulfate by hemodialysis. J Am Soc Nephrol 2005;16:3430–3436.
14 De Loor H, Bammens B, Evenepoel P, De Preter V, Verbeke K: Gas chromatographic-mass spectrometric analysis for measurement of p-cresol and its conjugated metabolites in uremic and normal serum. Clin Chem 2005;51:1535–1538.
15 Schepers E, Meert N, Glorieux G, et al: p-Cresylsulphate, the main in vivo metabolite of p-cresol, activates leucocyte free radical production. Nephrol Dial Transplant 2007;22:592–596.
16 De Smet R, Van Kaer J, Van Vlem B, et al: Toxicity of free p-cresol: a prospective and cross-sectional analysis. Clin Chem 2003;49:470–478.
17 Bammens B, Evenepoel P, Keuleers H, Verbeke K, Vanrenterghem Y: Free serum concentrations of the protein-bound retention solute p-cresol predict mortality in hemodialysis patients. Kidney Int 2006;69:1081–1087.
18 Bammens B, Evenepoel P, Verbeke K, Vanrenterghem Y: Removal of middle molecules and protein-bound solutes by peritoneal dialysis and relation with uremic symptoms. Kidney Int 2003;64:2238–2243.
19 Eloot S, Torremans A, De Smet R, et al: Kinetic behavior of urea is different from that of other water-soluble compounds: the case of the guanidino compounds. Kidney Int 2005;67:1566–1575.

20   Cohen G, Glorieux G, Thornalley P, et al: Review on uraemic toxins III – recommendations for handling uraemic retention solutes in vitro: towards a standardized approach for research on uraemia. Nephrol Dial Transplant 2007;22:3381–3390.

21   Vanholder R, Meert N, Schepers E, et al: Review on uraemic solutes II Variability in reported concentrations: causes and consequences. Nephrol Dial Transplant 2007;22:3115–3121.

22   Meert N, Schepers E, De Smet R, et al: Inconsistency of reported uremic toxin concentrations. Artif Organs 2007;31:600–611.

23   Witko-Sarsat V, Friedlander M, Capeillere-Blandin C, et al: Advanced oxidation protein products as a novel marker of oxidative stress in uremia. Kidney Int 1996;49:1304–1313.

24   Valli A, Suliman ME, Meert N, et al: Overestimation of advanced oxidation protein products in uremic plasma due to presence of triglycerides and other endogenous factors. Clin Chim Acta 2007;379:87–94.

25   Selmeci L, Szekely M, Soos P, et al: Human blood plasma advanced oxidation protein products correlates with fibrinogen levels. Free Radic Res 2006;40:952–958.

26   Fliser D, Novak J, Thongboonkerd V, et al: Advances in urinary proteome analysis and biomarker discovery. J Am Soc Nephrol 2007;18:1057–1071.

27   Eknoyan G, Beck GJ, Cheung AK, et al: Effect of dialysis dose and membrane flux in maintenance hemodialysis. N Engl J Med 2002;347:2010–2019.

28   Cheung AK, Levin NW, Greene T, et al: Effects of high-flux hemodialysis on clinical outcomes: results of the HEMO study. J Am Soc Nephrol 2003;14:3251–3263.

29   Delmez JA, Yan G, Bailey J, et al: Cerebrovascular disease in maintenance hemodialysis patients: results of the HEMO Study. Am J Kidney Dis 2006;47:131–138.

30   Cheung AK, Rocco MV, Yan G, et al: Serum β_2-microglobulin levels predict mortality in dialysis patients: results of the HEMO study. J Am Soc Nephrol 2006;17:546–555.

31   Locatelli F, Hannedouche T, Jacobson S, et al: The effect of membrane permeability on ESRD: design of a prospective randomised multicentre trial. J Nephrol 1999;12:85–88.

32   Canaud B, Bragg-Gresham JL, Marshall MR, et al: Mortality risk for patients receiving hemodiafiltration versus hemodialysis: European results from the DOPPS study. Kidney Int 2006;69:2087–2093.

33   Jirka T, Cesare S, Di Benedetto A, et al: Mortality risk for patients receiving hemodiafiltration versus hemodialysis. Kidney Int 2006;70:1524–1525.

Raymond Vanholder
Nephrology Section, Department of Internal Medicine
University Hospital, 0K12, De Pintelaan, 185
BE–9000 Gent (Belgium)
Tel. +32 9240 4525, Fax +32 9240 4599, E-Mail raymond.vanholder@ugent.be

Ronco C, Cruz DN (eds): Hemodialysis – From Basic Research to Clinical Trials.
Contrib Nephrol. Basel, Karger, 2008, vol 161, pp 132–137

· ·

Oxidative Stress in Hemodialysis

Jonathan Himmelfarb

Department of Medicine, Division of Nephrology and Renal Transplantation, Maine
Medical Center, Portland, Me., USA

Abstract

Patients with advanced chronic kidney disease are at a greatly increased cardiovascular
risk that cannot be explained entirely by traditional cardiovascular risk factors. An increase in
oxidative stress is proposed as a non-traditional cardiovascular risk factor in this patient population. Many laboratories have now unequivocally demonstrated that uremia is an increased
oxidative stress state. Uremic oxidative stress is characterized biologically by an increase in
lipid peroxidation products and reactive aldehyde groups as well as by increased retention of
oxidized thiols. The pathophysiology of increased oxidative stress in uremia is multifactorial,
but the retention of oxidized solute by the loss of kidney function is probably a major
contributor.

Pathways of Increased Oxidative Stress

Oxidative stress has historically been defined as an imbalance between
oxidant production and antioxidant defense. This definition emphasizes the significance of the overall redox status. More recently, the identification of the role
of oxidants in redox regulation of cell signaling and gene expression through
discrete redox pathways rather than through global redox balance has led to the
development of a new definition of oxidative stress. This definition focuses on
as a disruption of redox signaling and control, recognizing the occurrence of
compartmentalized redox circuits within the cell [1]. Although the definition
and pathophysiological processes leading to an increase in oxidative stress may
seem clearcut, unfortunately the use of the terms 'oxidative stress' and 'oxidant
stress' are relatively non-specific, and few biological systems are in redox equilibrium. In most biological systems, reducing equivalents are constantly being
generated and converted and interconverted, indicating that a major component

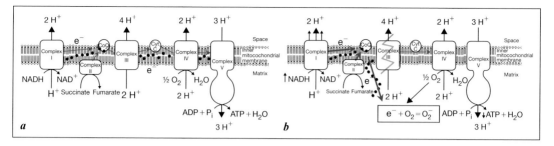

Fig. 1. *a* Coupled electron transport and oxidative phosphorylation. *b* Uncoupled electron transport and oxidative stress.

of 'antioxidant balance' has to do with how extensively fed the cell or organism is at any moment. Limitations on the definition of oxidative stress require that mechanisms thought to contribute to increased oxidative stress in vivo should be investigated utilizing a series of detailed biochemical assays. In vivo, during increased oxidative stress states, the major sources of excess oxidant production derive either from the mitochondria, or from mixed-functional intracellular oxidases such as the NADPH oxidase or myeloperoxidase. The mitochondrial cytochrome oxidase enzyme complex accounts for the majority of the oxygen humans metabolize. The cytochrome oxidase enzyme complex transfers four electrons to oxygen in a coordinated reaction that produces two molecules of water as a byproduct. The enzyme complex contains four redox centers, each of which stores a single electron. The simultaneous reduction of the four redox centers results in the transfer of results in no detectable reactive oxygen intermediates, and thereby limits the production of reactive oxygen species (fig. 1a). Nevertheless, mitochondrial oxygen can leak through the electron transport chain, resulting in the formation of reactive oxygen intermediates and free radicals, which can then diffuse out of the mitochondria and be a source of oxidant stress (fig. 1b) [2, 3].

An additional important in-vivo source of excess oxidants occurs through the action of the enzyme complex, nicotinamide adenine dinucleotide phosphate (NADPH) oxidase. NADPH oxidase generates reactive oxygen intermediates within the endothelium and in phagocytic cells [4, 5]. The reactive oxygen intermediate superoxide anion produced by NADPH oxidase reacts extremely rapidly with nitric oxide, resulting in the loss of nitric oxide activity. During an inflammatory response, phagocytes deliberately use high levels of oxygen and the generation of reactive oxygen intermediates for a host defense against pathogens via the NADPH respiratory burst. Phagocytes contain other enzymes (including superoxide dismutase, nitric oxide synthase, and myeloperoxidase), which also contribute to the production of hydrogen peroxide, nitric oxide, peroxynitrite and hypochlorous acid, respectively [6, 7]. A novel additional oxidative pathway within phagocytes has been described, whereby nitrite is converted to nitryl chloride and nitrogen dioxide via the myeloperoxidase enzyme or via hypochlorous acid [8]. Ozone derived from singlet oxygen in inflammatory cells may also be a byproduct of oxidative stress that contributes to atherosclerosis [9].

Stimulated leukocytes generate the reactive oxygen intermediate superoxide and its dismutation product hydrogen peroxide and secrete the heme enzyme MPO. MPO is one of the most abundant proteins in leukocytes, constituting approximately 5% of neutrophil protein and 1% of monocyte protein. MPO has the unique property of converting chloride in the presence of hydrogen peroxide to hypochlorous acid. MPO can also directly modulate vascular inflammatory responses by functioning as a vascular nitric oxide oxidase, thereby regulating nitric oxide availability. Because MPO is released during acute inflammation, MPO-catalyzed oxidative injury and endothelial nitric oxide regulation can provide a direct mechanistic linkage between inflammation, oxidative stress, and endothelial dysfunction.

Oxidative Stress in the Pathogenesis of Atherosclerosis

Oxidative stress and inflammation contribute to the pathogenesis of atherosclerosis [10]. Hypercholesterolemia, diabetes mellitus, tobacco use, and uremia are also commonly associated with increased oxidative stress, reduced vascular availability of nitric oxide, and inflammation and are important independent risk factors for cardiovascular disease. Steinberg first suggested that oxidative modification of low-density lipoproteins (LDL) greatly increases atherogenecity. Oxidatively modified LDL is taken up by a family of scavenger receptors such as SR-A1, thereby initiating conversion into foam cells, an early step in the development of atherosclerosis. Reactive oxygen species can directly promote LDL oxidation, stimulate vascular smooth muscle cell proliferation and migration, and potentiate the production of proinflammatory cytokines. Reactive oxygen species can also activate several matrix metalloproteinases, thereby contributing to atherosclerotic plaque instability and rupture, and precipitating acute coronary syndromes.

Reactive oxygen species increase the production of proinflammatory cytokines such as interleukin-6 and acute-phase proteins such as C-reactive protein (CRP) through activation of the transcription nuclear factor-κB (NF-κB). NF-κB is a ubiquitous rapid-response transcription factor involved in inflammatory reactions through its action on expression of cytokines, chemokines, and cell-adhesion molecules and has been identified in situ in human atherosclerotic plaques. CRP itself can potently increase the expression of NF-κB, thereby constituting a positive feedback loop that contributes to ongoing proatherosclerotic risk. CRP itself may directly contribute to the atherosclerotic process by leukocyte activation, by induction of endothelial dysfunction, and by attenuating endothelial progenitor cell survival, differentiation, and function. NF-κB activation is controlled by the redox status of the cell, and intracellular reactive oxygen species may be common to all of the signaling pathways that lead to activation of NF-κB.

Prevalence of Oxidative Stress in Kidney Disease

Biomarkers of oxidative stress in kidney disease have been best studied in ESRD patients receiving dialysis therapy. LDL from uremic patients has greater susceptibility to in vitro copper-induced lipid peroxidation than plasma LDL isolated from healthy subjects. Numerous studies have shown that biomarkers of oxidative stress are altered in uremic patients. These include alterations in concentration of lipid peroxidation products, reactive aldehydes, and oxidized thiols all of which are postulated play in the atherosclerotic process. In particular, the formation of α,β-unsaturated aldehydes are important as the formation of two sites of reactivity frequently leads to the formation of cyclic adducts or crosslinks with other macromolecules. α,β-Unsaturated aldehydes are also capable of reacting with protein nucleophiles to form advanced glycation end products. Many reactive aldehyde compounds, including glyoxal, methylglyoxal, malondialdehyde, acrolein, and hydroxynonenal, are detectable at higher concentrations in uremia compared to healthy individuals.

Thiol groups are important antioxidants. Intracellular thiols, including glutathione and thioredoxin, which are found in millimolar concentrations, are crucial for maintaining the highly reduced environment within the cell. Extracellular thiols also constitute an important component of antioxidant defense. The plasma protein-reduced thiols (located primarily on albumin) are depleted in hemodialysis patients and are thus not able to participate in antioxidant defense, serving as redox buffers. In addition, there are diminished plasma glutathione levels and a profound decrease in glutathione peroxidase function in hemodialysis patients. Oxidized thiols that include homocysteine and cysteine accumulate in uremia and may have proatherogenic effects. In uremic patients, lipid peroxidation can also contribute to atherosclerosis through the oxidation of LDL. The detection of free and esterified plasma F_2-isoprostanes has been used to demonstrate an increase in lipid peroxidation in uremic individuals. In addition, another family of highly reactive electrophiles can be generated by the free radical-induced lipid oxidation of arachidonic acid with the production of isolevuglandins. Isolevuglandin adducts to plasma proteins are elevated in ESRD patients compared with healthy individuals. Levels of breath ethane, which results from the scission of lipid hydroperoxides, are also higher in hemodialysis patients than in healthy individuals.

Oxidative Stress and Inflammation Are Linked in Uremic Patients through Myeloperoxidase

A substantial body of evidence has accumulated to suggest that MPO is involved in inflammation and oxidative stress in patients with kidney disease. Catalytically active MPO can be released during the hemodialysis procedure, and 3-chlorotyrosine, an oxidative stress biomarker highly specific for MPO-catalyzed oxidation through hypochlorous acid, has been demonstrated in the plasma proteins of dialysis patients but not in that of healthy subjects. Uremic plasma containing advance oxidation protein products can induce MPO-dependent oxidation activity ex vivo in leukocytes. A recent study also suggests that thiocyanate is yet another substrate for MPO. Oxidation of thiocyanate results in the formation of cyanate, which can then covalently modify protein and lipoprotein lysine residues to form homocitrulline. The resulting ε-carbamyllysine is frequently referred to as carbamylated protein, which can also occur after dissociation of cyanate from urea. Carbamylated LDL is potently atherogenic. MPO- catalyzed protein carbamylation may link inflammation, smoking, kidney disease, and cardiovascular disease [11, 12]. These data strongly suggest that MPO may be a critical link between acute-phase inflammation, oxidative stress, and atherosclerosis in the uremic patient population.

References

1   Jones DP: Redefining oxidative stress. Antioxid Redox Signal 2006;8:1865–1879.
2   Marnett LJ, Riggins JN, West JD: Endogenous generation of reactive oxidants and electrophiles and their reactions with DNA and protein. J Clin Invest 2003;111:583–593.
3   Papa S, Skulachev VP: Reactive oxygen species, mitochondria, apoptosis, and aging. Mol Cell Biochem 1997;174:305–319.
4   Babior BM: The NADPH oxidase of endothelial cells. IUBMB Life 2000;50:267–269.
5   Babior BM: The respiratory burst oxidase. Adv Enzymol Relat Areas Mol Biol 1992;65:49–95.
6   Winterbourn CC, Vissers MC, Kettle AJ: Myeloperoxidase. Curr Opin Hematol 2000;7:53–58.
7   Koppenol WH, Moreno JJ, Pryor WA, Ischiropoulos H, Beckman JS: Peroxynitrite, a cloaked oxidant formed by nitric oxide and superoxide. Chem Res Toxicol 1992;5:834–842.
8   Eiserich JP, Hristova M, Cross CE, Jones AD, Freeman BA, Halliwell B, van der Vliet A: Formation of nitric oxide-derived inflammatory oxidants by myeloperoxidase in neutrophils. Nature 1998;391:393–397.
9   Wentworth P Jr, Nieva J, Takeuchi C, Galve R, Wentworth AD, Dilley RB, DeLaria GA, Saven A, Babior BM, Janda KD, Eschenmoser A, Lerner RA: Evidence for ozone formation in human atherosclerotic arteries. Science 2003;302:1053–1056.

10 Libby P: Inflammation in atherosclerosis. Nature 2002;420:868–874.
11 Rader DJ, Ischiropoulos H: 'Multipurpose oxidase' in atherogenesis. Nat Med 2007;13:1146–1147.
12 Wang Z, Nicholls SJ, Rodriguez ER, Kummu O, Horkko S, Barnard J, Reynolds WF, Topol EJ, DiDonato JA, Hazen SL: Protein carbamylation links inflammation, smoking, uremia and athero-genesis. Nat Med 2007;13:1176–1184.

Dr. Jonathan Himmelfarb
Department of Medicine, Division of Nephrology and Renal Transplantation
Maine Medical Center, 22 Bramhall Street
Portland, Maine 04102 (USA)
Tel. +1 207 662 2417, Fax +1 207 662 6306, E-Mail himmej@mmc.org

Ronco C, Cruz DN (eds): Hemodialysis – From Basic Research to Clinical Trials.
Contrib Nephrol. Basel, Karger, 2008, vol 161, pp 138–144

....

Determinants of Insulin Resistance and Its Effects on Protein Metabolism in Patients with Advanced Chronic Kidney Disease

Edward D. Siew, T. Alp Ikizler

Vanderbilt University Medical Center, Department of Medicine,
Division of Nephrology, Nashville, Tenn., USA

Abstract

Insulin resistance (IR) and its associated metabolic derangements are known complications of advanced chronic kidney disease (CKD). The etiology of IR in CKD is multifactorial with likely contributions from vitamin D deficiency, obesity, metabolic acidosis, inflammation, and accumulation of 'uremic toxins' leading to acquired defects in the insulin-receptor signaling pathway. An important consequence in end-stage renal disease (ESRD) is its role in the pathogenesis of uremic protein energy wasting, a commonly observed state of metabolic derangement characterized by loss of somatic and visceral protein stores not entirely accounted for by inadequate nutrient intake. In the general population, IR has been associated with accelerated protein catabolism. Among ESRD patients, enhanced muscle protein breakdown has been observed in patients with type 2 diabetes mellitus (DM) compared to ESRD patients without DM. In the absence of DM or severe obesity, IR is detectable in dialysis patients and strongly associated with increased muscle protein breakdown, even after controlling for inflammation. This process appears to be mediated by the ubiquitin-proteasome pathway. Given the high prevalence of protein energy wasting in ESRD and its unequivocal association with adverse clinical outcomes, IR may represent an important modifiable target for intervention in the ESRD population.

Despite recent advances in the care of chronic dialysis patients, mortality rates remain unacceptably high with life expectancy 20–25 years less than in age-, sex- and race-matched controls from the US population over the age of 45 [1]. Moreover, the healthcare cost of treating the US end-stage renal disease

(ESRD) program exceeds 17 billion US dollars annually [1]. One of the most potent predictors of poor outcome in this population is the presence of uremic protein energy wasting, a unique metabolic abnormality present in 20–25% of dialysis patients characterized by an insidious loss of somatic protein stores (lean body mass), and to a lesser extent, visceral protein stores (reflected by serum albumin and prealbumin). Although the mechanisms behind this syndrome are complex and poorly understood, it is clear that factors beyond simple nutritional intake are responsible. Insulin resistance (IR) has become an increasingly recognized complication of chronic kidney disease (CKD) with emerging evidence critically implicating it in the pathogenesis of both uremic wasting and cardiovascular disease progression.

Insulin Resistance Is Associated with Kidney Disease

Derangement of insulin action in the setting of CKD has been noted for decades [2]. Compensatory increases in renal tubular uptake and excretion of insulin in the setting of diminished glomerular filtration rate were specifically reported in 1970 [3]. Seminal observations by DeFronzo et al. [4] of uremic IR in chronic hemodialysis (CHD) patients were characterized using euglycemic insulin clamp techniques. These investigators demonstrated alterations in glucose metabolism in the face of hyperinsulinemia and diminished tissue sensitivity to insulin partially correctable by maintenance hemodialysis. The primary site of this altered insulin sensitivity appears to be a post-receptor defect altering primarily skeletal muscle (peripheral) rather than hepatic (central) glucose uptake. The precise mechanism for IR in CKD remains to be elucidated. However, recent in vitro and animal studies implicate impaired insulin signaling via phosphatidylinositol 3-kinase (PI$_3$-kinase) as the most likely cause of IR and associated glucose intolerance in advanced CKD [5, 6].

Observational data from large population-based cohorts have also established a link between IR and earlier CKD. A cross-sectional study involving patients from the Third National Health and Nutrition Examination Survey (NHANES III) found the odds of having kidney disease increased with the number of metabolic syndrome components accrued. Prospective data from the Atherosclerosis Risk in Communities (ARIC) cohort examined by Kurella et al. established the metabolic syndrome as an independent risk factor for CKD in non-diabetic adults. Their data confirmed a stepwise increase in risk for the development of CKD with the number of metabolic syndrome criteria met, even after controlling for the development of diabetes and hypertension.

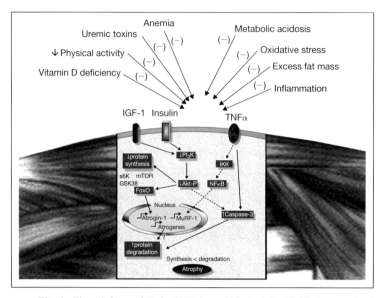

Fig. 1. The etiology of IR in CKD is multifactorial with likely contributions from vitamin D deficiency, obesity, metabolic acidosis, inflammation, and accumulation of 'uremic toxins' leading to acquired defects in the insulin-receptor signaling pathway. [Adapted from Lecyer SH, et al. J Am Soc Nephrol 2006;17:1807–1819].

Factors Affecting Insulin Resistance in CKD

Insulin-mediated glucose metabolism in skeletal muscle is predicated on normal downstream function of the insulin-receptor substrate PI_3-K-Akt pathway which is subject to influence from factors associated with the uremic milieu including inflammation, acidosis, vitamin D status, anemia, and accumulation of 'uremic toxins' (fig. 1).

Like other chronic diseases characterized by cachexia and IR, patients with CKD demonstrate low-grade systemic inflammation marked by elevated levels of pro-inflammatory cytokines such as C-reactive protein, tumor necrosis factor-α, and interleukin-1β. Factors responsible for the accumulation of these cytokines include decreased renal clearance, activation of complement in response to certain dialytic factors such as hemodialysis membrane, endotoxin transfer, peritoneal dialysate bio-incompatibility and vascular access (grafts, catheters), and the presence of co-morbidities such as chronic infections (periodontal, peritonitis), diabetes mellitus (DM), atherosclerosis and congestive heart failure [7]. A recent study demonstrated that tumor necrosis factor-α

infusion in healthy humans induces IR by direct suppression of glucose uptake and metabolism in skeletal muscle. The mechanism appears to be related to impaired phosphorylation of Akt substrate 160 leading to dysfunction of GLUT4 translocation and glucose uptake.

Intriguing data have begun to emerge linking the known vitamin D deficiency observed with CKD and IR. A recent large cross-sectional analysis of 14,679 subjects, also from NHANES III, revealed that serum 25-hydroxyvitamin D levels and loss of renal function have an independent and inverse relationship with IR as measured by homeostatis model assessment (HOMA), an established surrogate for IR (HOMA-IR). Active vitamin D compounds are distinguished by their ability to bind with high affinity to vitamin D receptors not only in the parathyroid glands, but in cells throughout the body indicating a role for significant systemic effects. One important non-classical function of 1,25-dihydroxyvitamin D_3 is a modulator of insulin release from pancreatic islets [8]. Intravenous vitamin D_3 corrects glucose intolerance and stimulates insulin secretion in response to a glucose challenge in 1,25 $(OH)_2D_3$-deficient animals [9]. In line with these in vitro and in vivo animal data, Mak [8] showed that intravenous vitamin D_3 administration corrected glucose intolerance, IR, hypoinsulinemia as well as hypertriglyceridemia in 8 relatively young CHD patients in the absence of PTH suppression. The precise mechanisms by which these effects are mediated remain unclear.

Metabolic acidosis is a common complication of advanced uremia and may represent yet another factor associated with increased IR. Correction of this acidosis with bicarbonate supplementation has been demonstrated to improve IR in animal models of uremia as well as in humans. Mak [8] demonstrated that 2 weeks of oral bicarbonate replacement significantly improved IR in 8 CHD patients as measured by hyperinsulinemic euglycemic clamp. The mechanism remains unclear but may be mediated through upregulation of vitamin D 1,25$(OH)_2D_3$ levels potentially via enhanced renal 1α-hydroxylase activity.

As in the general population, increased fat mass appears to also be an important risk factor for IR in CKD. Our laboratory recently reported that body mass index, specifically fat mass, was the principle determinant of IR as measured by HOMA-IR in non-obese, non-diabetic stage III–IV CKD patients after adjustment for potential confounders including glomerular filtration rate. Similarly in a limited analysis of ESRD, we demonstrated that body mass index was correlated with HOMA-IR scores in a cohort of 18 non-diabetic CHD patients without severe obesity.

Other factors which have been implicated in the pathogenesis of increased IR include anemia, physical inactivity, and numerous potential uremic toxins, particularly of the middle molecule variety.

The Role of Insulin in Protein Turnover

Multiple in vitro and in vivo studies have demonstrated the anabolic effects of insulin extend beyond simple carbohydrate metabolism. The earliest observations of the insulinopenic condition in humans (i.e. uncontrolled type 1 DM) were hallmarked by negative nitrogen balance, lean tissue atrophy, and hyperaminoacidemia easily reversed through the provision of insulin. Investigations using tracer kinetic models and insulin clamp techniques in healthy individuals have detailed that it remains the blunting of proteolysis rather than enhanced protein synthesis that belies the net protein anabolic effect of insulin in the fasting state. The lack of effect on protein synthesis is probably due to the insulin-mediated decrease in amino acid release into the bloodstream. Biolo et al. [10] examined protein metabolism in insulin-dependent DM patients and healthy subjects and found no differences in protein turnover in the fasting or fed state between the two groups. However, several other studies indicated that muscle protein synthesis is sensitive to both insulin and concomitant increase in amino acid concentrations induced by intravenous infusion [11].

The underlying proteolytic mechanism, elegantly demonstrated by Mitch and colleagues [12] in an animal model of insulin deficiency, appears to involve a decrease in the activity of PI_3K leading to enhanced activation of the ubiquitin-proteasome pathway. Specifically, a decrease in PI_3K activity is expected to lower the activity of Akt and a low phosphorylated Akt activity has been shown to stimulate the expression of specific E3 ubiquitin-conjugating enzymes, atrogin-1/MAFbx and MuRF1, in muscle. They also reported that a decrease in muscle PI_3K activity will activate Bax leading to stimulation of caspase-3 activity and increased protein degradation [13].

Insulin Resistance and Protein Turnover

Experimental observations have been made suggesting that enhanced protein catabolism not only applies to insulin-deficient states, but also to insulin resistant ones. In patients with CKD, we have reported that patients with ESRD secondary to DM have a higher incidence of uremic protein energy wasting as compared with CHD patients who are not diabetic. Specifically, CHD patients with type 2 DM had significantly increased (83%) skeletal muscle protein breakdown compared with their non-diabetic counterparts. There was no significant difference in muscle protein synthesis between groups, resulting in significantly negative net protein balance in the muscle compartment of the DM group. A similar trend was observed in whole-body protein synthesis and breakdown. We subsequently examined whether this unfavorable metabolic state could lead to accelerated loss of lean body mass over a period of 12 months [14, 15]. Our results showed that chronic dialysis patients with DM had significantly accelerated loss of LBM compared to non-diabetic chronic dialysis patients during the first year of maintenance dialysis (3.4 ± 0.6 kg vs. 1.1 ± 0.2 kg, $p < 0.05$). Multivariate linear regression analysis revealed that the presence of DM was the strongest predictor of LBM loss independently of several clinically relevant variables such as age, gender, serum albumin, presence of malnutrition, presence of inflammation, and renal replacement therapy modality.

These observations led us to hypothesize that the degree of IR would significantly contribute towards the enhanced protein catabolism. We examined the relationship between HOMA-IR and whole-body and skeletal muscle protein turnover in 18 non-diabetic CHD patients (median [IQR] HOMA for the group 1.6 [1.4, 3.9]). Using simple linear regression, a positive correlation was observed between HOMA and skeletal muscle protein synthesis ($R^2 = 0.28$; $p = 0.024$), and breakdown ($R^2 = 0.49$; $p = 0.001$). An inverse association between net skeletal muscle protein balance and HOMA was also observed that approached significance ($R^2 = 0.20$; $p = 0.066$). After adjustment for C-reactive protein, only the relationship between HOMA score and skeletal muscle protein breakdown remained significant ($R^2 = 0.49$; $p = 0.006$). The results demonstrated that even in the absence of overt glucose intolerance or severe obesity, IR is evident in the dialysis population, is associated with enhanced skeletal muscle protein breakdown, and represents a novel target for intervention in uremic wasting.

References

1   US Renal Data System: Excerpts from the USRDS 2001 Annual Data Report. Am J Kidney Dis 2001;38:S1–S248.
2   Zubrod CG, Eversole SL, Dana GW: Amelioration of diabetes and striking rarity of acidosis in patients with Kimmelstiel-Wilson lesions. N Engl J Med 1951;245:518–528.
3   Rabkin R, Simon NM, Steiner S, Colwell JA: Effect of renal disease on renal uptake and excretion of insulin in man. N Engl J Med 1970;282:182–187.
4   DeFronzo RA, Smith D, Alvestrand A: Insulin action in uremia. Kidney Int Suppl 1983;16: S102–S114.
5   Price SR, Du JD, Bailey JL, Mitch WE: Molecular mechanisms regulating protein turnover in muscle. Am J Kidney Dis 2001;37:S112–S114.
6   Lee SW, Dai G, Hu Z, Wang X, et al: Regulation of muscle protein degradation: coordinated control of apoptotic and ubiquitin-proteasome systems by phosphatidylinositol 3-kinase. J Am Soc Nephrol 2004;15:1537–1545.
7   Bergstrom J, Lindholm B, Lacson E Jr, Owen W Jr, et al: What are the causes and consequences of the chronic inflammatory state in chronic dialysis patients? Semin Dial 2000;13:163–175.
8   Mak RH: 1,25-Dihydroxyvitamin D_3 corrects insulin and lipid abnormalities in uremia. Kidney Int 1998;53:1353–1357.

9   Cade C, Norman AW: Vitamin D_3 improves impaired glucose tolerance and insulin secretion in the vitamin D-deficient rat in vivo. Endocrinology 1986;119:84–90.
10 Biolo G, Inchiostro S, Tiengo A, Tessari P: Regulation of postprandial whole-body proteolysis in insulin-deprived IDDM. Diabetes 1995;44:203–209.
11 Bohe J, Rennie MJ: Muscle protein metabolism during hemodialysis. J Ren Nutr 2006;16:3–16.
12 Lee SW, Dai G, Hu Z, Wang X, et al: Regulation of muscle protein degradation: coordinated control of apoptotic and ubiquitin-proteasome systems by phosphatidylinositol 3-kinase. J Am Soc Nephrol 2004;15:1537–1545.
13 Du J, Wang X, Miereles C, Bailey JL, et al: Activation of caspase-3 is an initial step triggering accelerated muscle proteolysis in catabolic conditions. J Clin Invest 2004;113:115–123.
14 Pupim LB, Flakoll PJ, Majchrzak KM, Aftab Guy DL, et al: Increased muscle protein breakdown in chronic hemodialysis patients with type 2 diabetes mellitus. Kidney Int 2005;68:1857–1865.
15 Pupim LB, Heimburger O, Qureshi AR, Ikizler TA, et al: Accelerated lean body mass loss in incident chronic dialysis patients with diabetes mellitus. Kidney Int 2005;68:2368–2374.

T. Alp Ikizler, MD
Vanderbilt University Medical Center
1161 21st Ave. S. & Garland, Division of Nephrology, S-3223 MCN
Nashville, TN 37232-2372 (USA)
Tel. +1 615 343 6104, Fax +1 615 343 7156, E-Mail alp.ikizler@vanderbilt.edu

Ronco C, Cruz DN (eds): Hemodialysis – From Basic Research to Clinical Trials.
Contrib Nephrol. Basel, Karger, 2008, vol 161, pp 145–153

· ·

What Is Important in Dialysis? The Frequency of Treatment Sessions

Robert M. Lindsay

The University of Western Ontario and London Health Sciences Centre,
London, Ont., Canada

Abstract

Outcomes from conventional thrice-weekly hemodialysis (CHD) are disappointing for a lifesaving therapy. The results of the HEMO Study show that the recommended minimum dose (Kt/V) for adequacy is also the optimum attainable with CHD. Interest is therefore turning to alternative therapies exploring the effects of increased frequency and time of hemodialysis treatment. This paper is mainly concerned with frequency. The rationale for daily hemodialysis is discussed and a short history of its use given. The results of studies of more frequent hemodialysis indicate the potential for health and quality of life improvement in a number of areas. Blood pressure control is improved and this appears to be associated with improvement in left ventricular geometry and mass. At face value the studies suggest that increased frequency (and/or time) improve intermediate outcomes that may be associated with survival. The need for well-designed, randomized prospective trials is indicated and these are underway. An international registry has also been established. Results from these initiatives will tell whether the improvement potential is realized.

Copyright © 2008 S. Karger AG, Basel

The current paradigm of providing thrice-weekly dialysis to patients with end-stage renal failure has been followed worldwide for over 30 years. In North America, treatment times tend to be within 3–4 h but they are often longer in Europe. The hemodialysis (HD) treatment is so conducted to remove all excess fluid that is accumulated within the interdialytic period and to deliver a targeted Kt/V_{urea}. It is certainly a paradigm not based on optimizing physiology. At best, it can be seen as being an unhappy compromise between what we have come to know about the adequacy of therapy, the acceptance of the therapy by patient and provider alike, and finally, the economics of the therapy. It is often felt that these three factors pull in different directions. A decrease in funding, for example, being translated into a reduction in treatment time and the provision of an inferior treatment with potentially poor outcomes including patient quality of life. The treatment outcomes are poor at best, with annual mortality rates of around 20% in countries that do not select and provide treatment for all that need it. In 2002 the results of the HEMO Study were reported [1]. This study showed that increasing Kt/V_{urea} beyond the minimum recommended by NKF-K/DOQI [2] does not improve outcomes with thrice-weekly HD as practiced in the USA today. In essence, the HEMO Study provided objective evidence that the established minimum dose is also the optimum.

Why then does more dialysis not help? If uremia is a toxic state caused by the accumulation of dialyzable solutes, then its severity should correlate with toxin level and lowering this level by dialysis should progressively improve health. However, clearance does not correlate linearly with solute levels (for example, creatinine is a hyperbolic function of native kidney clearance) and presumably concentrations of toxin do not necessarily correlate linearly with a toxic effect, e.g. death. It is more likely that there will be a sigmoidal survival curve where there exists a threshold toxic level above which some (animals) begin to die and a threshold lethal level above which all die. Toxin removal presumably inverts this sigmoidal curve and when applied to the results of the HEMO study, this likely implies that the dose/mortality curve has reached a plateau so there is no further benefit in increasing the dose. If one examines the results of the National Cooperative Dialysis Study (NCDS) one might have predicted that HEMO was not going to show benefit. The mechanistic analysis by Gotch and Sargent [2] showed a discontinuous downward step in the relative probability of failure; patients dialyzed with a Kt/V <0.9 had almost a fivefold increment in the probability of failure than patients dialyzed with Kt/V >0.9 and that there was no difference between a Kt/V of 0.09 and 1.5. It is for this reason that nephrologists are now exploring the barriers of time and frequency to ascertain whether better outcomes may be obtained. This article is mainly concerned with frequency.

Rationale for Daily Hemodialysis

The rationale for daily HD appears straightforward. If one were comparing three times 4-hour dialysis sessions with six times 2-hour sessions, one could be persuaded that more urea (and other small molecules) were removed per week with the more frequent therapy. Because of the bi-exponential fall in urea during treatment with a dialyzer of modest efficiency, approximately 60% of the urea is removed during the first 2 h of the 4-hour dialysis. Thus, limiting the session to 2 h decreases the removal capacity by approximately 40% per treatment.

However, with 6 days of therapy, there would be a weekly increment of 20%. Higher gains are likely with high efficiency dialyzers. The favorable effect is obviously blunted by reduction in the pre-dialysis blood levels and a new steady state will be realized. Nevertheless, the time average concentrations of solutes become reduced, as are their time average deviations, thereby improving the 'unphysiology' of dialysis [3]. Several dialysis dose measurements have been designed to allow comparison of different dialysis regimens. The most popular is the standard weekly Kt/V (Std Kt/V) introduced by Gotch [4]. Dialysis regimens with the same mid-week pre-dialysis urea (or steady state with CAPD) have the same Std Kt/V and perhaps (speculative) provide the same clinical outcomes. A Std Kt/V of 2 corresponds to the minimum NKF-K/DOQI recommended level of adequacy of Kt/V of 2 for CAPD and single pool Kt/V (sp Kt/V) of 1.2 for thrice-weekly HD. Thus, with more frequent dialysis it is possible to have a Std Kt/V of 2 with shorter treatments and lower per treatment single pool or equilibrated Kt/V (e Kt/V).

The History of Daily Hemodialysis

A review of the history is given elsewhere with detailed references [5]. The first report on daily dialysis in patients with chronic renal failure was from DePalma in Los Angeles. Patients who had problems with dialysis disequilibrium, hypertension, and severe intradialytic hypotensive episodes were treated. With daily dialysis, their symptoms improved and it was noted that appetite increased and weight gained. Blood pressure came under control both during and between dialyses. Unfortunately, equipment proved unreliable, cost of treatment became unsupportable and the program was abandoned. Schneider's group in Brooklyn subsequently treated 10 patients with five 2-hour dialyses weekly for periods ranging from 2 months to over 7 years. It was noted that these patients had fewer complications and they required neither transfusions nor hospitalizations. Again this program was discontinued because of inadequate reimbursement. In 1979, Bonomoni (Bologna, Italy) reported similar benefits in patients treated for 3–5 h five times per week. In 1982, Buonocristiani and colleagues started a daily HD program in Perugia selecting patients with medical and social indications. Despite low values of Kt/V, these patients showed marked improvements in well-being, muscle strength, hematocrit, blood pressure control, cardiovascular stability and quality of life. More recently, long nightly home HD was stimulated by the work of Uldall, continued by Pierratos and co-workers in Toronto. This program, with 15 years of experiences, has reported extensively on the benefits, issues and problems associated with this treatment. Ting in California treated patients with serious medical problems and dialysis intolerance by doing in-center short hours daily HD and showed marked improvement of the medical conditions, tolerance of dialysis and quality of life. Lockridge in Virginia (providing home nocturnal HD) and the Northwest Kidney Centers in Seattle (doing home short hours daily HD) have added to the experience. Finally, our own group in London, Ontario, has a large program using more frequent HD and has published the first and very extensive report on a prospective cohort-matched trial comparing short daily and long nightly HD with conventional three times weekly treatment [6].

In Europe a number of physicians outside Italy have also developed programs providing more frequent HD. These include Traeger and Galland in France and Koistra and Vos in the Netherlands. There are now numerous reports in the world literature on all aspects of more frequent (and/or longer) hemodialyses. The numbers of programs and of patients treated are increasing slowly but steadily.

Results of More Frequent Hemodialysis: The London Study

The details and results of the London Study have been reported [6]. The study was a prospective observational study whereby 11 patients on short hours daily and 12 patients on long hours nocturnal HD therapy were followed for up to 18 months. Control data were obtained from these patients during their last week on conventional HD therapy (thrice weekly) before starting the quotidian therapy as well as from control patients treated with conventional thrice-weekly HD throughout the study period. The outcomes evaluated in the study are shown in table 1. The results of the study show much better blood pressure control and maintenance of hemoglobin in spite of increased dialytic blood losses without the necessity for increased erythropoietin. With nocturnal but not short hours daily dialysis, perfect control of phosphate and calcium/phosphorus product was possible without the need for phosphate binders. Nutritional parameters appear to improve with at least the short hours daily HD group and improvement in quality of life was recorded using a number of established assessment tools. In particular, it was noted that levels of fatigue declined significantly in both the short hours daily and the nocturnal HD groups while they remained unchanged in the controls. Furthermore, the average amount of time taken to recover from an individual dialysis session decreased dramatically and significantly for both the short hours daily and nocturnal patients (to as low as 2 min). Control patients showed virtually no change in this parameter with mean time to dialysis recovery ranging from 375 to 460 min throughout the study (fig. 1). The data from this study have been used to validate the 'minutes to recovery' as an assessment tool for use in HD-related research [7].

Table 1. Outcomes evaluated in the London Daily/Nocturnal Hemodialysis Study [reprinted with permission]

Parameters	Study data collected
Volume control	Blood pressure, mean arterial pressure, antihypertensive therapy, interdialytic weight gain, homocysteine
Anemia management	Hemoglobin, hematocrit, serum ferritin, transferrin saturation, EPO dose, blood loss, oral/IV iron
Calcium/phosphorus control	Pre- and post-dialysis calcium and phosphorus, bone alkaline phosphatase, Ca×P product, iPTH
Nutrition	Albumin, pre-albumin, nPNA, weight, body mass index, anthropometrics, cholesterol, triglycerides, HDL, LDL
Quality of life	Dialysis symptomatology, uremic symptomatology, psychosocial stress, SF-36, Health Utilities Index, time trade-off
Adequacy	Urea, percent reduction urea,, nPNA Kt/V, sp Kt/V, Std Kt/V, e Kt/V, efficiency of dose delivery
Economics	Total operating costs, set-up costs, total operating costs/QALY
Nursing issues	Training time, vascular access parameters (survival, complications, cannulation techniques)
Monitoring and alarms	Number and changes in number of alarms, causes of alarms, analysis of monitoring experience and costs
Equipment and water treatment considerations	Assessment of home environment, installation of HD equipment, analysis of water treatment systems

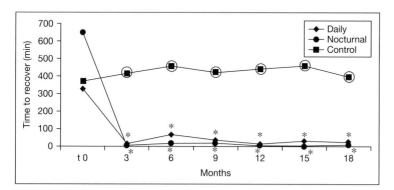

Fig. 1. Time to recover (min) shown at time zero (t_0) and at 3 monthly intervals for the daily/nocturnal and control HD patients. Statistical significance shown both within group (* = different from baseline at $p < 0.05$)) and between groups (○ = between group difference at $p \leq 0.05$) [reprinted with permission].

Table 2. HD prescription received [reprinted with permission]

	Daily HD	Nocturnal HD	Conventional HD
Time, min	126 ± 16[†]	430 ± 42[†]	226 ± 26[†]
K_d, ml/min	305 ± 10[†]	150 ± 18*,[†]	263 ± 15*
Q_d, ml/min	800 ± 0[†]	300 ± 0[†]	500 ± 0[†]
Q_b, ml/min	465 ± 35[†]	234 ± 44*,[†]	417 ± 55*
Frequency, days/week	5.8 ± 0.6[†]	5.6 ± 0.5*	3 ± 0*,[†]

Values are given ± SD. K_d = Dialyzer clearance; Q_d = dialyzer flow rate; Q_b = blood flow rate.
*and [†]denote that $p < 0.05$ between groups.

Concerning urea kinetic data, the HD prescriptions used are shown in table 2 and a summary of the delivered HD doses in table 3. The ideal method of measuring adequacy in daily/nocturnal HD regimens has not been established. Theoretically, Std Kt/V is the best method to compare regimens of differing frequency because it was developed for this purpose [4]. However, validation of Std Kt/V against direct dialysate quantification is required to determine whether Std Kt/V accurately quantifies clearances delivered with quotidian HD regimens.

Finally, the economic analysis carried out demonstrated a decrease of total annualized cost per quality adjusted life year for both the daily and nocturnal HD groups reflecting both improved quality of life and reduced costs for these patients. This was in spite of a doubling of per treatment costs.

Other Studies

There are now many reports in the literature from other groups all over the world. Generally they have similar results to those of the London Study. Uniformly the studies report on reduction in blood pressure with the use of fewer antihypertensive agents. This improvement in blood pressure is associated with an improvement in left ventricular geometry and mass [8] and improvement in symptoms and left ventricular ejection fraction in patients who have had congestive heart failure [9].

At face value, the studies would suggest that both short hours daily and nightly HD regimens improve intermediate outcomes that may be associated with survival. It must be recognized that to date all of the studies are small and underpowered to detect mortality or morbidity. Two systematic reviews have been carried out. One relating to nocturnal HD carried out by the Calgary group

Table 3. Summary of delivered HD dose

	Conventional HD		Daily HD		Nocturnal HD	
	t_0	t_1	t_0	t_1	t_0	t_1
Single session PRU	73.7 ± 1.5	73.1 ± 0.83*	73.8 ± 2.1	57.0 ± 2.1*	74.7 ± 1.5	67.3 ± 1.9*
Single session sp Kt/V	1.84 ± 0.11	1.73 ± 0.04*	1.57 ± 0.14	0.93 ± 0.04*,†	1.73 ± 0.11	1.64 ± 0.05†
Single session e Kt/V	1.59 ± 0.09	1.42 ± 0.06§	1.36 ± 0.12	0.82 ± 0.04§,‡	1.51 ± 0.10	1.45 ± 0.08‡
Weekly sp Kt/V	5.51 ± 0.33	5.18 ± 0.12*,‡	4.70 ± 0.42	5.55 ± 0.23*	5.18 ± 0.34	9.08 ± 0.32‡
Weekly e Kt/V	4.78 ± 0.28	4.26 ± 0.17§	4.07 ± 0.35	4.79 ± 0.51‡	4.52 ± 0.30	8.11 ± 0.46§,‡
Weekly Std Kt/V	2.36 ± 0.05	2.35 ± 0.04*,‡	2.37 ± 0.08	3.01 ± 0.27*,~	2.42 ± 0.06	4.65 ± 0.28†,~

Data are presented as mean ± SE. t_0 = Baseline (all patients on conventional HD); t_1 = longitudinal mean over 1–18 months' follow-up for PRU and sp Kt/V values; t_1 = cross-sectional mean at 10-month follow-up for e Kt/V and Std Kt/V values; PRU = percent reduction urea.
  * and †denote that p < 0.05 between these two study groups.
  §, ‡, and ~denote that p < 0.001 between these two study groups.

[10], the other on short hours daily HD by our London group [11]. Both reviews emphasized that the need for rigorous randomized control studies. The Calgary group has recently reported on the first randomized controlled trial examining the effect of frequent nocturnal HD versus conventional HD. They showed that frequent HD improved left ventricular mass, reduced the need for blood pressure medications, improved some measures of mineral metabolism and improved measures of quality of life [12]. The National Institutes of Health (USA) have ongoing two randomized trials; one comparing in-center short hours six times per week HD versus conventional three times per week and the second, examining six nights per week versus three conventional dialyses, all at home. The results of these studies will not be available until approximately 2010. It must be realized that the Calgary study and the NIH nocturnal study are not just examining frequency but overlap frequency with increased time. Data regarding hard outcomes such as hospitalizations and mortality are likely to come from the International Quotidian Hemodialysis Registry [13] and its planned cohort controlled studies. Even the NIH studies are not powered enough to detect such hard outcomes which are necessary for dialysis providers.

Conclusion

More frequent dialysis regimens offer the potential for better patient outcomes than the current paradigm of intermittent therapies. This potential has not yet been proven. In spite of this, some providers have already approved and funded quotidian therapies. The results of the NIH and Quotidian Registry studies are awaited by others. A major paradigm shift might then occur.

References

1   Eknoyan G, Beck GJ, Cheung AK, et al: Effect of dialysis dose and membrane flux in maintenance hemodialysis. N Engl J Med 2002;347:2010–2019.
2   National Kidney Foundation: K/DOQI Clinical Practice Guidelines for Hemodialysis Adequacy: Update 2000. Am J Kidney Dis 2001;37(suppl 1):S7–S62.
3   Kjellstrand CM, Evans RL, Peterson RJ, et al: The 'unphysiology' of dialysis. A major cause of dialysis side effects? Kidney Int Suppl 1975;2:S30–S34.
4   Gotch FA: The current place of urea kinetic modelling with respect to different dialysis modalities. Nephrol Dial Transplant 1998;13:10–14.
5   Blagg CR, Ing TS, Berry D, Kjellstrand CM: The history and rationale of daily and nightly hemodialysis; in Lindsay RM, Buonocristiani U, Lockridge RS, Pierratos A, Ting GO (eds): Daily and Nocturnal Hemodialysis. Contrib Nephrol. Basel, Karger 2004, vol 145, pp 1–9.
6   Blagg CR, Lindsay RM (eds): The London Daily/Nocturnal Hemodialysis Study. Am J Kidney Dis 2003;42;1(suppl 1):S1–S70.
7   Lindsay RM, Heidenheim AP, Nesrallah G, Garg AX, Suri R, and Daily Hemodialysis Study Group London Health Sciences Centre: Minutes to recovery after a hemodialysis session: a simple

health-related quality of life question that is reliable, valid, and sensitive to change. Clin J Am Soc Nephrol 2006;1:952–959.

8   Chan C, Floras J, Miller J, et al: Regression of left ventricular hypertrophy after conversion to nocturnal hemodialysis. Kidney Int 2002;61:2235–2239.

9   Chan C, Floras JS, Miller JA, Pierratos A: Improvement in ejection fraction by nocturnal hemodialysis in end-stage renal failure patients with co-existing heart failure. Nephrol Dial Transplant 2002;17:1518–1521.

10 Walsh M, Culleton B, Tonelli M, Manns B: A systematic review of the effect of nocturnal hemodialysis on blood pressure, left ventricular hypertrophy, anemia, mineral metabolism and health-related quality of life. Kidney Int 2005;67:1500–1508.

11 Suri RS, Nesrallah GE, Mainra R, et al: Daily hemodialysis: a systemic review. Clin J Am Soc Nephrol 2006;1:33–32.

12 Culleton BF, Walsh M, Klarenbach SW, et al: Effect of frequent nocturnal hemodialysis vs. conventional hemodialysis on left ventricular mass and quality of life. A randomised controlled trial. JAMA 2007;298:1291–1299.

13 Nesrallah GE, Suri RS, Carter ST, et al: The International Quotidian Dialysis Registry: Annual Report 2007. Hemodial Int 2007;11:271–277.

Prof. Robert M. Lindsay, MD, FRCPC, FRCP
Room A2-345, London Health Sciences Centre
800 Commissioners Road East, London, Ont N6A 4G5 (Canada)
Tel. +1 519 685 8349, Fax +1 519 685 8395, E-Mail Robert.lindsay@lhsc.on.ca

Ronco C, Cruz DN (eds): Hemodialysis – From Basic Research to Clinical Trials.
Contrib Nephrol. Basel, Karger, 2008, vol 161, pp 154–161

· ·

Treatment Time

Charles Chazot, Guillaume Jean

Centre de Rein Artificiel, Tassin, France

Abstract

The session duration for hemodialysis (HD) patients has become an old-fashioned issue since the blooming debate on dialysis frequency. However, all over the dialysis community, the most frequent scheme of HD treatment remains three-weekly sessions. Pursuing long dialysis strategy 3 times/week for ESRD patients in Tassin after the retirement of the historical leaders relies on the wisdom pillars of dialysis clinical adequacy that are survival, session tolerance, blood pressure control, nutrition and phosphate control. Recent data, including those of the large-scale DOPPS, clearly indicate that survival is associated with the length of the HD session and the ultrafiltration (UF) rate. The UF rate is the key factor for session tolerance and long dialysis reduces dramatically the incidence of significant intradialytic hypotension episodes. The corollary result is the easier and efficient control of extracellular volume overload and its complications, hypertension, left ventricular hypertrophy and acute pulmonary edema. Whereas conventional HD patients present with progressive nutritional impairment, like in the HEMO study, stability of nutritional markers is obtained with long dialysis. It also allows a significant reduction of hyperphosphatemia and phosphate-binder prescriptions when compared to DOPPS data. All these clinical markers that represent the essence of dialysis adequacy, favor strongly the strategy of a sequential long-hour dialysis program that may clinically and economically challenge with daily programs.

Copyright © 2008 S. Karger AG, Basel

Historical Background

When a dying Clyde Shields started hemodialysis (HD) in 1960 under Scribner's supervision [1], nothing was known about the required duration of the dialysis session. The first dialysis session lasted for 76 h! Progressively, the prescription reached a consensus by the end of the 1990s at three weekly sessions of 8–12 h [2]. Because of this successful new therapy, with the rising number of patients requiring dialysis, and with the resource scarcity, decreasing session time was used to increase dialysis availability for end-stage renal disease (ESRD) patients. During the second decade of dialysis practice, dialysis patient outcomes became a matter of thoughts and the first prospective trial of the dialysis history, the National Cooperative Dialysis Study (NCDS) was designed [3]. In this trial, blood urea nitrogen level and dialysis time were used to categorize patients in four different groups included in the study follow-up. Treatment time was considered as non-significant for the outcome, whereas the p value for this relationship was 0.056, and was then unfairly forgotten for years [4]. The mathematicians then took over the dialysis field and described the concept of 'dialysis dose' using urea as a marker of uremia modeled in the Kt/V_{urea} formula. This concept became so popular that HD treatment adequacy remained restricted for two decades on the ability to clear low molecular uremic toxins. A minimum target dose of Kt/V_{urea} was recommended in several guidelines with the hope of improving patients' outcomes.

The NCDS conclusions helped to design the second prospective trial called the HEMO study. Its ambition was to explore the ability of a high level of Kt/V_{urea} and/or high-flux membrane to improve patient survival. With significant disappointment in the dialysis community, this last study failed to show a clear survival advantage with either a higher dialysis dose for small molecules or a high permeability membrane [5]. As in the peritoneal dialysis study ADEMEX, the conclusion is that increasing Kt/V_{urea} is of no benefit on HD patient outcomes. Moreover, for 10 years, the Dialysis Outcome and Practice Patterns Study (DOPPS) has provided large-scale clinical data of HD patients in different areas of the world treated with various practice patterns. Recently it has shown that the dialysis dose assessed from Kt/V_{urea} meets the target recommendation in 80% of the HD patients and even more in the USA [6]. However, significant clinical complications reported in table 1 remain frequent and unsolved in HD patients despite reaching the recommended target of Kt/V_{urea} in most of the cases. This clearly demonstrates that this last index is of limited value to define dialysis adequacy because HD patients do not fulfill targets of optimal HD treatment.

Even if not controlled, the Tassin experience with long dialysis has reported interesting observational data in survival, hypertension, nutrition, and bone mineral metabolism [7–11]. Because its effect goes far beyond the small molecule clearance, treatment time remains one of the most efficient parameters in dialysis practice to improve HD adequacy.

Treatment Time and Survival

Recently, the DOPPS has significantly contributed to highlight the effect of treatment time on HD patient survival. Saran et al. [12] have reported the survival analysis of 22,000 patients according to dialysis dose and treatment time in

Table 1. Clinical complications reported in HD patients

Complications (n)	HD patients, %
Hypertension (20)	56–83
Congestive heart failure (20)	6–46[1]
Serum phosphate > DOQI target (6)	47
Malnutrition criteria (28)	20–36[2]
Yearly mortality rate (20)	6.6–21.7[3]

[1]The presence of congestive heart failure varies according to the area of the DOPPS study: 6% in Japan, 25% in Europe and 46% in the USA.

[2]The four criteria used to define malnutrition are: BMI $<20\,kg/m^2$, serum prealbumin $<0.3\,g/l$, serum albumin $<35\,g/l$, protein intake assessed from nPCR $<1\,g/kg/day$.

[3]From DOPPS. The lower mortality rate is reported in Japan and the highest in the USA. The mortality rate in Europe is 15.6%.

7 countries involved in the DOPPS. When compared to those receiving $>240\,min/session$ 3 times/week, patients receiving $<211\,min/session$ have a significantly higher relative risk of mortality at 1.34, and those between 211 and 240 a relative risk at 1.19. This effect of treatment time on survival is synergic with dialysis dose, the lower mortality being observed in patients receiving sessions lasting 270 min and a Kt/V_{urea} at 1.6. These data confirm previous reports. In Japan, Shinzato et al. [13] found that, after adjustment for dialysis dose, patients receiving 5–5.5 h sessions had the longer survival. Recently from the ANZA registry the lower mortality was observed in patients treated with at least 4.5 h/session and Kt/V_{urea} >1.3 [14]. Therefore, a higher treatment time is associated with better survival in HD patients. However, we lack controlled studies to confirm this. Nevertheless, several features related to patient survival are influenced by treatment time and explain the beneficial effect of this parameter.

The Overlooked Importance of the Ultrafiltration Rate

Ultrafiltration (UF) rate is directly related to the interdialytic weight gain and treatment time. In several studies, interdialytic weight gain is positively associated with nutritional markers and survival [15, 16]. However, recent data stress the deleterious effect of a high UF rate. The previously quoted DOPPS study [12] has reported that mortality is increased in patients with an UF rate $>10\,ml/h/kg$ with a 30% increase of intradialytic hypotension episodes. This

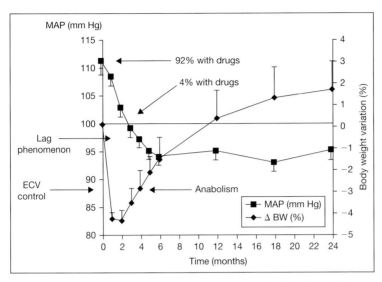

Fig. 1. Extracellular fluid overload correction in 61 incident HD patients treated with long-hour HD 3 times/week. After a 4% decrease of body weight (BW) during the first 2 months of treatment (the 'dry weight quest'), it progressively increased later on because of restored appetite and anabolism. Blood pressure (predialysis mean arterial pressure (MAP)) decreases progressively despite tapering the antihypertensive drugs. It reaches a plateau at 6 months, a delay related to the lag phenomenon [adapted from 29].

has been recently confirmed by Movilli et al. [17] who found in a 5-year prospective study and after multiparameter adjustment the same relationship between increased mortality and an UF rate >12.4 ml/h/kg. If patient survival is positively influenced by interdialytic weight gain and negatively by UF rate, session time is the key factor to conciliate both.

Intradialytic hypotension related to a high UF rate prompts a number of decisions such as UF stop, saline infusion, dry weight prescription or sodium dialysate concentration increases. The direct consequence is that the prescribed dry weight is not achieved leading to extracellular fluid overload [18]. Inability to reach and maintain the dry weight exposes the patient to hypertension, left ventricular hypertrophy and congestive heart failure, conditions known to be associated with decreased patient survival [7, 19]. Congestive heart failure is an important comorbid condition in many patients in Europe and the USA (25–46% in the DOPPS report) [20]. Inadequate handling of extracellular fluid excess is probably responsible for this worrying finding. Increasing session time allows better session tolerance [21], easier correction of extracellular fluid overload and hypertension [9]. Evolution of blood pressure and body weight in incident patients with long-hour dialysis is reported in figure 1. However,

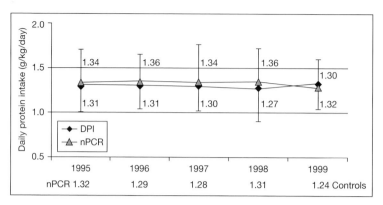

Fig. 2. Protein intake in 53 HD patients during a 5-year follow-up. 33 patients filled out a yearly food record and 23 patients who did not fill out the food record are quoted as a 'control group' [10]. The protein intake meets the recommendations for HD patients, whatever the method of quantification (food record or nPCR calculation).

Ozkahya et al. [22] have been able to correct extracellular volume and hypertension in a large group of patients treated with conventional short HD sessions using low salt diet and a tight UF policy to reach the dry weight prescription. This report shows that the doctor's will is as important as the treatment time itself to reach the correction of fluid excess.

Treatment Time and Nutrition

During the HEMO study and the 3-year follow-up, a progressive decline has been observed for body weight, serum albumin and protein intake assessed from normalized protein catabolic rate (nPCR) calculation [23] in the four patient groups, even for those who remained alive until the end of the study. These data clearly indicate that the nutritional status progressively deteriorates with standard dialysis. On the contrary, we have been able to show a 5-year stability of body weight, protein intake (fig. 2) and energy intakes in 53 patients treated with long dialysis and who remained alive during the follow-up [10]. Moreover, improvement of nutritional parameters by increasing treatment time has been also reported in observational studies [24, 25]. The hypothesis for the mechanism of this result is the increased clearance or decreased exposure to middle molecules inducing anorexia which have been described by Bergstrom [26].

Table 2. Proportion of patients over DOQI targets for serum phosphate and prescribed phosphate binders in the DOPPS and in Tassin patients treated with sequential (3 times/week) long-hour dialysis [adapted from 11]

	Europe (%)	USA (%)	Japan (%)	Tassin (5–6 h) (%)	Tassin (7–8 h) (%)
Phosphate level >5.5 mg/dl	50	54	52	18	10
Phosphate-binder prescription		←77–83→		39	29

Treatment Time and Phosphate Balance

There is a contradiction between the recommendation of a large protein intake for HD patients to maintain nutritional status and the recommendation for phosphate intake that comes mainly from proteins, with a significant risk of positive phosphate balance. Gotch and Levin's group [27] have described models for phosphate removal with different dialysis techniques. Phosphate balance depends on phosphate intake, intestinal absorption and phosphate removal by the dialysis technique. During dialysis, phosphate removal depends on the phosphate clearance of the filter and the time spent on dialysis. It is obvious that with sequential dialysis 3 times/week, a short treatment (3–4 h) with 1.2 g/kg/day of protein intake leads to a positive phosphate balance and requires a phosphate-binder prescription, whereas a longer treatment removes enough phosphate to avoid this prescription. We have reported the proportion of patients treated with sequential long-hour dialysis above the DOQI target for phosphate levels, with data issued from the DOPPS [11] (table 2). Whereas around 50% of DOPPS patients are beyond this target despite a large proportion of phosphate-binder prescriptions, only 10% of the patients treated with long-hour dialysis presents with high phosphate level whereas only 30% of these patients require a phosphate-binder prescription.

Conclusions

Hence even in the absence of randomized controlled studies, observational data clearly indicate that treatment time is critical for optimal dialysis in a large number of patients. Recent years have focused the efficiency of increased frequency rather than prolonged time to improve patient outcomes. At least two randomized controlled trials are on the way to compare conventional HD treatment either with in-center short or home long daily HD. Unfortunately, one arm including long dialysis 3 times/week is lacking. Both patient outcomes, quality of life and global costs should be analyzed with this technique against conventional and daily HD modalities.

Looking further, we can say there is no 'ideal' treatment time and it is for sure not uniform for all the patients. We have enough indicators of dialysis adequacy beyond small molecule clearance to guide and individualize dialysis prescription. The roles of the nephrologists and the staff are essential to provide the patient the information she or he may need to accept the proposed improvement in his therapy. Moreover, individualization of dialysis prescription is conflicting with the unit organization, with the staff and patient schedules. Important research on medical topics and deep thoughts on organization of dialysis units are necessary to improve dialysis patient care and outcomes.

References

1   Scribner BH, Buri R, Caner JE, Hegstrom R, Burnell JM: The treatment of chronic uremia by means of intermittent hemodialysis: a preliminary report. Trans Am Soc Artif Intern Organs 1960;6:114–122.
2   Pendras J, Pollard T: Eight years' experience of a community dialysis center: The North West Kidney Center. Trans Am Soc Art Int Organs 1970;16:77–84.
3   Lowrie EG, Laird NM, Parker TF, Sargent JA: Effect of the hemodialysis prescription of patient morbidity: report from the National Cooperative Dialysis Study. N Engl J Med 1981;305: 1176–1181.
4   Twardowski ZJ: Treatment time and ultrafiltration rate are more important in dialysis prescription than small molecule clearance. Blood Purif 2007;25:90–98.
5   Eknoyan G, Beck GJ, Cheung AK, Daugirdas JT, Greene T, Kusek JW, Allon M, Bailey J, Delmez JA, Depner TA, Dwyer JT, Levey AS, Levin NW, Milford E, Ornt DB, Rocco MV, Schulman G, Schwab SJ, Teehan BP, Toto R: Effect of dialysis dose and membrane flux in maintenance hemodialysis. N Engl J Med 2002;347:2010–2019.
6   Port FK, Pisoni RL, Bommer J, Locatelli F, Jadoul M, Eknoyan G, Kurokawa K, Canaud BJ, Finley MP, Young EW: Improving outcomes for dialysis patients in the international Dialysis Outcomes and Practice Patterns Study. Clin J Am Soc Nephrol 2006;1:246–255
7   Charra B, Calemard E, Ruffet M, Chazot C, Terrat JC, Vanel T, Laurent G: Survival as an index of adequacy of dialysis. Kidney Int 1992;41:1286–1291.
8   Chazot C, Charra B, Laurent G, Didier C, Vo Van C, Terrat JC, Calemard E, Vanel T, Ruffet M: Interdialysis blood pressure control by long haemodialysis sessions. Nephrol Dial Transplant 1995;10:831–837.
9   Chazot C, Charra B, Vo Van C, Jean G, Vanel T, Calemard E, Terrat JC, Ruffet M, Laurent G: The Janus-faced aspect of 'dry weight'. Nephrol Dial Transplant 1999;14:121–124.
10 Chazot C, Vo VC, Blanc C, Hurot JM, Jean G, Vanel T, Terrat JC, Charra B: Stability of nutritional parameters during a 5-year follow-up in patients treated with sequential long-hour hemodialysis. Hemodial Int 2006;10:389–393.
11 Jean G, Chazot C, Charra B: Hyperphosphataemia and related mortality. Nephrol Dial Transplant 2006;21:273–280.
12 Saran R, Bragg-Gresham JL, Levin NW, Twardowski ZJ, Wizemann V, Saito A, Kimata N, Gillespie BW, Combe C, Bommer J, Akiba T, Mapes DL, Young EW, Port FK: Longer treatment time and slower ultrafiltration in hemodialysis: associations with reduced mortality in the DOPPS. Kidney Int 2006;69:1222–1228.

13   Shinzato T, Nakai S, Akiba T, Yamazaki C, Sasaki R, Kitaoka T, Kubo K, Shinoda T, Kurokawa K, Marumo F, Sato T, Maeda K: Survival in long-term haemodialysis patients: results from the annual survey of the Japanese Society for Dialysis Therapy. Nephrol Dial Transplant 1997;2:884–888.

14   Marshall MR, Byrne BG, Kerr PG, McDonald SP: Associations of hemodialysis dose and session length with mortality risk in Australian and New Zealand patients. Kidney Int 2006;69:1229–1236.

15   Kimmel PL, Varela MP, Peterson RA, Weihs KL, Simmens SJ, Alleyne S, Amarashinge A, Mishkin GJ, Cruz I, Veis JH: Interdialytic weight gain and survival in hemodialysis patients: effects of duration of ESRD and diabetes mellitus. Kidney Int 2000;57:1141–1151.

16   Lopez-Gomez JM, Villaverde M, Jofre R, Rodriguez-Benitez P, Perez-Garcia R: Interdialytic weight gain as a marker of blood pressure, nutrition, and survival in hemodialysis patients. Kidney Int Suppl 2005;93:S63–S68.

17   Movilli E, Gaggia P, Zubani R, Camerini C, Vizzardi V, Parrinello G, Savoldi S, Fischer MS, Londrino F, Cancarini G: Association between high ultrafiltration rates and mortality in uraemic patients on regular haemodialysis. A 5-year prospective observational multicentre study. Nephrol Dial Transplant 2007;22:3547–3552.

18   Charra B: Control of blood pressure in long slow hemodialysis. Blood Purif 1994;12:252–258.

19   Goodkin DA, Young EW, Kurokawa K, Prutz KG, Levin NW: Mortality among hemodialysis patients in Europe, Japan, and the United States: case-mix effects. Am J Kidney Dis 2004;44:16–21.

20   Goodkin DA, Bragg-Gresham JL, Koenig KG, Wolfe RA, Akiba T, Andreucci VE, Saito A, Rayner HC, Kurokawa K, Port FK, Held PJ, Young EW: Association of comorbid conditions and mortality in hemodialysis patients in Europe, Japan, and the United States: the Dialysis Outcomes and Practice Patterns Study (DOPPS). J Am Soc Nephrol 2003;14:3270–3277.

21   Laurent G, Charra B: The results of an 8-hour thrice weekly haemodialysis schedule. Nephrol Dial Transplant 1998;13:125–131.

22   Ozkahya M, Toz H, Unsal A, Ozerkan F, Asci G, Gurgun C, Akcicek F, Mees EJ: Treatment of hypertension in dialysis patients by ultrafiltration: role of cardiac dilatation and time factor. Am J Kidney Dis 1999;34:218–221.

23   Rocco MV, Dwyer JT, Larive B, Greene T, Cockram DB, Chumlea WC, Kusek JW, Leung J, Burrowes JD, McLeroy SL, Poole D, Uhlin L: The effect of dialysis dose and membrane flux on nutritional parameters in hemodialysis patients: results of the HEMO Study. Kidney Int 2004;65:2321–2334.

24   Alloatti S, Molino A, Manes M, Bonfant G, Pellu V: Long nocturnal dialysis. Blood Purif 2002;20:525–530.

25   Charra B, Laurent G, Chazot C, Jean G, Terrat JC, Vanel T: Hemodialysis trends in time, 1989–1998, independent of dose and outcome. Am J Kidney Dis 1998;32:S63–S70.

26   Bergstrom J: Why are dialysis patients malnourished? Am J Kidney Dis 1995;26:229–241.

27   Gotch FA, Panlilio F, Sergeyeva O, Rosales L, Folden T, Kaysen G, Levin NW: A kinetic model of inorganic phosphorus mass balance in hemodialysis therapy. Blood Purif 2003;21:51–57.

28   Aparicio M, Cano N, Chauveau P, Azar R, Canaud B, Flory A, Laville M, Leverve X: Nutritional status of haemodialysis patients: a French national cooperative study. French Study Group for Nutrition in Dialysis. Nephrol Dial Transplant 1999;14:1679–1686.

29   Charra B, Bergstrom J, Scribner BH: Blood pressure control in dialysis patients: importance of the lag phenomenon. Am J Kidney Dis 1998;32:720–724.

Dr. C. Chazot
Centre de Rein Artificiel
FR–69160 Tassin (France)
Tel. +33 66 22 33 130, Fax +33 47 83 48 703, E-Mail chchazot@club-internet.fr

Ronco C, Cruz DN (eds): Hemodialysis – From Basic Research to Clinical Trials.
Contrib Nephrol. Basel, Karger, 2008, vol 161, pp 162–167

....

Membrane Characteristics

Sara M. Viganò, Salvatore Di Filippo, Celestina Manzoni,
Francesco Locatelli

Department of Nephrology, Dialysis and Renal Transplantation, A. Manzoni Hospital,
Lecco, Italy

Abstract

Dialysis membrane characteristics are important for an effective and biocompatible dialysis. The properties of a membrane determine the size range of uremic toxins that are eliminated, but are also associated to patient morbidity and mortality. In this paper we describe dialysis the membrane characteristics that could influence the choice of a different type of dialysis.

Copyright © 2008 S. Karger AG, Basel

Semipermeable membranes have been produced since the early 1900s. In the dialysis field, membranes are classified into two groups: cellulosic or synthetic. Permeability and biocompatibility are the two major features of dialysis membranes that may be implicated in the outcome of patients undergoing maintenance hemodialysis (HD). The purpose of this review is to describe membrane and dialyzer technology, with a general overview of membrane-related determinants of dialyzer.

Hollow-Fiber Membrane Characteristics

Hollow-Fiber Dimensions

An individual hollow fiber is a solid cylinder in which the central region has been removed, forming the blood compartment. From a structural perspective, a lot of hollow fibers have a standard blood compartment diameter (180–220 μm) and length (20–24 cm). These parameters are dictated essentially by the operating conditions used during HD and are the result of a compromise between opposing forces. A relatively small blood compartment diameter is desirable because it provides a short diffusive distance for solute mass transfer. At a given blood flow rate, a lower inner diameter also provides a higher shear rate, resulting in greater attenuation of blood-side boundary layer effects [1]. However, a decrease inner diameter also has undesirable effects. Fluid flow along the length of a cylinder (i.e., the axial flow) in many situations is governed by the Hagen-Poiseuille equation [2]: $Q_B = \Delta P/(8\,\mu l/\pi r^4)$.

In this equation, Q_B is blood flow rate, ΔP is axial pressure drop, μ is blood viscosity, L is fiber length, and r is hollow-fiber radius.

A more general form of equation is: $Q_B = \Delta P/R$, with $R = 8\,\mu l/\pi r^4$.

Due to the inverse relationship between R and r^4, a small decrease in hollow-fiber inner diameter induces a large increase in flow resistance. Increases in fiber length and hematocrit (μ) are associated with an increase in flow resistance (R). So, an increase in R results in an increase in axial pressure drop at a constant blood flow rate.

Patients with progressively rising hematocrits are commonly treated with large surface area dialyzers of high water permeability. These dialyzers require relatively high blood flow rates (at least 350 ml/min) to derive maximum benefit from a solute removal perspective. The high flow resistance and associated large axial pressure drop in this specific scenario result in significant backfiltration of dialysate under normal HD operating conditions [3]. The combination of significant backfiltration and contaminated dialysate increases the likelihood of cytokine-inducing substance transfer [4].

Surface Area

The inner annular surface represents the blood compartment surface area and is the theoretically maximal area available for blood contact. For the entire group of fibers forming a dialyzer, total nominal surface area then depends on fiber length, inner diameter, and overall number (that varies from 7,000 to 14,000).

Membrane Pore-Related Characteristics

The rate of ultrafiltrate flow is directly related to the fourth power of the pore radius (r^4) at a constant transmembrane pressure. Thus, although the number of pores also influences water permeability, the membrane characteristic that most directly influences water permeability is mean pore size.

The diffusive properties of a dialysis membrane are determined mainly by the porosity (pore density) and the pore size. Membrane porosity is directly proportional to both the number of pores and the square of the pore radius (r^2). The major pore-related determinants of flux (r^4) and diffusive permeability (number of pores, r^2) differ sufficiently that the two properties can be independent of one another for a particular HD membrane. For example, cellulosic high-efficiency dialyzers have high diffusive permeability values for small solutes but low water permeability. There are examples of high-flux dialyzers that have significantly lower small solute diffusive permeabilities than comparably sized dialyzers of much lower water permeability.

Non-Membrane-Related Determinants of Dialyzer Performance

The membrane is a key determinant of overall dialyzer function, but the manner in which the membrane interacts with other components of the dialyzer is also very important. Manufacturing steps for the production of dialyzer are the sequent: after removal of glycerin (used in the hollow-fiber preparation), fibers are covered with spacer yarns, which are filaments designed to create optimal spacing between fibers [5]. Subsequently the fibers are assembled ('bundled') and inserted in the dialyzer casing. The fiber bundle is then 'potted' (encapsulated) at both ends with silicone rubber and cut. Finally, the dialyzer is placed in a pouch and the entire unit is sterilized, usually by ethylene oxide, γ-rays, or steam.

Several of these steps may have a direct effect on dialyzer function and performance. Fiber bundle configuration and spacing have a major impact on mass transfer. Dialyzer's packing density is the ratio of the area comprised of fibers to the total area, based on a transverse cut through the dialyzer. Empirically, packing densities less than approximately 50% imply insufficient membrane surface area for an appropriate set of flow rates. On the other hand, values greater than approximately 60% are associated with a high risk of dialysate flow maldistribution in which dialysate is 'channeled' to the peripheral aspect of the fiber bundle, at the expense of flow to the inner bundle area. Finally, the sterilization technique may influence the dialyzer performance through an effect on mean membrane pore size [6].

Dialyzer Classification by Membrane Composition

Unmodified Cellulosic Dialyzers

The constituent component of cellulosic membranes is cellobiose, a saccharide found in a number of natural substances. These membranes have a homogeneous, symmetric structure and have good performance for small solute removal. The performance is poorer with respect to solutes of medium/high molecular weight. The use of these membranes is therefore limited to standard HD.

With respect to biocompatibility, cellobiose has a high density of hydroxyl groups, which are very susceptible toward chemical reaction, forming esters and ethers. The abundance of hydroxyl groups makes the activation of the alternative complement pathway particularly pronounced for these dialyzers. This characteristic was considered clinically undesirable when first reported and has contributed to the progressive decline in unmodified cellulosic use.

Modified Cellulosic Dialyzers

Modified cellulosic membranes are characterized by low wall thickness values, typically in the 6- to 15-μm range, and symmetric structures. However, dialyzers composed of these membranes cause less pronounced complement activation and generally have a larger mean pore size [7] than their unmodified cellulosic counterparts. This characteristic determines a higher water permeability and middle molecule clearances.

Various types of modified cellulosic membrane include the following:

(1) *Cellulose acetate membranes (rigorously cellulose diacetate):* Approximately 75% of the hydroxyl groups on the cellulosic backbone are replaced with an acetate group that does not bind to C3 molecule to initiate activation of the complement cascade. Consequently, complement activation is attenuated, as is the leukopenic response.

(2) *Hemophan:* Only a small percentage (<5%) of the hydroxyl groups are actually replaced. However, the tertiary amine replacement group is bulky and effectively shields a significantly greater percentage of hydroxyl groups by a steric mechanism. The attenuation in the degree of complement activation and leukopenia with Hemophan dialyzers is similar to that observed with cellulose acetate dialyzers.

(3) *Synthetically modified cellulose:* A small percentage of hydroxyl groups are covalently replaced with neutrally charged aromatic benzyl groups. This characteristic determines a better biocompatibility, especially the thrombogenicity.

Synthetic Dialyzers

Synthetic membranes were developed essentially in response to concerns related to the narrow scope of solute removal and the pronounced complement activation associated with unmodified cellulosic dialyzers. The large mean pore size and thick wall structure of these membranes allowed the high ultrafiltration rates necessary in hemofiltration to be achieved at relatively low transmembrane pressures. Dialyzers with these highly permeable membranes were used subsequently in the diffusive mode as high-flux dialyzers.

An obvious difference between synthetic and cellulosic membranes is chemical composition. Synthetic membranes are manufactured polymers that are classified as thermoplastics. Another feature differentiating cellulosic and synthetic membranes is wall thickness. Synthetic membranes have wall thickness values of at least 20 μm and may be structurally symmetric or asymmetric. In the latter category, a very thin 'skin' (approx. 1 μm) contacting the blood compartment lumen acts primarily as the membrane's separative element with regard to solute removal. The structure of the remaining wall thickness, which determines a synthetic membrane's thermal, chemical, and mechanical properties, varies considerably among the various synthetic membranes [8]. Takeyama and Sakai [9] have suggested an effective mean pore radius of 5–8 nm achieves the appropriate balance between β_2-microglobulin removal and albumin loss.

Many of the synthetic polymers composing these membranes are hydrophobic and require the addition of a hydrophilic agent (PVP) to avoid excessive protein adsorption upon blood exposure. In addition to imparting hydrophilicity, PVP influences membrane pore size distribution through its effects on pore surface tension, and its content may vary considerably across a synthetic membrane's wall thickness.

In order to provide greater clearances of low-molecular-weight proteins and small protein-bound solutes than conventional high-flux dialysis membranes, a new class of membranes has been developed (super-flux membranes). Many trials have suggested that protein-leaking membranes improve anemia correction, decrease plasma total homocysteine concentrations, and reduce plasma concentrations of glycosylated and oxidized proteins [10]. The problems are that it is unclear yet whether these membranes offer benefits beyond those obtained with conventional high-flux membranes and the amount of albumin loss in dialysate that can be tolerated by patients on a long-term therapy has yet to be determined.

References

1   Colton CK, Lowrie EG: Hemodialysis: physical principles and technical considerations; in Brenner BM, Rector FC (eds): The Kidney, ed 2. Philadelphia, Saunders, 1981, pp 2425–2489.
2   Bird RB, Stewart WE, Lightfoot EN: Velocity distributions in laminar flow; in Bird RB, Stewart WE, Lightfoot EN (eds): Transport Phenomena, ed 1. New York, Wiley, 1960, pp 34–70.
3   Clark WR: Quantitative characterization of hemodialyzer solute and water transport. Semin Dial 2001;14:32–36.

4 Lonnemann G: Chronic inflammation in hemodialysis: the role of contaminated dialysate. Blood Purif 2000;18:214–223.

5 Clark WR, Hamburger RJ, Lysaght MJ: Effect of membrane composition and structure on performance and biocompatibility in hemodialysis. Kidney Int 1999;56:2005–2015.

6 Clark WR, Gao D: Properties of membranes used for hemodialysis therapy. Semin Dial 2002;15:191–195.

7 Varela MP, Kimmel PL, Phillips TM, Mishkin GJ, Lew SQ, Bosch JP: Biocompatibility of hemodialysis membranes: interrelations between plasma complement and cytokine levels. Blood Purif 2001;19:370–379.

8 Mishkin GJ: What clinically important advances in understanding and improving dialyzer function have occurred recently? Semin Dial 2001;14:170–173.

9 Takeyama T, Sakai Y: Polymethylmethacrylate: one biomaterial for a series of membrane. Contrib Nephrol. Basel, Karger, 1999, vol 125, pp 9–24.

10 Ward RA: Protein-leaking membranes for hemodialysis: a new class of membranes in search of an application? J Am Soc Nephrol 2005;16:2421–2430.

Prof. Francesco Locatelli
Department of Nephrology, Dialysis and Renal Transplantation
A. Manzoni Hospital, Via dell'Eremo 9/11
IT–23900 Lecco (Italy)
Tel. +39 0341 489 850, Fax +39 0341 489 860, E-Mail f.locatelli@ospedale.lecco.it

Ronco C, Cruz DN (eds): Hemodialysis – From Basic Research to Clinical Trials.
Contrib Nephrol. Basel, Karger, 2008, vol 161, pp 168–177

....

What Is Important in Dialysis? Efficiency: Blood Flow, KoA and Kt/V?

Frank Gotch

Renal Research Institute, New York, N.Y., USA

Abstract

The relationships of clinical outcome to Kt/V and treatment time (t) in the two large randomized controlled trials of dialysis (National Cooperative Dialysis Study, NCDS, and the Hemodialysis Study, HEMO) were reviewed and compared to several major observational studies (OS). The HEMO study was originally conceived to determine whether outcome was improved by increasing Kt/V to 1.40, 40% higher than spKt/V >1.00 which was concluded to be adequate in the NCDS. However, OS suggested improvement in outcome up to and higher than Kt/V 1.40, so the HEMO dose targets were changed to 1.40 and 1.70. HEMO showed there was no change in outcome over this dose range but when the data were analyzed as a dose targeting OS, there was spurious improvement in outcome over the total range studied. Thus it cannot be concluded that Kt/V >1.0 results in improvement in clinical outcome since the range 1.00–1.40 has not been studied and both levels found adequate in randomized controlled trials. The borderline inverse correlation of outcome to treatment time in NCDS was shown to be meaningless because Kt/V was not successfully separated from t.

Copyright © 2008 S. Karger AG, Basel

This session frames the general question 'What is important in dialysis?' The factors considered are dialysis frequency, treatment time, efficiency and Kt/V, membrane characteristics and membrane flux. I have been asked to address the importance of efficiency and Kt/V.

The established rational of intermittent dialysis therapy for ESRD is removal of accumulated low-molecular-weight toxic catabolites of protein (urea, H^+, K^+, inorganic phosphorus and Ca^{2+} and Na^+ and H_2O, all of which are normally eliminated by the kidneys. Thus virtually all of the solutes targeted for removal with intermittent dialysis therapy are of low molecular weight and cleared by diffusive transport across the dialyzer except Na^+ and H_2O which are removed by ultrafiltration. There is a big inventory of larger molecular weight solutes that accumulate in uremia but the only one with clearly established organ system toxicity is β_2-microglobulin although there are no well-established guidelines to target safe concentration or magnitude of removal.

Dialysis Prescription

The only widely accepted method to quantify the dose of dialysis is the fractional clearance of urea from body water or $K \cdot t/V_U$, where K is dialyzer urea clearance, t is treatment time, and V is the urea distribution volume (KDOQI) which is considered to be a dose surrogate for removal of low-molecular-weight toxins. There have been only two prospectively randomized controlled trials (RCT) of dialysis dose [1, 2] and in both of these trials the dialysis dose was tightly controlled with urea kinetic modeling (UKM). A third RCT of more frequent dialysis is now underway in the USA and the dose is again targeted with UKM.

The dialysis prescription and Kt/V have also been highly controversial for a quarter of a century. It has been argued that: (1) The National Cooperative Dialysis Study (NCDS) [1] was incorrectly interpreted and that spKt/V = 1.0 was not an adequate dose of dialysis; (2) the adverse effect of treatment time (t) on outcome in the NCDS was incorrectly rejected because of a marginal p = 0.06; (3) Kt/V does not account for middle molecules in the prescription, and (4) Kt/V neglects the importance of Na and water removal in adequate dialysis. My purpose here will be to briefly explore these controversies concerning Kt/V and treatment time.

Was the NCDS Incorrectly Interpreted with Respect to an Adequate spKt/V?

The NCDS was guided by UKM [3] with the basic design shown in figure 1a. UKM was used to control BUN at two nominal levels of 70 ± 10 and 120 ± 10 mg/dl with protein intake (normalized protein catabolic rate or NPCR, g/kg) controlled to $0.80 \le NPCR \le 1.40$. The protocol also called for short and long treatment times for both low and high BUN groups as shown in figure 1a. The short treatment times were targeted at 2.5–3.5 h and long treatment times 4.5–5.5 h and the mean times achieved were 3.2 and 4.5 h, so a substantial difference in treatment time was in fact observed.

Clinical outcome in the NCDS for the 160 patients, each expressed as *success* or *failure*, and plotted on BUN, NPCR coordinates is shown in figure 1b [4]. Groups II and IV with high BUN had a 56% incidence of *failure* while

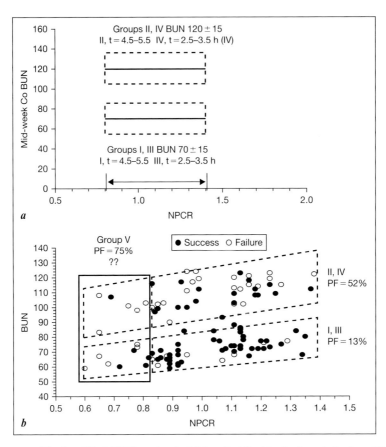

Fig. 1. *a* The NCDS protocol which called for identical control of pre-BUN irrespective of NPCR (low and high BUN) with short and long treatment times in each group. *b* With respect to clinical outcome there was a group V with very high failure rate irrespective of BUN when NPCR <0.80.

groups I and III with low BUN had 13% failure which was thought to confirm the hypothesis that high BUN resulted in poor outcome. However, a fifth group (V) of patients was identified with NPCR <0.80 and a very high incidence of *failure* = 75% irrespective of BUN. In an attempt to understand group V, the urea kinetic model used to guide the study was solved for BUN over a wide range of spKt/V and NPCR with results shown in figure 2a. When spKt/V is held constant, BUN is a linear function of NPCR as depicted by the family of lines in figure 2a over the range $0.4 \le spKt/V \le 2.0$. Analysis of the NCDS data with the UKM grid is shown in figure 2b where it can be seen that spKt/V <1.0 clearly separated the patients in groups II, IV and V with high failure rate

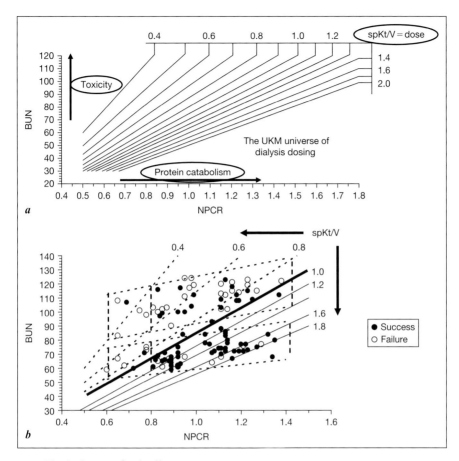

Fig. 2. See text for details.

from groups I and III with low failure rate. The analysis in figure 2b is portrayed in figure 3a as relative probability of failure (RPF) and plotted as a function of spKt/V. These data were interpreted to show that the mechanism by which dialysis controls uremia can be quantified as the magnitude of dialyzer urea clearance (Kt) normalized to urea distribution (V) or Kt/V and it was concluded that an adequate dose of dialysis was achieved with spKt/V = 1.00 and no improvement was seen with higher doses up to spKt/V 1.45. This conclusion is also illustrated in figure 3b on BUN, PCR and spKt/V coordinates.

In addition to the step function outcome plot, we also reported linear and exponential dependence of RPF on spKt/V as shown by curves (2) and (3) in

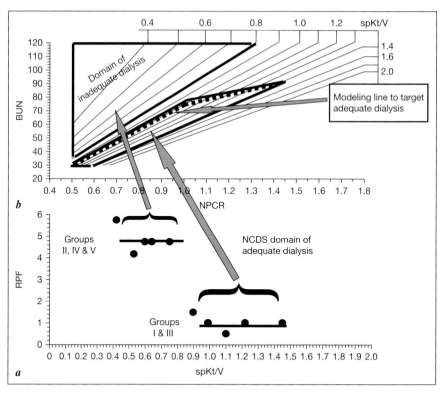

Fig. 3. Results of mechanistic analysis of NCDS outcome.

figure 4a. Some championed both of these functions [5] resulting in a 20-year controversy about an adequate dose.

The NCDS Dosing Controversy and HEMO

The exponential outcome function as shown in figure 4b was strongly supported by accumulating observational studies (OS) which indicated continuing improvement in outcome up to spKt/V 1.40 [6]. The HEMO study [2] was subsequently undertaken to evaluate the benefit of higher dialysis doses in a RCT. The HEMO study design developed in the pilot phase called for a standard arm with spKt/V 1.0–1.2 and high dose arm spKt/V 1.4–1.5. As shown in figure 4b, this design would have overlapped the high dose arm in NCDS and provided an evaluation of dose from these combined RCTs ranging from 0.45 to 1.50.

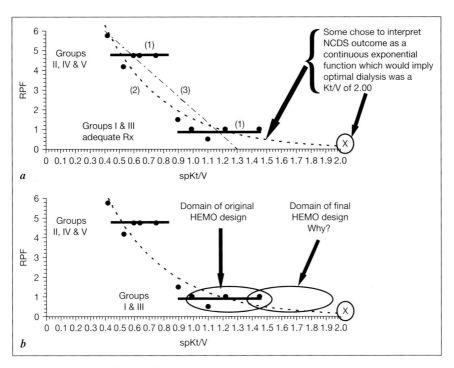

Fig. 4. See text for details.

By the time the pilot phase of HEMO was finished there was clinical consensus in the nephrology community that OS had shown the minimum adequate dose was spKt/V = 1.40 and consequently the standard dose arm was moved up to spKt/V = 1.40 as shown in figure 4b. The increase of standard arm to 1.40 eliminated any evaluation with HEMO of the validity of the NCDS conclusion, spKt/V >1.0 does not improve outcome. Much to the surprise of many, there was no difference in outcome in the standard arm vs. high dose arm in HEMO and we still do not know if spKt/V = 1.4 is better therapy than spKt/V = 1.0 since the NCDS remains the only comparative study of dosage in that range.

Reconciliation of RCT Results with OS Results

Many patients recruited for HEMO had to have a reduction of dose to fit the spKt/V = 1.40 target for the standard arm of HEMO. This caused concern about inadequate dialysis in view of the OS, especially in patients who did not

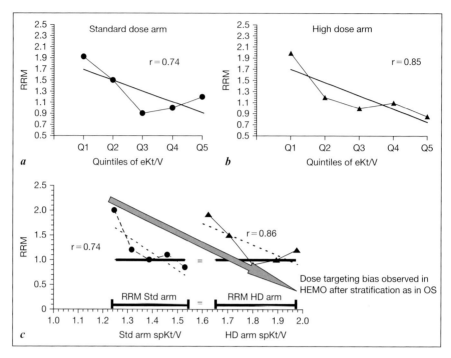

Fig. 5. Reconciliation of OS with randomized trials.

quite reach the spKt/V goal of 1.40. Consequently, the HEMO safety committee instructed the Data Coordinating Center (DCC) to stratify the standard arm by quintiles of Kt/V and monitor outcome over this range in the standard arm [7]. The results of these analyses are shown in figure 5a where a highly significant decrease in RRM was observed as the stratified spKt/V increased in the standard arm. This observation might well have resulted in early termination of the study and a conclusion that the minimum adequate spKt/V is 1.65 if the DCC had not done the same analysis in the high dose arm and found exactly the same relationship as in figure 5b. This striking dose targeting bias found in both arms of HEMO reveals a serious flaw in OS – they are in a sense self-fulfilling prophecies in that the optimal dose found always increases as the dose range studied increases. Figure 5c shows the HEMO dose stratification results expressed as approximate values of spKt/V in the two arms. The two arms had equal outcomes but using OS techniques it would have been spuriously concluded from the combined outcomes that there was a continuous decrease in mortality over the whole range of dosage despite that fact that very little more

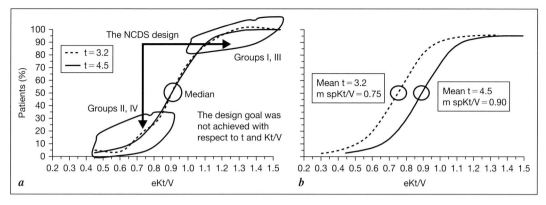

Fig. 6. See text for details.

solute is being removed as spKt/V increases from 1.0 to 2.0 with thrice-weekly dialysis.

Effect of Treatment Time (t) on Patient Outcome in the NCDS

A very frequent commentary about the NCDS is that the slightly increased mortality with shorter treatment time was highly significant clinically but falsely interpreted as not significant because p = 0.06 and therefore the nephrology community was misled about the importance to t in the dialysis prescription [8–11]. In fact, the contrary argument is more defensible: the marginal effect seen actually may suggest that short time was beneficial in the study because the study design goal of separating Kt/V from t was not achieved and Kt/V was significantly lower in the short time groups compared to long time groups. The study design planned is schematically illustrated in figure 6a where it can be seen that the median eKt/V should be 0.90 for both groups and the eKt/V distributions identical in both short and long time groups. The actual distributions are shown in figure 6b where the spKt/V distribution is substantially lower in the short time patients compared to long time patients with median 0.75 vs. 0.91. This means that 52% of the short time patients were in the Kt/V region of 56% probability of failure while only 18% of the long time patients fell into the high probability of failure region. It is surprising that there was not a more significant relationship between probability of failure and t in view of the 5-fold increase in risk of failure in the low Kt/V group. The effect of Kt/V was never tested in the initial analysis of the NCDS [1] but, rather, a surrogate, TAC urea, which is a very poor substitute for Kt/V since it cannot distinguish the effect of PCR.

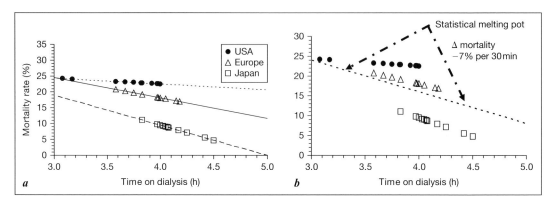

Fig. 7. Mortality rate as function of treatment time in DOPPS data. *a* The regression of mortality rate on t is extremely variable across different geographic regions. These curves are not convincing evidence of a generalizable inverse dependence of mortality on treatment time. *b* The DOPPS data after statistical analysis showed mortality rate decreases 7% per 30 min increase in t. This looks a bit like adding oranges, apples and onions!

Effect of Treatment Time on Outcome in Recent DOPPS Studies

It was recently reported that longer treatment reduced mortality in the DOPPS data base for three large geographic areas: USA, Europe and Japan [8]. The authors concluded the data supported the generalized conclusion that mortality rate fell by 7% for each 30 min increase in t. The data reported for each region adjusted for co-morbidities are plotted in figure 7a and the statistical conclusion of 7% decrease in mortality for each 30 min increase in t is shown in figure 7b. It is not reasonable to generalize these data with such striking geographic differences in the effect of t. The effect of t is almost negligible in the USA and quite striking in Japan while mortality is much lower in Japan at all levels of t. It was also concluded in the DOPPS paper that slower ultrafiltration rates correlated with lower mortality. This is difficult to understand when in DOPPS II [3, and table 1 therein] the mean UFR was 9.9 in Japan and 9.8 in the USA.

Thus it has not been possible to clearly show an effect of treatment time on mortality despite many efforts over the years while it has been quite easy to show an effect of Kt/V on morbidity and mortality. Dialysis is an imperfect therapy and it is not appropriate to add to patient burdens with undue elongation of treatment time. The optimal treatment time is that required to (1) deliver an adequate Kt/V with highly efficient dialyzers and (2) remove accumulated Na and H_2O without inducing hypotension. We reported a comparison of mortalities some years ago [12] and found the two lowest mortalities were observed with the longest and shortest treatment times.

References

1   Lowrie EG: History and organization of the National Cooperative Dialysis Study (NCDS). Kidney Int 1983;13(suppl):S1–S221.
2   Eknoyan G, Beck G, Cheung A, et al: Effect of dialysis dose and membrane flux in maintenance dialysis. N Engl J Med 2002;347:2010–2019.
3   Sargent JA: Control of dialysis by a single pool urea model: the National Cooperative Dialysis Study. Kidney Int 1983;13(suppl):S19–S25.
4   Gotch FA, Sargent JA: A mechanistic analysis of the National Cooperative Dialysis Study. Kidney Int 1985;28:526–534.
5   Keshaviah PR: Urea kinetic and middle molecule approaches to assessing the adequacy of hemodialysis and CAPD. Kidney Int Suppl 1993;40:S228–S238.
6   Held P, Port F, Wolf R, Stannard D, Carroll D, Daugirdas J, Bloembergen W, Greer J, Hakim R: The dose of hemodialysis and patient mortality. United States Renal Data System, University of Michigan, Ann Arbor, USA.
7   Greene T, Daugiordas J, Depner T, Allon M, et al, Hemodialysis Study Group: Association of achieve dialysis dose with mortality in the hemodialysis study: an example of 'dose targeting bias'. J Am Soc Nephrol 2005;11:3371–3380.
8   Saran R, Brago-Gresham J, Levin N, Twardowski Z, et al: Longer treatment time and slower ultra-filtration in hemodialysis: associations with reduced mortality with treatment time in the DOPPS. Kidney Int 2006;69:1222–1228.
9   Marshall MR, Byrne BG, Kerr PG, McDonald SP: Associations of hemodialysis dose and session length with mortality risk in Australian and New Zealand patients. Kidney Int 2006;69:1229–1236.
10 Twardowski ZL: Short, thrice-weekly hemodialysis is inadequate regardless of small molecule clearance. Int J Artif Organs 2004;27:452–467.
11 Kurella M, Chertow G: Dialysis session length (t) as a determinant of the adequacy of dialysis. Semin Nephrol 2005;2:90–95.
12 Gotch F, Uehlinger D: Mortality rate in US dialysis patients. Dial Transplant 1991;20:255057.

Frank Gotch, MD
144 Belgrave Ave.
San Francisco, CA 94117(USA)
Tel. +1 415 661 6191, Fax +1 415 731 7876, E-Mail frank.gotch.md@fmc-na.com

Ronco C, Cruz DN (eds): Hemodialysis – From Basic Research to Clinical Trials.
Contrib Nephrol. Basel, Karger, 2008, vol 161, pp 178–184

....

Cross-Membrane Flux Is a Major Factor Influencing Dialysis Patient Outcomes

Bernard Canaud[a,b], *Leila Chenine*[a], *Delphine Henriet*[a], *Hélène Leray*[a]

[a]Lapeyronie Hospital – Nephrology, and [b]Renal Research and Training Institute, Montpellier, France

Abstract

Conventional diffusive-based dialysis modalities including high-flux hemodialysis are limited in their capacity to clear middle and large size uremic toxins. Middle molecule substances are recognized as pathogenic substances implicated in the genesis of accelerated atherosclerosis. Convective methods, mimicking glomeruli filtration of native kidneys, are required to enlarge the molecular weight spectrum of solutes removed. By combining diffusive and convective solute clearances, HDF offers at the present time the highest dialysis efficiency method with the more biocompatible profile. Instantaneous dialyzer clearance does not reflect solute mass removal when body clearance is concerned. Intracorporeal resistance to solute clearance is the main barrier to solute removal. Increasing treatment time and/or frequency of sessions in hemodiafiltration is the only way to overcome body barriers generated from patient/dialysis interaction. A dialysis dose based on normalized middle molecules clearance using β_2-microglobulin as surrogate marker should be considered as a new adequacy target.

Copyright © 2008 S. Karger AG, Basel

Recent prospective randomized studies exploring the specific role of 'dialysis dose' and 'membrane permeability' on hemodialysis (HD) patient mortality have reported conflicting results. In the HEMO study, high dialysis dose (Kt/V 1.7 vs. 1.3) and/or high permeable membrane had no significant effects on patient mortality [1]. On the contrary, in the MPO study patient survival was significantly improved by using high-flux membranes, particularly in hypoalbuminemic and/or diabetics patients [2, 3]. Secondary post-hoc analyses of the HEMO study are suggesting now that high-flux membrane is beneficial for HD patients. Mortality is reduced in high-flux-treated patients after about 3 years of treatment suggesting that a certain time exposure to this type of membrane is needed. Survival improvement has been associated in the HEMO study to the reduction of the predialysis circulating β_2-microglobulin (β_2M) concentrations, which is associated with the use of high-flux membrane [4].

In addition, the European Uremic Toxin Work Group (EUTox) group has made a comprehensive inventory of uremic toxins, separating them into three categories from small molecules, to middle molecules and protein-bound solutes [5]. Toxicity of middle molecules and protein-bound solutes is strongly supported by experimental data. Unifying hypothesis for interpreting these discordant results, suggest that conventional 'dialysis dose' based on small molecules clearance (urea) is meaningless, provided a minimal dose 1.3 has been delivered, while 'dialysis dose' based on middle molecules clearance (e.g. β_2M) would be more powerful in predicting patient outcomes [6].

Cross-Membrane Flux and Middle-Molecule Removal

Conventional diffusive-based dialysis modalities including high-flux HD are limited in their capacity to clear middle and large size uremic toxins [7, 8]. Convective methods, mimicking glomeruli filtration of native kidneys, are required to enlarge the molecular weight spectrum of solutes removed [9–12].

Convective-based methods include a large range of renal replacement modalities applicable in clinic, lying from pure convection methods (hemofiltration, HF) to mixed diffusive and enhanced convective methods (hemodiafiltration, HDF) [13]. Due to the solvent drag effect, solute clearance is virtually independent from their molecular weight in HDF. In these methods, solute clearances are governed by the sieving coefficient of the membrane. All these methods share the need for substituting isovolumetrically the fluid removed to the patient but they differ by the mode of substituting fluid (post-, pre- or mixed mode dilution) [14, 15]. 'Online' production of substitution fluid by cold sterilization process gives access to virtually unlimited amount of sterile non-pyrogenic substitution fluid [16, 17]. By combining diffusive and convective solute clearances, HDF offers at the present time the highest dialysis efficiency method. Over the last decade, it has been shown that on-line HDF was a safe, reliable and very efficient renal replacement modality for clearing middle molecules [18] and improving survival of dialysis patients [19, 20].

Convective-Based Modalities Increases Instantaneous Solute Mass Transfer of Middle Molecules and Protein-Bound Solutes

Enhanced efficiency of high-flux convective therapies is one of the best documented aspects of the method. HDF provides significantly higher instantaneous clearances than high-flux HD both for small and middle molecule solutes [21, 22]. Enhancement in solute mass removal results in a significant decline of blood middle molecules concentrations over time.

Phosphate removal is increased with HDF methods. Based on 3 sessions weekly, phosphate removal averaged 1,200 mg/session in HDF as compared to 900 mg/session in high-flux HD [23]. Phosphate removal is still not adequate to restore phosphate balance in a uremic patient, but that permits to reduce use of oral phosphate binders [24].

β_2M is effectively removed by high-flux convective therapies. Online HDF is significantly more effective than high-flux HD to remove β_2M. The reduction ratio of β_2M is between 70 and 80% in HDF while it is comprised between 40 and 50% in HD. β_2M mass removal per session range between 180 and 220 mg while it is 70–100 mg in high-flux HD [25, 26]. Several prospective controlled studies have confirmed that the enhancement of β_2M clearance by HDF was accompanied by a significant decline of blood β_2M concentrations on a mid-term period [27, 28]. However, no long-term study allows us to assume that this method will reduce the incidence of β_2M amyloidosis in long-term dialysis patients.

Leptin (16 kDa) levels are elevated in chronic kidney disease patient. They are suspected to negatively affect food intake and energy expenditure. Predialysis blood leptin concentrations are reduced by the long-term use of HDF [29, 30]. Effective removal of free leptin by HDF may favor the improvement of patient nutritional status.

3-Carboxy-4-methyl-5-propyl-2-furanpropionic acid, a protein-bound erythropoietic inhibitor, can be reduced with protein-leaking high-flux membranes [31, 32]. Removal of this erythropoietic inhibitor may facilitate the anemia correction in EPO-resistant patients.

Several circulating *AGEs and AGE precursors* suspected of being involved in dialysis-related amyloidosis are effectively reduced in diabetic and non-diabetic ESRD patients treated with high- and super-flux membranes used in HDF [33]. These beneficial effects may be due to a reduction of the oxidative stress associated with HDF methods [34]. Beneficial effects and clinical relevance of this capacity remains unclear.

p-Cresol, a protein-bound solute, which accumulates during uremia, is implicated in uremic immunodeficiency and endothelial dysfunction. Serum *p*-cresol concentrations are also associated with the relative risk of mortality [35]. ol-HDF has superior clearances than high-flux HD for removing free *p*-cresol and reduces circulating free *p*-cresol [36].

Homocysteine plasma levels, a known cardiovascular risk factor, are significantly reduced by the use of HDF [37]. Due to almost complete protein binding of homocysteine, its reduction has been attributed to the removal of larger molecular inhibitors of homocysteine metabolism.

Body Transfer Resistance Reduces Solute Mass Transfer of Middle Molecules and Protein-Bound Solutes during Dialysis

Effective clearance and removal of middle molecules and protein-bound solutes is restricted by body transfer resistance. Intracorporeal kinetic of solute is complex during HD sessions depending on several factors that include solute characteristics (molecular size, protein-binding capacity, molecule charges), site (superficial or remote compartment) and rate of solute production and tissue perfusion (well vs. poorly perfused). Intracorporeal solute mass transfer coefficient (MTC), a surrogate for body clearance, integrates this biological complexity. It may serve to illustrate the fact that solute removal limitation is generated by the patient/dialysis interaction.

Phosphate and $\beta_2 M$ are two uremic toxins that are particularly useful to illustrate the gap that exists between dialyzer clearance and body clearance.

Phosphate mass transfer per session remains desperately low despite the extensive use of high-flux and high-efficiency dialysis modalities. Phosphate removal limitation is mainly due to its low body MTC (PO_4 MTC $\cong 30\,ml/min$) [38]. Reduced body clearance of inorganic phosphate is due to the intracellular and mitochondrial location of this compound. This phenomenon has been well documented in a recent kinetic-modeling analysis showing that phosphate kinetic fits a four-compartment model with a biphasic concentration changes during high-efficiency dialysis methods [39].

$\beta_2 M$ removal remains low despite the use of highly efficient convective modalities. Limitation in $\beta_2 M$ mass removal during post-dilutional HDF is mainly due to patient body mass transfer resistance rather than hemodiafilter clearance per se. High resistance of body mass transfer reduces access to $\beta_2 M$ stores in the remote poorly perfused compartment. $\beta_2 M$ concentration gradient built during the dialysis session within these two compartments is referred to as the 'compartmentalization' effect. This apparent sequestration of $\beta_2 M$ within the patient's body occurs during high-efficiency HDF and resolves in post-dialysis by the rebound phenomenon. A recent $\beta_2 M$ kinetic analysis has shown that $\beta_2 M$ MTC ($\beta_2 M \cdot MTC \cong 87\,ml/min$) is closed to hemodiafilter clearance.

Treatment Time Is the Main Factor to Overcome Body Solute Mass Transfer Resistance

Extending session treatment time and/or session frequency are the only means to overcome body solute mass transfer resistance generated by patient/dialysis interaction. Recent clinical studies have shown that long duration and more frequent dialysis sessions enhanced mass solute removal and reduced blood concentration levels of middle molecules substances. This is particularly well documented for inorganic phosphate and $\beta_2 M$.

Daily (short, long or nocturnal) high-flux HD is associated with a better control of blood phosphate concentrations and a reduction of phosphate binders [40]. Few studies have addressed the specific role of convective-based therapies on these markers. Based on a daily post-dilutional HF program (20 liters) it has been shown that $\beta_2 M$ concentrations were significantly reduced over time reaching lower concentration equilibrium [41]. According to the results of this study it was evaluated that daily HF program exchanging 70–90 liters would be necessary to normalize circulating $\beta_2 M$. More recently, converting a group of 8 patients from a conventional (4–5 h session) thrice-weekly session HDF program to a short (2–2.5 h) daily HDF program, it has been shown that solute mass removed weekly was significantly increased by 50–70% and blood solute concentrations were reduced consequently [42].

All these studies confirm that body patient clearance is the second main barrier restricting middle molecules mass removal during dialysis. Extended time and frequency are required to overcome body resistance to solutes transfer.

Conclusions

Convective-based modalities (HDF) are the most efficient modalities of treatment since they act both on small and middle molecules toxins. Instantaneous dialyzer clearance does not reflect solute mass removal when body clearance is concerned. Intracorporeal resistance to solute clearance is the main barrier to solute removal. Increasing treatment time and/or frequency of sessions in HDF patients is the only way to overcome body barriers generated from patient/dialysis interaction [43]. A dialysis dose based on normalized middle molecules clearance using $\beta_2 M$ as surrogate marker should be considered as a new adequacy target 4.

References

1   Eknoyan G, Beck GJ, Cheung AK, Daugirdas JT, Greene T, Kusek JW, Allon M, Bailey J, Delmez JA, Depner TA, Dwyer JT, Levey AS, Levin NW, Milford E, Ornt DB, Rocco MV, Schulman G, Schwab SJ, Teehan BP, Toto R, Hemodialysis (HEMO) Study Group: Effect of dialysis dose and membrane flux in maintenance hemodialysis. N Engl J Med 2002;347:2010–2019.
2   Locatelli F, Gauly A, Czekalski S, Hannedouche T, Jacobson SH, Loureiro A, Martin-Malo A, Papadimitriou M, Passlick-Deetjen J, Ronco C, Vanholder R, Wizemann V, Membrane Permeability Outcome (MPO) Study Group: The MPO study: just a European HEMO study or something very different? Blood Purif 2008;26:100–104.
3   Locatelli F, et al, Membrane Permeability Outcome (MPO) Study Group. ERA-EDTA, Barcelona 2007 (oral presentation).

4   Cheung AK, Rocco MV, Yan G, Leypoldt JK, Levin NW, Greene T, Agodoa L, Bailey J, Beck GJ, Clark W, Levey AS, Ornt DB, Schulman G, Schwab S, Teehan B, Eknoyan G: Serum β_2-microglobulin levels predict mortality in dialysis patients: results of the HEMO study. J Am Soc Nephrol 2006;17:546–555.

5   Cohen G, Glorieux G, Thornalley P, Schepers E, Meert N, Jankowski J, Jankowski V, Argiles A, Anderstam B, Brunet P, Cerini C, Dou L, Deppisch R, Marescau B, Massy Z, Perna A, Raupachova J, Rodriguez M, Stegmayr B, Vanholder R, Hörl WH, European Uremic Toxin Work Group (EUTox): Review on uraemic toxins. III. Recommendations for handling uraemic retention solutes in vitro – towards a standardized approach for research on uraemia. Nephrol Dial Transplant 2007;22:3381–3390.

6   Saran R, Canaud BJ, Depner TA, Keen ML, McCullough KP, Marshall MR, Port FK: Dose of dialysis: key lessons from major observational studies and clinical trials. Am J Kidney Dis 2004; 44(suppl 2):47–53.

7   Henderson LW: Dialysis in the 21st century. Am J Kidney Dis 1996;28:951–957.

8   Clark WR, Gao D: Low-molecular-weight proteins in end-stage renal disease: potential toxicity and dialytic removal mechanisms. J Am Soc Nephrol 2002;13(suppl 1):S41–S47.

9   Vanholder R, Glorieux G, De Smet R, et al: New insights in uremic toxins. Kidney Int Suppl 2003;84:S6.

10   Vanholder R, Glorieux GL, De Smet R: Back to the future: middle molecules, high-flux membranes, and optimal dialysis. Hemodial Int 2003;7:52.

11   Henderson LW, Clark WR, Cheung AK: Quantification of middle molecular weight solute removal in dialysis. Semin Dial 2001;14:294–299.

12   Leypoldt JK, Cheung AK, Carroll CE, Stannard DC, Pereira BJ, Agodoa LY, Port FK: Effect of dialysis membranes and middle molecule removal on chronic hemodialysis patient survival. Am J Kidney Dis 1999;33:349–355.

13   Leber HW, Wizemann V, Goubeaud G, Rawer P, Schutterle G: Hemodiafiltration: a new alternative to hemofiltration and conventional hemodialysis. Artif Organs 1978;2:150–153.

14   Feliciani A, Riva MA, Zerbi S, Ruggiero P, Plati AR, Cozzi G, Pedrini LA: New strategies in haemodiafiltration (HDF): prospective comparative analysis between on-line mixed HDF and mid-dilution HDF. Nephrol Dial Transplant 2007;22:1672–1679.

15   Tiranathanagul K, Yossundharakul C, Techawathanawanna N, Katavetin P, Hanvivatvong O, Praditpornsilp K, Tungsanga K, Eiam-Ong S: Comparison of middle-molecule clearance between convective control double high-flux hemodiafiltration and on-line hemodiafiltration. Int J Artif Organs 2007;30:1090–1097.

16   Henderson LW, Beans E: Successful production of sterile pyrogen-free electrolyte solution by ultrafiltration. Kidney Int 1978;14:522–525.

17   Henderson LW, Sanfelippo ML, Beans E: 'On-line' preparation of sterile pyrogen-free electrolyte solution. Trans Am Soc Artif Intern Organs 1978;24:465–467.

18   Canaud B, Bosc JY, Leray-Moragues H, Stec F, Argiles A, Leblanc M, Mion C: On-line haemodiafiltration. Safety and efficacy in long-term clinical practice. Nephrol Dial Transplant 2000;15 (suppl 1):60–67.

19   Canaud B, Bragg-Gresham JL, Marshall MR, Desmeules S, Gillespie BW, Depner T, Klassen P, Port FK: Mortality risk for patients receiving hemodiafiltration versus hemodialysis: European results from the DOPPS. Kidney Int 2006;69:2087–2093.

20   Panichi V, Rizza GM, Paoletti S, Bigazzi R, Aloisi M, Barsotti G, Rindi P, Donati G, Antonelli A, Panicucci E, Tripepi G, Tetta C, Palla R, on behalf of the RISCAVID Study Group: Chronic inflammation and mortality in haemodialysis: effect of different renal replacement therapies. Results from the RISCAVID study. Nephrol Dial Transplant 2008 (in press).

21   Canaud B, Bosc JY, Leblanc M, Garred LJ, Vo T, Mion C: Evaluation of high-flux hemodiafiltration efficiency using an on-line urea monitor. Am J Kidney Dis 1998;31:74–80.

22   Shinzato T, Kobayakawa H, Maeda K: Comparison of various treatment modes in terms of β_2-microglobulin removal: hemodialysis, hemofiltration, and push/pull HDF. Artif Organs 1989;13:66–70.

23   Lornoy W, De Meester J, Becaus I, Billiouw JM, Van Malderen PA, Van Pottelberge M: Impact of convective flow on phosphorus removal in maintenance hemodialysis patients. J Ren Nutr 2006; 16:47–53.

24   Zehnder C, Gutzwiller JP, Renggli K: Hemodiafiltration – a new treatment option for hyperphosphatemia in hemodialysis patients. Clin Nephrol 1999;52:152.

25   Lornoy W, Becaus I, Billiouw JM, et al: On-line haemodiafiltration. Remarkable removal of β_2-microglobulin. Long-term clinical observations. Nephrol Dial Transplant 2000;15(suppl 1):49.

26   Maduell F, del Pozo C, Garcia H, et al: Change from conventional haemodiafiltration to on-line haemodiafiltration. Nephrol Dial Transplant 1999;14:1202.

27   Locatelli F, Mastrangelo F, Redaelli B, et al, The Italian Cooperative Dialysis Study Group: Effects of different membranes and dialysis technologies on patient treatment tolerance and nutritional parameters. Kidney Int 1996;50:1293.

28   Ward RA, Schmidt B, Hullin J, Hillebrand GF, Samtleben W: A comparison of on-line hemodiafiltration and high-flux hemodialysis: a prospective clinical study. J Am Soc Nephrol 2000;11:2344–2350.

29   Widjaja A, Kielstein JT, Horn R, et al: Free serum leptin but not bound leptin concentrations are elevated in patients with end-stage renal disease. Nephrol Dial Transplant 2000;15:846.

30   Mandolfo S, Borlandelli S, Imbasciati E: Leptin and β_2-microglobulin kinetics with three different dialysis modalities. Int J Artif Organs 2006;29:949–955.

31   Niwa T, Asada H, Tsutsui S, et al: Efficient removal of albumin-bound furancarboxylic acid by protein-leaking hemodialysis. Am J Nephrol 1995;15:463.

32   Kawano Y, Takaue Y, Kuroda Y, et al: Effect of alleviation of renal anemia by hemodialysis using the high-flux dialyzer BK-F. Kidney Dial 1994:200.

33   Stein G, Franke S, Mahiout A, et al: Influence of dialysis modalities on serum AGE levels in end-stage renal disease patients. Nephrol Dial Transplant 2001;16:999.

34   Tomo T, Matsuyama K, Nasu M: Effect of hemodiafiltration against radical stress in the course of blood purification. Blood Purif 2004;22(suppl 2):72–77.

35   Bammens B, Evenepoel P, Keuleers H, Verbeke K, Vanrenterghem Y: Free serum concentrations of the protein-bound retention solute *p*-cresol predict mortality in hemodialysis patients. Kidney Int 2006;69:1081–1087.

36   Bammens B, Evenepoel P, Verbeke K, Vanrenterghem Y: Removal of the protein-bound solute *p*-cresol by convective transport: a randomized crossover study. Am J Kidney Dis 2004;44:278–285.

37   Righetti M, Ferrario GM, Serbelloni P, Milani S, Tommasi A: Homocysteine reduction rate in internal haemodiafiltration – a comparison with other mixed dialysis therapies. Nephrol Dial Transplant 2006;21:2034–2035.

38   Schindhelm K, Farrell PC: Patient-hemodialyzer interactions. Trans Am Soc Artif Intern Organs 1978;24:357–366.

39   Spalding EM, Chamney PW, Farrington K: Phosphate kinetics during hemodialysis: evidence for biphasic regulation. Kidney Int 2002;61:655–667.

40   Ayus JC, Achinger SG, Mizani MR, Chertow GM, Furmaga W, Lee S, Rodriguez F: Phosphorus balance and mineral metabolism with 3 h daily hemodialysis. Kidney Int 2007;71:336–342.

41   Canaud B, Assounga A, Kerr P, Aznar R, Mion C: Failure of a daily haemofiltration programme using a highly permeable membrane to return β_2-microglobulin concentrations to normal in haemodialysis patients. Nephrol Dial Transplant 1992;7:924–930.

42   Maduell F, Navarro V, Torregrosa E, Rius A, Dicenta F, Cruz MC, Ferrero JA: Change from three times a week on-line hemodiafiltration to short daily on-line hemodiafiltration. Kidney Int 2003;64:305–313.

43   Clark WR, Leypoldt JK, Henderson LW, Mueller BA, Scott MK, Vonesh EF: Quantifying the effect of changes in the hemodialysis prescription on effective solute removal with a mathematical model. J Am Soc Nephrol 1999;10:601–609.

Prof. Bernard Canaud
Nephrology, Dialysis and Intensive Care, Hôpital Lapeyronie
CHU Montpellier, 371, Av du Doyen G. Giraud
FR–34925 Montpellier Cedex 05 (France)
Tel. +33 467 338 955, Fax +33 467 603 783, E-Mail b-canaud@chu-montpellier.fr

Ronco C, Cruz DN (eds): Hemodialysis – From Basic Research to Clinical Trials.
Contrib Nephrol. Basel, Karger, 2008, vol 161, pp 185–190

························

Inflammatory Pattern in Hemodiafiltration

Vincenzo Panichi, Sabrina Paoletti, Cristina Consani

Department of Internal Medicine, University of Pisa, Pisa, Italy

Abstract

Chronic inflammation may play an important role in early morbidity and mortality in hemodialysis (HD) patients. Interleukin-6 (IL-6) production is enhanced in long-term HD patients and this activated phase response has been shown to be a predictor of cardiovascular disease in the uremic syndrome as well as in the general population. Furthermore, IL-6 and C-reactive protein (CRP) have been negatively related to low serum albumin levels (MIA syndrome). Several studies have attempted to address the question as to whether the type of the dialysis membrane, the quality of the dialysate, and the dialysis technique may be responsible for the induction of a chronic inflammatory state. Recently, the Dialysis Outcomes and Practice Patterns Study (DOPPS) has shown that high-efficiency hemodiafiltration (HDF)-treated patients had a better survival than HD-treated patients accounting for sex, dialysis dose, co-morbid condition and country specificities. Here we report data from the RISCAVID study, an observational and prospective trial including the whole chronic HD population in the north-west part of Tuscany (1,235 million people). The aim of the study was to elucidate the relevance of traditional and non-traditional risk factors on mortality and morbidity in HD patients as well as the impact of different HD modalities. Data at 30 months from this study showed the synergic effect of CRP and pro-inflammatory cytokines as the strong predictors of overall and cardiovascular mortality. HDF was associated to an improved cumulative survival independently of dialysis dose.

Cardiovascular (CV) disease is the primary cause of morbidity in the western world and the clinical impact of atherosclerosis is even more dramatically present in chronic uremic patients. Moreover, chronic kidney disease has been associated with a high prevalence of CV complications [1].

In uremic patients, traditional risk factors such as hypertension, dyslipidemia, obesity and smoking seem to be less important than other additional 'non-traditional' factors such as uremic toxins or chronic inflammation [2]. Several papers have reported that most chronic kidney disease patients have a subclinical microinflammatory state with high serum levels of some pro-inflammatory/pro-atherogenic cytokines and accumulation in peripheral blood of activated mononuclear cells that prolong their lifespan [3]. This activated acute phase response has been shown to be a predictor of CV disease in the general population and in the uremic syndrome [4]. Furthermore, interleukin-6 (IL-6) production is enhanced in long-term hemodialysis (HD) patients [5], and in these patients both IL-6 and C-reactive protein (CRP) have been negatively related to low serum albumin levels. These events have been linked in a new fascinating syndrome – the so-called MIA syndrome [6]. Moreover, elevated CRP plasma values have been shown in patients on HD but not in patients on peritoneal dialysis, suggesting the role of monocyte activation and IL-6 production in the increased CRP generation due to back-filtered dialysate contaminants or blood membrane interaction [7].

Chronic Inflammation in HDF

Several studies have attempted to address the question as to whether the type of dialysis membrane, the quality of the dialysate and the dialytic technique may be responsible for the induction of a chronic inflammatory state [8, 9]. At this time, however, it is not known whether high convective transport may have a beneficial role in modulating the chronic inflammation of HD patients. Improved biocompatibility and reduced inflammation have been reported with on-line HDF based on sensitive markers of the acute phase reaction or pro-inflammatory cell population such as monocyte-derived CD14+ and CD16+ cells [10, 11]; several prospective studies have shown that the behavior of these markers remains stable over time in all HDF patients. More recently in a prospective randomized study it was shown in all HDF patients that there was a less damaging and better repair effect of the endothelial cells [12]. These positive effects results from the combined use of a synthetic biocompatible membrane, ultrapure dialysis fluid and increased removal of some putative uremic toxins. However, in spite of these improvements in dialysis technology and better clinical care, the annual mortality rate of patients with end-stage renal disease undergoing dialysis remains unacceptably high (15–22%) and mortality is the most hard endpoint used to compare the efficacy of renal replacement therapy modalities [13, 14].

Few cohort studies have shown that mortality was reduced in each HDF-treated group [15]. The European Section of International Dialysis and Outcomes Practice Pattern Study (DOPPS) has shown that high efficiency HDF-treated patients had a better survival than regularly HD-treated patients accounting for each sex, dialysis dose, co-morbid condition and country specificities. Despite the fact that the relative risk of death was reduced in both HDF-treated groups, only the high-efficiency HDF group (substitution volume 15–25 liters/session) had a significant benefit marked by a 35% reduction of death risk compared to patients treated with low-flux HD. However, in the DOPPS, only surrogate markers of inflammation were measured, i.e. albumin and ferritin, since the measurements of CRP and cytokines were not included in the data collection [16].

The RISCAVID Study

In June 2004, a prospective observational study (RISCAVID, 'RISchio CArdiovascolare nei pazienti afferenti all'Area Vasta In Dialisi') was started with the aim to investigate the link between traditional and non-traditional risk factors on mortality and morbidity in a large and homogenous HD population [17]. A total of 757 HD patients (mean age 66 ± 14 years, mean dialytic age 70 ± 76 months, diabetes 19%) representing the whole HD population of 1,235,062 inhabitants were included and prospectively followed up for 30 months; overall mortality, CV mortality and non-fatal CV events (acute myocardial infarction, stroke and ictus) were registered. At the time of enrolment, demographic, clinical, laboratory data of the whole population were entered into a centralized database; each of the 15 dialysis facilities of this area provided at the start of the study blood samples from all patients for the centralized determination of inflammatory markers. Patients were stratified into three groups according to the HD modality: standard bicarbonate hemodialysis (BHD) (n = 424), hemodiafiltration (HDF) with sterile bags (n = 204) and on-line HDF (n = 129).

As main results, this study confirmed the high mortality rate in HD (all-cause mortality 12.9%/year; CV mortality 5.9%/year). Patients with combined high levels of CRP and pro-inflammatory cytokines showed an increased risk for CV (RR 1.9, $p < 0.001$) and overall mortality (RR 2.57, $p < 0.001$). Multivariate analysis adjusted for co-morbidity and demographic data showed CRP as the most powerful mortality predictor ($p < 0.001$) followed by IL-6.

Furthermore, our study also provides information on the effect association of different HD modalities on chronic inflammation and consequently on cumulative survival. The evaluation of the inflammatory state in patients categorized according to the different HD modality showed that IL-6 was statistically reduced in on-line HDF vs. BHD and HDF.

HDF with sterile bags and on-line HDF had lower crude overall mortality rates than standard HD even after adjustment for age, gender, diabetes, dialytic vintage, albumin levels, hemoglobin levels, use of epoetin, blood pressure, use

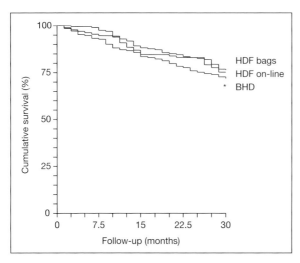

Fig. 1. Cumulative survival and dialytic techniques. Cumulative survival curves estimated from the Cox model according to dialytic techniques. On-line HDF (n = 129) and
HDF on bags (n = 204) patients showed lower overall mortality rates than standard HD
(n = 424) even after adjustment for co-morbidity after 30 months of follow-up (*p < 0.01).

of antihypertensive medications and dialytic efficiency (relative risk = 0.78,
p = 0.01) (fig. 1), as shown by Kaplan-Meier survival curve.

The enhanced cumulative survival of patients receiving HDF in comparison to standard bicarbonate dialysis observed in the RISCAVID Study extends
the results of Canaud et al. [16] who recently compared the mortality of
patients receiving HDF to that of patients receiving HD in a large cohort
prospectively followed for 3 years in the DOPPS. In respect to the DOPPS, the
RISCAVID population differed from other existing studies for the high incidence of mixed convective-diffusive techniques (HDF 44% of the entire population). This equaled 333 patients being followed for 30 months in respect to
the 89 over 443 Italian patients of the DOPPS. Of interest in the RISCAVID
Study is the difference in cumulative survival started after 15 months of observation after adjustment for age, dialysis vintage and co-morbidities (fig. 1). At
variance with the paper of Canaud et al., this study was not able to establish a
relationship between mortality and volume exchange. Despite this limitation,
HDF using sterile bags is customarily prescribed using 10–15 liters/session of
reinfusion fluid while on-line HDF is performed with at least 22–25 liters/
session [17].

Conclusions

Pro-inflammatory cytokines and CRP are independently associated with all-cause and CV mortality in dialysis patients, and the combined determination of CRP and IL-6 seems to be the best option for risk stratification in dialysis patients, particularly in the context of clinical studies. The effect on cumulative survival by HDF provides compelling evidence that adoption of appropriate technologies in HD may benefit patients at a higher risk of morbidity and mortality. Future randomized clinical trials will need to better discern the effects of on-line HDF and the patients to treat based on a risk stratification.

References

1   Reiss AB, Glass AD: Atherosclerosis: immune and inflammatory aspects. J Invest Med 2006; 54:123–131.
2   Arici M, Walls J: End-stage renal disease, atherosclerosis, and cardiovascular mortality: is C-reactive protein the missing link? Kidney Int 2001;59:407–414.
3   Roberts MA, Hare DL, Ratnaike S, Ierino FL: Cardiovascular biomarkers in CKD: pathophysiology and implications for clinical management of cardiac disease. Am J Kidney Dis 2006;48: 341–360.
4   Kaysen GA: The microinflammatory state in uremia: causes and potential consequences. J Am Soc Nephrol 2001;12:1549–1557.
5   Bologa RM, Levine DM, Parker TS, Cheigh JS, Serur D, Stenzel KH, Rubin A: Interleukin-6 predicts hypoalbuminemia, hypocholesterolemia, and mortality in hemodialysis patients. Am J Kidney Dis 1998;32:107–114.
6   Stenvinkel P, Heinburger O, Paultre F, et al: Strong associations between malnutrition, inflammation and atherosclerosis in chronic renal failure. Kidney Int 1999;55:1899–1911.
7   Panichi V, De Pietro S, Andreini B, Migliori M, Tessore V, Taccola D, Rindi P, Palla R, Tetta C: Cytokine production in haemodiafiltration: a multicentre study. Nephrol Dial Transplant 1998; 13:1737–1744.
8   Schouten WEM, Grooteman MPC, van Houte AJ, et al: Effects of dialysers and dialysate on the acute phase reaction in clinical bicarbonate dialysis. Nephrol Dial Transplant 2000;15:379–384.
9   Kerr PG, Sutherland WH, de Jong S, Vaithalingham I, Williams SM, Walker RJ: The impact of standard high-flux polysulfone versus novel high-flux polysulfone dialysis: membranes on inflammatory markers: a randomized, single-blinded, controlled clinical trial. Am J Kidney Dis 2007;49: 533–539.
10 Ollson J, Dadfar E, Paulsson J, Laundahl J, Moshfegh A, Jacobson SH: Preserved leukocyte CD1b expression at the site of interstitial inflammation in patients with high-flux hemodiafiltration. Kidney Int 2007;71:582–588.
11 Carracedo J, Merino A, Nogueras S, Carretero D, Berdud I, Ramirez R, Tetta C, Rodriguez M, Martin-Malo A, Aljama P: On-line hemodiafiltration reduces the proinflammatory CD14+CD16+ monocyte-derived dendritic cells: a prospective, crossover study. J Am Soc Nephrol 2006;17: 2315–2321.
12 Ramirez R, Carracedo J, Merino A, Nogueras S, Alvarez-Lara MA, Rodriguez M, Martin-Malo A, Tetta C, Aljama P: Microinflammation induces endothelial damage in hemodialysis patients: the role of convective transport. Kidney Int 2007;72:109–113.
13 Ganesh SK, Hulbert-Shearon T, Port FK, Eagle K, Stack AG: Mortality differences by dialysis modality among incident ESRD patients with and without coronary artery disease. J Am Soc Nephrol 2003;14:415–424.

14   Rayner HC, Pisoni RL, Bommer J, Canaud B, Hecking E, Locatelli F, et al: Mortality and hospitalization in haemodialysis patients in five European countries: results from the Dialysis Outcomes and Practice Patterns Study (DOPPS). Nephrol Dial Transplant 2004;19:108–120.

15   Shiffl H: Prospective randomized cross-over long-term comparison of online hemodiafiltration and ultrapure high-flux hemodialysis. Eur J Med Res 2007;12:26–33.

16   Canaud B, Bragg-Gresham JL, Marshall MR, Desmeules S, Gillespie BW, Depner T, Klassen P, Port FK: Mortality risk for patients receiving hemodiafiltration versus hemodialysis: European results from the DOPPS. Kidney Int 2006;69:2087–2093.

17   Panichi V, Manca-Rizza G, Paoletti S, Bigazzi R, Aloisi M, Barsotti G, Rindi P, Donati G, Antonelli A, Panicucci E, Tripepi G, Tetta C, Palla R: Chronic inflammation and mortality in hemodialysis: effects of different renal replacement therapies. Results from the RISCAVID study. Nephrol Dial Transplant 2008 (in press).

Vincenzo Panichi, MD
Dipartimento Medicina Interna
Via Roma 67, IT–56100 Pisa (Italy)
Tel. +39 050 992887, Fax +39 050 553414, E-Mail vpanichi@med.unipi.it

Ronco C, Cruz DN (eds): Hemodialysis – From Basic Research to Clinical Trials.
Contrib Nephrol. Basel, Karger, 2008, vol 161, pp 191–198

....

Online Hemodiafiltration: A Multipurpose Therapy for Improving Quality of Renal Replacement Therapy

Bernard Canaud[a,b], Leila Chenine[a], Delphine Henriet[a], Hélène Leray[a]

[a]Lapeyronie Hospital – Nephrology, and [b]Renal Research and Training Institute, Montpellier, France

Abstract

By combining diffusive and enhanced convective clearances, hemodiafiltration (HDF) offers the most efficient and biocompatible renal replacement therapy modality at the present time. HDF increases solute mass transfer and enlarges the molecular weight spectrum of uremic toxins, and reduces the microinflammation profile of dialysis patients. Online (ol) production of substitution fluid by 'cold sterilization' of dialysis fluid gives access to virtually an unlimited amount of sterile and non-pyrogenic solution. ol-HDF provides a multipurpose platform that permits to develop and customize HDF options (HDF, post-, pre-, mixed-, mid-dilution) to patients' needs. With these unique features, ol-HDF should be considered as a dialysis platform permitting to develop new options such as feedback-controlled volemia, automation of priming and restitution and daily treatment schedule. At the present time, ol-HDF offers major options to enhance dialysis efficacy and to improve global care of patients.

Copyright © 2008 S. Karger AG, Basel

Introduction

By combining diffusive and enhanced convective clearances, hemodiafiltration (HDF) offers the most efficient instantaneous solute clearances at the present time. HDF increases instantaneous solute mass transfer and enlarges the molecular weight spectrum of uremic toxins removed [1–4]. By improving the hemocompatibility of the dialysis system, HDF reduces the microinflammation profile of dialysis patients [5, 6]. Online HDF (ol-HDF) is now an established treatment modality that tends to gain in popularity in chronic renal disease patients [7–9].

Online production of substitution fluid by 'cold sterilization' of dialysis fluid gives access to virtually an unlimited amount of sterile and non-pyrogenic solutions [10–12]. Implementing the ol-HDF module onto the hemodialysis machine has several advantages: it simplifies the handling procedure for the nursing staff and technicians; it secures the process by coupling the infusion module to the safety regulation of the HDF monitor; it permits regular control of ultrafilters' integrity [13]. ol-HDF provides a multipurpose platform that permits to develop and customize HDF options (HDF, post-, pre-, mixed-, mid-dilution) to patients' needs [14–16].

Technical Prerequisite and Basic Hygienic Rules for ol-HDF

Safety of the ol-HDF relies on very strict rules of use. Strict compliance with guidelines warrants success of the ol-HDF therapy program.

The use of ultrapure water (UPW) to feed the HDF machine is a basic requirement for online HDF [17]. UPW is high-grade quality water which has been developed mainly to satisfy the needs of the semiconductor industry. For HDF purposes, UPW refers to reverse osmosis-treated water (two stages of reverse osmosis in series) with a resistivity in the range of $10–20\,M\Omega$ with a very low level of bacterial and endotoxin contamination ($\geq 100\,CFU/l$, endotoxin *Limulus* amebocyte lysate $<0.03\,EU/ml$). Distribution pipes must be adequately designed to prevent stagnation, to eliminate dead arms and other recontamination sites. Permanent recirculation of treated water through a closed loop circuit with a microfiltration system is required when a buffer tank is used.

The use of specifically designed HDF- and European Community (EC)-certified machines is necessary. Several ol-HDF-certified machines are presently available on the European market. Basically, these ol-HDF machines share common features that include an infusion pump with a flow-measuring system, a dialysate ultrafilter module (usually two certified ultrafilters in series) placed onto the hydraulic circuit of the machine and controlled by the dialysis machine-monitoring system. The infusate module is a captive part of the machine which is disinfected simultaneously with each process of the HDF machine. The infusate module consists in an adjustable pump running up to 200 ml/min with a counter calculating the total amount of fluid infused to the patient. Ultrapure dialysate flowing into the dialysate compartment of the hemodiafilter is produced through an ultrafilter (UF1) placed just at the exit site of the dialysate [18, 19]. A fraction of the fresh dialysate (100/800 ml/min) produced by the proportioning HDF system is diverted by the infusion pump and infused into the blood of the patient (either post- or pre-filter). Ultrapurity of the infusate is then secured by a second stage ultrafiltration (UF2) placed just before the infusion site located close to the patient. Infusate flow diverted from the inlet dialysate is compensated by an equivalent ultrafiltration flow dragged from the patient thanks to the fluid-balancing module. Ultrafilters are an integral part of the HDF machine that are disinfected after each run and changed periodically.

Hygiene handling is a crucial measure to ensure permanent safety of the HDF system. Frequent disinfection of the water treatment system and dialysis machine, destruction of biofilm by chemical agents and/or thermochemical disinfection, change of filters at regular interval, maintenance of a permanent circulation of water, are among basic measures requested to ensure ultrapurity of water and dialysis fluid.

Quality monitoring of the dialysate and the infusate is mandatory to detect early microbiologic contamination of the system. A microbiologic inventory of water, dialysate and infusate should be performed according to best practice guidelines and pharmacopeia regulation [20, 21].

Prerequisite and Technical Options for ol-HDF

Vascular Access

Patients treated with ol-HDF require a vascular access capable of delivering a blood flow of 350–400 ml/min. High blood flow facilitates ultrafiltration rate and reduces transmembrane pressure (TMP) during the session.

Hemodiafilter

The use of highly permeable dialyzers is mandatory. High hydraulic permeability ($K_{UF} \geq 50$ ml/h/mm Hg) and high solute permeability (K_oA urea >600 and β_2-microglobulin >60 ml/min) with large surface area (1.50–2.10 m²) dialyzers are needed.

Conventional ol-HDF: ol-HDF relies on the combination of diffusive and forced convective clearances in the same hemodiafilter module. Basically, the substitution fluid (infusate) is a sterile non-pyrogenic solution produced extemporaneously from fresh dialysate by double ultrafiltration (cold sterilization process) and infused directly into the patient's blood on the venous site. Infusate diverted from the inlet dialysate is extemporaneously compensated by the fluid-balancing system of the dialysis machine which ultrafilters the same amount of fluid from the patient's blood. High ultrafiltration rate is achieved by the dialysis machine by increasing adequately the TMP applied to the hemodiafilter. Weight loss required to correct patient fluid overload and is taken out in addition by increasing consequently the ultrafiltration rate.

Depending on the infusion site of fluid substitution, several HDF modalities have been described: *post-dilution HDF* (infusion after the hemodiafilter) [22]; *pre-dilution HDF* (infusion before the hemodiafilter), and *mixed HDF* (infusion simultaneous pre- and post-hemodiafilter) [23, 24].

HDF requires use of a high-flux dialyzer and high blood flow (350–450 ml/min) with high dialysate flow (600–800 ml/min). It is recommended to couple the infusion rate to the effective blood flow to optimize filtration fraction (20–30% maximum). Typical infusion flow rates are 100 ml/min (24 liters for a 4-hour session) in post-dilution HDF and 200 ml/min (48 liters for a 4-hour session) in pre-dilution HDF mode, respectively to match urea clearance. Mixed pre- and post-dilution HDF represents a recently introduced technical option. The ratio of pre- to post-infusion flow is feedback-controlled by the HDF monitor (programmed HDF) in order to maintain the TMP in a safe range.

Alternative based convective HDF methods: Several variants of ol-HDF methods have been described over the last decade. They are briefly described in the next section.

Push/pull HDF is based on a double-cylinder piston pump (push/pull pump) implemented on the effluent dialysate line of the dialysis machine. Based on this alternate pump device, 25 alternate cycles of 20 ml of ultrafiltration (pull) and backfiltration (push) are performed through the hemodialyzer per minute, meaning that 120 liters of ultrafiltered plasma water are backfiltered from the fresh inlet dialysate in a 4-hour treatment [25].

Double high-flux HD consists in two high-flux dialyzers assembled in series while the dialysis fluid irrigates countercurrently the two dialyzers [26]. By means of an adjustable clamp restriction placed on the dialysis fluid pathway between the two dialyzers, ultrafiltration is promoted in the first dialyzer and backfiltration in the second dialyzer [27].

Paired hemofiltration is a double-chamber HDF technique that was initially proposed to separate convective and diffusive solute fluxes in two modules [28]. This method is based on the association of two high-flux dialyzers in series, one with a small surface (e.g. 0.4 m^2) that permits the infusion of substitution fluid (backfiltration) and the second high-flux hemodialyzer (1.8 m^2) that allows convective and diffusive exchange from dialysate. The substitution fluid produced by cold sterilization from the fresh dialysis fluid is infused either on pre-dilution mode or on post-dilution mode according to the position of the dialyzer [29].

HDF with endogenous reinfusion (HFR) derives from paired hemofiltration. The main feature of HFR is the online regeneration of the ultrafiltrate by an adsorbing multilayer device [30, 31]. The regenerated ultrafiltrate is then reinfused as an endogenous substitution fluid [32]. HFR has been evaluated in several clinical trials and appears to be beneficial on inflammatory and oxidative stress markers [33, 34].

Mid-dilution HDF is the last option that relies on a newly designed hemodiafilter consisting of two high-flux fiber bundles built in one dialyzer housing [35]. Blood is run countercurrently (ultrafiltration in the first bundle and diffusion in the second bundle) with an infusion performed on the distal head (mid-part of the two bundles). In this version the first part of the module ensures the convective transport (ultrafiltration) and the second part of the module ensures the diffusive transport countercurrently with the dialysate after blood has been diluted in the opposite head of the dialyzer. In order to improve ultrafiltration performances and to reduce TMP, a reverse version of the blood circulation within the filter has been tested successfully in clinic [36].

ol-HDF Prescription in Practice

A conventional ol-HDF treatment schedule based on 3 dialysis sessions per week of 4 h (12 h/week) requires high blood flow (400 ml/min) coupled with high dialysate and/or infusate flow to optimize solute exchange. Increasing frequency and/or duration of HDF sessions may help to enhance the effectiveness and physiological profile of intermittent dialysis.

ol-HDF-treated patients should be observed and monitored as those treated by conventional hemodialysis method. Dialysis adequacy targets are equivalents: extracellular fluid volume control, blood pressure control, minimum dialysis dose delivered (urea $Kt/V_{dp} > 1.2$), uremia control, acidosis and hyperkaliemia correction, phosphorus, calcium and PTH control, and anemia correction.

ol-HDF provides a higher solute removal rate for middle size uremic toxins including β_2-microglobulin (β_2M). Blood β_2M concentrations, considered as a surrogate of middle molecules, should be part of this long-term surveillance. Inflammation (CRP) and nutritional markers (albumin and transthyretin) should be monitored on a monthly basis in ol-HDF patients.

Handling and Microbial Monitoring of ol-HDF

Regular disinfection procedures and water and dialysis fluid monitoring are mandatory for conducting ol-HDF therapies. A complete disinfection of the ol-HDF machine (chemical, heat or mixed) is recommended after each run. Periodical changes of ultrafilters installed on inlet dialysate and infusate lines should be performed according to the manufacturer's instructions. Disinfection of the water treatment system and water distribution circuit should be performed as a minimum on a monthly basis. The type of disinfection (chemical, heat or mixed) and periodicity of disinfection procedures may vary from one center to another but should comply in any case with the manufacturer's recommendations and should be adapted to the microbiological results. More frequent disinfection procedures (daily or weekly) of the water distribution pipe using heat or mixed heat/chemical procedures appears to be the optimal way of preventing bacterial contamination and biofilm formation.

Monitoring the microbiology of the water treatment chain and ol-HDF machines should comply with best practice recommendations and country-specific rules. All recommendations have been reported in detail in the European Best Practices Guidelines. They represent the most comprehensive and update guidelines that should be applied to secure the ol-HDF method [37]. Water feeding the HDF machines should be checked weekly during the validation phase and at least monthly during the surveillance and maintenance period. Dialysate and infusate produced by proportioning ol-HDF machines should be performed at least every 3 months. Microbiological monitoring should include the culture of water and/or dialysate and the determination of endotoxin content. Sampling method, culture media and delay for observation have been published elsewhere. Membrane filtration and culture on a poor nutrient media (R2A) are strongly recommended [20, 38]. Cultures are maintained at room temperature (20–22°C) and observed for 7 days. Bacteria colony count and identification should be performed with appropriate methods. Endotoxin content (infusate and dialysate) should be performed with a sensitive *Limulus* amebocyte lysate assay with a threshold detection limit of 0.03 EU/ml.

Conclusions

At the present time, ol-HDF modalities offer the most effective renal replacement modality for CKD-5 patients [39–41]. By enhancing the convective fluxes, ol-HDF enlarges the spectrum and increases the uremic toxin mass removed. ol-HDF improves the hemocompatibility profile, reduces the cost of treatment and simplifies the technical aspect of the method. With these unique features, ol-HDF should be considered a dialysis platform permitting to develop new options such as feedback-controlled volemia and automation of priming and restitution. At present, ol-HDF offers major options to enhance dialysis efficacy and to improve global care of patients [42].

References

1   Sprenger KB: Haemodiafiltration. Life Support Syst 1983;1:127–136.
2   Ofsthun NJ, Leypoldt JK: Ultrafiltration and backfiltration during hemodialysis. Artif Organs 1995;19:1143–1161.
3   Leypoldt JK: Solute fluxes in different treatment modalities. Nephrol Dial Transplant 2000;1:3–9.
4   Ledebo I: On-line hemodiafiltration: technique and therapy. Adv Ren Replace Ther 1999;6:195–208.
5   Canaud B, Bosc JY, Leray H, Stec F, Argiles A, Leblanc M, Mion C: On-line haemodiafiltration: state of the art. Nephrol Dial Transplant 1998;5:3–11.
6   Canaud B, Wizemann V, Pizzarelli F, Greenwood R, Schultze G, Weber C, Falkenhagen D: Cellular interleukin-1 receptor antagonist production in patients receiving on-line haemodiafiltration therapy. Nephrol Dial Transplant 2001;16:2181–2187.
7   Leber HW, Wizemann V, Goubeaud G, Rawer P, Schutterle G: Hemodiafiltration: a new alternative to hemofiltration and conventional hemodialysis. Artif Organs 1978;2:150–153.
8   Passlick-Deetjen J, Pohlmeier R: On-line hemodiafiltration. Gold standard or top therapy? Contrib Nephrol. Basel, Karger, 2002, vol 137, pp 201–211.
9   Van Laecke S, De Wilde K, Vanholder R: Online hemodiafiltration. Artif Organs 2006;30:579–585.
10 Henderson LW, Sanfelippo ML, Beans E: 'On-line' preparation of sterile pyrogen-free electrolyte solution. Transactions ASAIO 1978;24:465–467.
11 Shinzato T, Sezaki R, Usuda M, Maeda K, Ohbayashi S, Toyota T: Infusion-free hemodiafiltration: simultaneous hemofiltration and dialysis with no need for infusion fluid. Artif Organs 1982;6;4: 453–456.
12 Canaud B, Flavier JL, Argilés A, Stec F, Nguyen QV, Bouloux C, Garred LJ, Mion C: Hemodiafiltration with on-line production of substitution fluid: long-term safety and quantitative assessment of efficacy. Contrib Nephrol. Basel, Karger, 1994, vol 108, pp 12–22.
13 Canaud B, Nguyen QV, Argilés A, Polito C, Polaschegg HD, Mion C: Hemodiafiltration using dialysate as substitution fluid. Artif Organs 1987;11:188–190.
14 Sterby J: A decade of experience with on-line hemofiltration/hemodiafiltration. Contrib Nephrol. Basel, Karger, 1994, vol 108, pp 1–11.
15 Lonnemann G, Behme TC, Lenzner B, Floege J, Schulze M, Colton CK, Koch KM, Shaldon S: Permeability of dialyzer membranes to TNF-α-inducing substances derived from water bacteria. Kidney Int 1992;42:61–68.
16 Canaud B, Imbert E, Kaaki M, Assounga A, Nguyen QV, Stec F, Garred LJ, Boström M, Mion C: Clinical and microbiological evaluation of a postdilutional hemofiltration system with in-line production of substitution fluid. Blood Purif 1990;8:160–170.
17 Canaud B, Peyronnet P, Armynot AM, et al: Ultrapure water: a need for future dialysis. Nephrol Dial Transplant 1986;1:110.
18 Schindler R, Lonnemann G, Schaffer J, Shaldon S, Koch KM, Krautzig S: The effect of ultrafiltered dialysate on the cellular content of interleukin-1 receptor antagonist in patients on chronic hemodialysis. Nephron 1994;68;2:229–233.
19 Mion CM, Canaud B: Should hemodialysis fluid be sterile? Semin Dial 1993;6:28–30.
20 Ward RA, Luehmann DA, Klein E: Are current standards for the microbiological purity of hemodialysate adequate? Semin Dial 1989;2:69–72.
21 Pass T, Wright R, Sharp B, Harding GB: Culture of dialysis fluids on nutrient-rich media for short periods at elevated temperatures underestimate microbial contamination. Blood Purif 1996;14: 136–145.
22 Canaud B, Lévesque R, Krieter D, Desmeules S, Chalabi L, Moragués H, Morena M, Cristol JP: On-line hemodiafiltration as routine treatment of end-stage renal failure: why pre- or mixed dilution mode is necessary in on-line hemodiafiltration today? Blood Purif 2004;22(suppl 2):40–48.
23 Pedrini LA, De Cristofaro V, Pagliari B, et al: Mixed predilution and postdilution online hemodiafiltration compared with the traditional infusion modes. Kidney Int 2000;58:2155.
24 Feliciani A, Riva MA, Zerbi S, Ruggiero P, Plati AR, Cozzi G, Pedrini LA: New strategies in haemodiafiltration (HDF): prospective comparative analysis between on-line mixed HDF and mid-dilution HDF. Nephrol Dial Transplant 2007;22:1672–1679.

25 Miwa M, Shinzato T: Push/pull hemodiafiltration: technical aspects and clinical effectiveness. Artif Organs 1999;23:1123.

26 Von Albertini B, Miller JH, Gardner PW, Shinaberger JH: Performance characteristics of the hemoflow F60 in high-flux hemodiafiltration. Contrib Nephrol. Basel, Karger, 1985, vol 46, pp 169–173.

27 Pisitkun T, Eiam-Ong S, Tiranathanagul K, Sakunsrijinda C, Manotham K, Hanvivatvong O, Suntaranuson P, Praditpornsilpa K, Chusil S, Tungsanga K: Convective-controlled double high-flux hemodiafiltration: a novel blood purification modality. Int J Artif Organs 2004;27:195–204.

28 Ghezzi PM, Botella J, Sartoris AM, et al: Use of the ultrafiltrate obtained in two-chamber (PFD) hemodiafiltration as replacement fluid. Experimental ex vivo and in vitro study. Int J Artif Organs 1991;14:327.

29 Pizzarelli F: Paired hemodiafiltration. Contrib Nephrol. Basel, Karger, 2007, 158, pp 131–137.

30 Marinez de Francisco AL, Ghezzi PM, Brendolan A, Fiorini F, La Greca G, Ronco C, Arias M, Gervasio R, Tetta C: Hemodiafiltration with online regeneration of the ultrafiltrate. Kidney Int Suppl 2000;76:S66–S71.

31 De Francisco AL, Pinera C, Heras M, Rodrigo E, Fernandez G, Ruiz JC, Tetta C, Arias M: Hemodafiltration with on-line endogenous reinfusion. Blood Purif 2000;18:231–236.

32 Marinez de Francisco AL, Ghezzi PM, Brendolan A, Fiorini F, La Greca G, Ronco C, Arias M, Gervasio R, Tetta C: Hemodiafiltration with online regeneration of the ultrafiltrate. Kidney Int Suppl 2000;76:S66–S71.

33 Panichi V, Manca-Rizza G, Paoletti S, Taccola D, Consani C, Filippi C, Mantuano E, Sidoti A, Grazi G, Antonelli A, Angelini D, Petrone I, Mura C, Tolaini P, Saloi F, Ghezzi PM, Barsotti G, Palla R: Effects on inflammatory and nutritional markers of haemodiafiltration with online regeneration of ultrafiltrate (HFR) vs. online haemodiafiltration: a cross-over randomized multicentre trial. Nephrol Dial Transplant 2006;21:756–762.

34 Calò LA, Naso A, Carraro G, Wratten ML, Pagnin E, Bertipaglia L, Rebeschini M, Davis PA, Piccoli A, Cascone C: Effect of haemodiafiltration with online regeneration of ultrafiltrate on oxidative stress in dialysis patients. Nephrol Dial Transplant 2007;22:1413–1419.

35 Krieter DH, Falkenhain S, Chalabi L, Collins G, Lemke HD, Canaud B: Clinical cross-over comparison of mid-dilution hemodiafiltration using a novel dialyzer concept and post-dilution hemodiafiltration. Kidney Int 2005;67:349–356.

36 Santoro A, Ferramosca E, Mancini E, Monari C, Varasani M, Sereni L, Wratten M: Reverse mid-dilution: new way to remove small and middle molecules as well as phosphate with high intrafilter convective clearance. Nephrol Dial Transplant 2007;22:2000–2005.

37 European Best Practice Guidelines for Haemodialysis (Part 1). Section IV. Dialysis fluid purity. Nephrol Dial Transplant 2002;1(suppl 7):45–62.

38 Pass T, Wright R, Sharp B, Harding GB: Culture of dialysis fluids on nutrient-rich media for short periods at elevated temperatures underestimate microbial contamination. Blood Purif 1996;14:136–145.

39 Golper TA: What technological advances will significantly alter the future care of dialysis patients? Semin Dial 1994;7:323–324.

40 Canaud B, Kerr P, Argilés A, Flavier JL, Stec F, Mion C: Is hemodiafiltration the dialysis modality of choice for the next decade? Kidney Int 1993;43(suppl 41):S296–S299.

41 Van der Weerd NC, Penne EL, van den Dorpel MA, Grooteman MP, Nube MJ, Bots ML, Ter Wee PM, Blankestijn PJ: Haemodiafiltration: promise for the future? Nephrol Dial Transplant 2008;23:438–443.

42 Henderson LW: Dialysis in the 21st century. Am J Kidney Dis 1996;28:951–957.

Prof. Bernard Canaud
Nephrology, Dialysis and Intensive Care
Hôpital Lapeyronie, CHU Montpellier, 371, Av du Doyen G. Giraud
FR–34925 Montpellier Cedex 05 (France)
Tel. +33 467 338 955, Fax +33 467 603 783, E-Mail b-canaud@chu-montpellier.fr

Ronco C, Cruz DN (eds): Hemodialysis – From Basic Research to Clinical Trials.
Contrib Nephrol. Basel, Karger, 2008, vol 161, pp 199–209

....

Biofeedback-Driven Dialysis: Where Are We?

Antonio Santoro, Emiliana Ferramosca, Elena Mancini

Malpighi Division of Nephrology, Dialysis, Hypertension, Policlinico
S.Orsola-Malpighi, Bologna, Italy

Abstract

The progressive increase in the mean age and the growing conditions of co-morbidity, especially of cardiovascular pathologies and diabetes, have significantly worsened the patients' clinical status and tolerance to the hemodialysis (HD) treatment. On the other hand, the demand for short treatment times enhances the risk for hemodynamic instability as well as for inadequate depuration. The traditional management of the dialysis session, setting of pre-defined treatment parameters, with active therapeutic interventions only in the event of complications, is definitely unsuitable for short-lasting treatments, often complicated by hemodynamic instability, especially in critical patients. The first step to improve the management of the dialysis session is the utilization of continuous and uninvasive monitoring systems for hemodynamic or biochemical parameters involved in the dialysis quality. Special sensors for the continuous measurement of blood volume, blood temperature, blood pressure, heart rate, electrolytes, have been realized throughout the last 10 years. As a second step, some of these devices have been implemented in the dialysis instrumentation, mainly with a view to preventing cardiocirculatory instability but also to control the dialysis efficiency (biofeedback control systems). The basic components of a biofeedback system are: the plant, the sensors, the actuators and the controller. The plant is the biological process that we need to control, while the sensors are the devices used for measuring the output variables. The actuators are the working arms of the controller. The controller is the mathematical model that continuously sets the measured output variable against the reference input and modifies the actuators in order to reduce any discrepancies. Yet, in practice there are a number of conceptual, physical and technological difficulties to be overcome. In particular, the behavior of what is to be controlled may be non-linear and time-varying, with interactions between the actuators and the controlled variable. In these cases, more sophisticated control systems are needed, which must be capable of identifying the behavior of the process, and continuously update information data while the control is on. These complex systems are called *adaptive controllers*. In dialysis, over the last few years, it has been relatively easy to realize some biofeedback systems since a series of sensors have been developed for online monitoring. Three biofeedback devices are routinely used with the aim of improving the cardiovascular instability, one of the main problems limiting the tolerance to treatment by the patient and the quality of HD in itself – the first is the biofeedback control of blood volume, the second is the biofeedback control of thermal balance, and the third is the biofeedback control of blood pressure.

Monitoring and Controlling Hemodiaysis

The progressive increase in the mean age and the growing conditions of co-morbidity, especially of cardiovascular pathologies and diabetes, has significantly increased the patients' critical status. On the other hand, the demand for short treatment times enhances the risk for hemodynamic instability as well as for inadequate depuration.

Over the past decade, dialysis industries have developed systems for *online intradialytic monitoring*, aiming to prevent critical situations and to continuously measure various hemodynamic and biochemical parameters of the patient [1]. The online monitoring systems have been most useful in high-efficiency, short-lasting dialysis techniques, since the risk of being 'unphysiological' is so much greater when the treatment times are shortened while at the same time increasing the efficiency. In such conditions there is the need to guarantee at least two objectives: (1) the adequacy of the *cardiocirculatory response* in terms of the progressive withdrawal of the fluids that guarantee a certain degree of hemodynamic stability, and (2) the overlapping of the *actually delivered dialysis dose* with the scheduled one.

It is thus necessary to dispose of adequate measurement devices and 'sensors' for continuous measures during the dialysis sessions, with essential characteristics such as simplicity of use, sterility and biocompatibility (for the sensors that come into direct contact with the blood), the possibility to interface the measurement system with a computer and, lastly, an acceptable cost. Another important prerequisite is its absolute non-invasiveness and tolerability on the part of the patient.

Some devices for continuous hemodynamic or biochemical monitoring can be implemented in the dialysis instrumentation in order to prevent cardio-circulatory instability (acute hypotension, arrhythmias) or control and improve the dialysis efficiency.

The feedback systems with a practical routine application are substantially three: the blood volume biofeedback, the thermal balance biofeedback, and the arterial pressure biofeedback.

Blood Volume Biofeedback

The blood volume (BV) behavior during dialysis has been extensively described mathematically [2] and several factors influencing and modifying BV

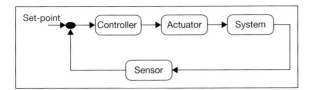

Fig. 1. Schematic representation of a closed-loop system. In a closed-loop system, the variable to be controlled is continuously measured by a sensor and the action on the controller is determined by the difference between the desired and the measured value of the system variables. In this case, it is not necessary to know in detail the model of the system to achieve the desired point. Often, only the knowledge of a simplified input-output relationship is sufficient. This way is in general much less sensitive to external noise as well as to internal system variations, because the deviations from the imposed set values are first measured then compensated for by the action of the controller on the system inputs.

changes throughout dialysis treatment have been identified [3]. Among these, ultrafiltration and changes in the dialysate sodium concentration are, however, the major and the most important dialysis variables in the control of volemia during dialysis treatment [4, 5]. On the other hand, ultrafiltration profiling can have a beneficial impact on blood pressure behavior during hemodialysis (HD).

We have recently modified, along with the Gambro-Hospal research group, our first automatic BV control system based on variable ultrafiltration [6]. This feedback control system is based on an adaptive controller, capable of forcing the spontaneous volemia trends along preselected trajectories by means of ultrafiltration and sodium. This model is *closed loop system* (fig. 1), with a dependent output variable or *controlled variable*, i.e. volemia, and two independent or *control variables*, i.e. ultrafiltration and conductivity [7].

The relative BV changes are measured continuously during dialysis by an optical absorbance system [8].

Simultaneously, the following parameters are continuously calculated: (1) the mathematical coefficients that link the controlled variable to the control variables; (2) the instantaneous errors in the actual BV trajectory as compared with the ideal one, and (3) the differences in the body weight loss first prescribed and then achieved and their relationships with BV reductions.

If substantial errors occur, the model automatically updates both the ultrafiltration rate and the conductivity, minimizing any possible discrepancies between the ideal volemia trajectories and the experimentally obtained ones, and any relevant errors in the patients' body weight reductions.

At the core of the system is a MIMO, multi-input, multi-output controller, in which all the branches are linearly controlled with adapted parameters (fig. 2). The adaptive controller manages three kinds of error: errors on the volemia, on

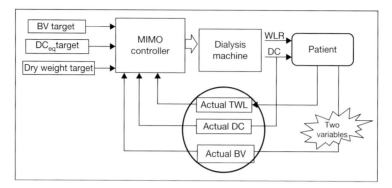

Fig. 2. The blood volume (BV) biofeedback with the multi-input and multi-output controller (MIMO controller). The BV biofeedback system consists in the setting of three clinical objectives: the total weight loss (TWL) for the restoration of the dry weight; the variation of the BV for the preservation of cardiovascular stability, and the equivalent dialysate conductivity (DC) to maintain a desired sodium balance. According to the biofeedback architecture, similar parameters are continuously measured: variations in the BV, total weight loss and equivalent conductivity. With this information the physiological controller adjusts continuously the ultrafiltration rate and the dialysate conductivity.

the total weight loss, and on dialysate conductivity. Ultrafiltration and conductivity can fluctuate only within a well-defined range, established at the start of the treatment according to the patients' clinical characteristics.

Moreover, the overall system allows to prescribe adequate ultrafiltration in order to achieve the ideal body weight in the individual patients along with personalized intradialytic sodium balance.

From a clinical point of view, biofeedback in BV regulation has several aims: (i) to avoid reaching serious and major contractions in BV; reductions over 25% should be avoided owing to the greater risk of intradialytic hypotension; (ii) modeling the volemia curves in patients with plasma refilling instability and non-homogeneous and non-linear plasma volume trends during dialysis; (iii) to avoid, in patients with cardiovascular instability, the reaching of critical hypovolemia thresholds independently of their absolute value, and (iv) to modulate the sodium balance and the patient's dehydration.

Biofeedback BV controlled HD is now possible with this system in routine dialysis, allowing the delivery of a more physiologically acceptable treatment.

Blood volume tracking (BVT) was validated by a multicenter cross-over study, involving our center and nine other Italian nephrology units, carried out in 36 patients with a high degree of cardiovascular co-morbidity and suffering from frequent dialysis-induced hypotensive episodes [9]. In this study the cardio-circulatory stability during dialysis was compared in two different treatments:

conventional dialysis (A) and dialysis with BVT (B). Each patient was randomly assigned either to a sequence A-B-A-B or B-A-B-A, each period lasting 4 weeks. At the end of the study a 30% reduction of dialysis hypotension incidence resulted in dialysis with the BVT system. The effect was particularly evident in patients with the highest number of hypotensive events in conventional dialysis (hypotension episodes reduction up to 65%). We also observed 10% overall reduction in interdialysis symptoms (thirst, cramps, fatigue, etc.). Body weight gain, pre-dialysis blood pressure, and Kt/V did not differ between the two treatments.

Our results were confirmed by Basile et al. [10] who also compared conventional HD with biofeedback equipped dialysis in 19 patients, in the short-medium term. They found out a reduction of both acute hypotension and muscle cramps and a significant difference in post-dialysis asthenia. The residual percentage reduction in BV divided by the percentage change in extracellular fluid volume (measured by a bioimpedance technique) was significantly higher during HD with biofeedback, suggesting a better capacity of refilling in dialysis with BV control.

Ronco et al. [11], besides observing similar results in terms of hypotension prevention, reported also better values of equilibrated Kt/V in BV controlled HD, with a striking reduction in post-dialysis percentage urea rebound (6.4 ± 2.3 vs. $14.2 \pm 2.7\%$, in BV controlled and standard HD, respectively). Hence, the better hemodynamic stability obtained with the biofeedback reflects positively in terms of HD efficacy: it reduces solute compartmentalization and favors a better blood flow distribution within the body. As a consequence, the amount of urea accessible to the dialyzer is greater, and greater is the amount actually removed.

Body Temperature Biofeedback

Since the thermal exchange processes between blood and heated dialysate may have an impact on different hemodynamic parameters of HD patients, intradialytic hemodynamics can also be improved with a blood temperature control.

The standard dialysate temperature setting of approximately 37°C does not take into account that most uremic patients tend to be slightly hypothermic. Consequently, in several HD treatments, an unwanted positive thermal energy balance is applied to the patient, which may provoke or contribute to symptomatic hypotension.

Maggiore et al. [12] observed an improved vascular response during cooled dialysate or during isolated ultrafiltration in comparison with conventional hemodialysis. Recently, Rosales et al. [13] have shown that the amount of thermal energy to be removed for an isothermic HD correlates with ultrafiltration. The prevalence of symptomatic hypotension is comparable in hemodialysis and isolated ultrafiltration, if the core temperature is stabilized.

There is some potential for thermal energy to accumulate *within* a hemodialysis treatment. Basically, there are three possibilities for intradialytic heat accumulation: (i) delivery of thermal energy by the extracorporeal system; (ii) increase in the metabolic rate; (iii) decreased dissipation of heat from the body surface during hemodialysis and ultrafiltration.

The reduced transfer of metabolic heat from the body core to the body shell is essentially caused by cutaneous vasoconstriction as a compensation for ultrafiltration-induced hypovolemia. However, if the heat accumulation increases beyond a critical threshold, the increase in the thermoregulatory drive will lead to an increase in cutaneous blood flow and BV which will reduce peripheral resistances, leading to a fall in blood pressure, and an increased risk of intradialytic morbid events.

This additional cardiovascular stress can be avoided by the controlled adaptation of dialysate temperature to the individual needs of an individual patient. The target should be a negative extracorporeal heat balance throughout the treatment. A manual adjustment of the dialysate temperature is not practical for routine application. In practice, it is necessary to realize a biofeedback system able to individualize and continuously adjust the dialysate temperature in order to keep a predefined patient temperature.

A practical realization is now available with the BTM *(blood temperature monitor)*, by Fresenius. Short sections of the extracorporeal circulation are inserted into arterial and venous measuring heads equipped with sensors to measure arterial and venous temperature. The body temperature control is exerted by a controller, that uses the error signals between the desired and actual changes in temperature to actuate a bounded change in dialysate temperature, which changes the temperature of the venous blood returning to the patient, thereby changing the extracorporeal heat flow.

Two active operational modes are possible with the BTM used as a closed-loop device: E-control and T-control. In the E-control modality the BTM controls the thermal energy balance of the extracorporeal circuit. The desired energy balances are keyed into the BTM by selecting a certain heat flux in kilojoules/hour over the treatment time (internal limits: -500 and $+200$ kJ/h). From the therapeutical point, E-control with a set parameter of 0 kJ/h is a useful tool, if the medical intention is to exclude any thermal influence from the extracorporeal circuit.

In T-control mode, the BTM tries to influence the patient's body temperature directly by assessing the body temperature of the patient and applying the respective dialysate temperature changes according to a preset temperature goal. This goal can be keyed into the BTM's panel by setting a certain body temperature change per time ($\pm \times$ °C/h; internal limits: -2 and $+1$°C/h). Setting the BTM goal to ± 0°C consequently stabilizes the patient's body temperature at the temperature level which was present when the active control program was started.

Maggiore et al. [14] have documented the benefits, in hypotension-prone HD patients, in terms of reduction of hypotension episodes of isoenergetic dialysis as compared with the thermoneutral treatment mode. In isoenergetic treatment the patient temperature was keep constant throughout the treatment.

Moreover, patients with left ventricular hypertrophy (LVH) seem to have more benefit from 'cold' HD compared to patients without. In fact, a reduction in the dialysis hypotension incidence was observed in as much as 86% of the patients with LVH (left ventricular mass >125 g/m^2), and in 62% of the patient without LVH, which was a statistically significant different [pers. unpubl. observations].

A hypothesis for this different effect could be seen in the fact that hypertrophic ventricle may present, during HD with concomitant UF, an inadequate filling, secondary to impaired relaxation. The reduced peripheral venous pooling, due to the cold-induced increase in venous tone, may favor the venous return to heart and the filling of the cardiac chambers, thereby maintaining an adequate cardiac output and blood pressure.

Different thermal balance characterizes convective and diffusive treatments, with the more negative one observed in cold hemodialysis (dialysate 35.5°C) and post-dilution hemofiltration (infusate 37°C) [15].

Arterial Blood Pressure Biofeedback

The arterial pressure control is definitely the most ambitious objective in the management of a dialysis session. So far, the continuous arterial pressure systems are invasive, so it is not thinkable to apply them in the routine dialysis.

B. Braun Co. have created a measuring system of arterial pressure that is a little more sophisticated than the normal cuff instruments, and a feedback control of arterial pressure based on ultrafiltration as the actuator. The feedback control measures arterial pressure and its trend during the treatment and an accurate regulation of ultrafiltration finalized to the maintenance of an adequate BV. The controller is based on fuzzy logic. Fuzzy logic does not work on the binary logic but allows for continuous and gradual transitions from 0 to 1. The fuzzy controller allows the modulation of ultrafiltration proportionally to the variation trend in the arterial pressure and so small variations in blood pressure

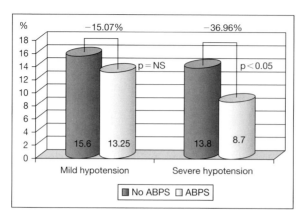

Fig. 3. Comparison of the frequency of hypotension episodes (severe and mild) in dialysis sessions without and with the automatic blood pressure stabilization system (ABPS). A significant difference between the two modalities was observed in the appearance severe hypotension events (−36.96% in ABPS dialysis).

are matched by small variations in ultrafiltration or the maintenance of a constant ultrafiltration, while large pressure variations are matched by large variations in the ultrafiltration. When the controller highlights a negative trend in the blood pressure it reduces the ultrafiltration to the extent of reducing it to zero when there is no pressure recovery.

We performed a clinical multicenter, prospective, controlled, randomized trial, based on the application of this system, known as APBS (Automatic Blood Pressure Stabilization System) in a group of patients with pressure instability. This system was efficacious in reducing the symptomatic intradialytic hypotension in 55 hypotension-prone HD patients (fig. 3); this is likely to be linked to the prevention of large reductions in the BV [16].

Biochemical Monitoring and Control

The need to verify the quality of the delivered treatment can only be satisfied by the use of systems aimed at the real-time monitoring of actual urea clearance (dialysis efficiency) and solute removal (dialyzer performance), using special biosensors.

An *indirect measurement* of the urea clearance can be obtained with the ionic dialysance *(total effective dialysance)* that can be measured *conducimetrically*. Conducimetric dialysance represents the effective dialyzer clearance, which does not take the vascular access and cardiopulmonary recirculation into account.

Further possibilities for monitoring dialysis efficiency can only be superseded by the real-time monitoring of urea concentration, by using dedicated urea sensors measuring urea directly on the extracorporeal circuit.

Continuous urea monitoring can now be carried out on the ultrafiltrate by means of a device that can only be used during *paired filtration dialysis*, where the urea concentration is wholly comparable to the plasma water concentration.

The measurement system consists of: (i) a conductivity cell measuring UF conductivity; (ii) a urea sensor containing urease, an enzyme inducing the complete hydrolysis of UF urea with production of ammonium ions, and (iii) a second conductivity cell which detects the UF conductivity changes induced by the ammonium ions.

The conductivity difference between the two cells correlates well to the UF urea concentration. The continuous intradialytic measurement of the urea concentration allows to calculate kinetic parameters, such as Kt/V and dialytic time-averaged urea concentration. Hence, this is a true 'quality control' of the treatment, with the possibility to check, in real-time, that the prescribed and the administered dialysis dose do actually overlap, and, eventually, modify the parameter prescription in order to avoid situations of underdialysis.

Conclusions

The technological innovation in the dialysis field in the past few years has allowed for the realization of sophisticated biofeedback systems, based on the continuous measurement of the physical variables such as body temperature or hemodynamic variables such as the BV and the arterial pressure. These systems have been implanted and used successfully in the day-to-day dialysis practice, above all in the management of the 'difficult' and unstable patients.

In our opinion, however, the future must look at an integration of the already existing system and the completion with other physical and chemical variables that are essential for a physiological dialysis (fig. 4). Only by means of a more accurate and complete monitoring and adaptive control of the patient during the dialysis session will it be possible to make the process of renal replacement therapy more physiological, with traditional times and methods. A similar system, integrated into the dialysis machine, is today impossible to create. Unfortunately, the continuous increase in demand for renal replacement therapies and the even lower availability of economic resources hamper the diffusion of long dialyses and extremely frequent ones, so it is quite likely that we should increasingly look at technology for a helping hand.

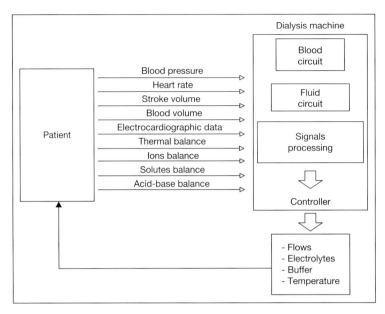

Fig. 4. Integrated adaptive control with a schematic view of the monitored variables and the controller dedicated to signal processing and dialysis machine control.

References

1   Santoro A: On-line monitoring. Nephrol Dial Transpl 1995;10:615–618.
2   Kimura G, Van Stone JC, Baven J: Model prediction of plasma volume change induced by hemodialysis. J Lab Clin Med 1984;104:932–938.
3   Scheneditz D, Roob J, Oswald M, Pogglitsch H: Nature and role of vascular refilling during hemodialysis and ultrafiltration. Kidney Int 1992;42:1425–1433.
4   Mancini E, Santoro A, Spongano M, Paolini F, Rossi M, Zucchelli P: Continuous on-line optical absorbance recording of blood volume changes during hemodialysis. Artif Organs 1993;17: 691–694.
5   Santoro A, Spongano M, Mancini E, Rossi M, Paolini F, Zucchelli P: Parameter estimator and adaptive controller to regulate intra-dialytic blood volume trends. Kidney Int 1992;41:1446.
6   Santoro A, Mancini E, Paolini F, Spongano M, Zucchelli P: Automatic control of blood volume trends during hemodialysis. ASAIO J 1994;40:M419–M422.
7   Santoro A, Mancini E, Paolini F, Cavicchioli G, Bosetto A, Zucchelli P: Blood volume regulation during hemodialysis. Am J Kidney Dis 1998;32:739–748.
8   Paolini F, Mancini E, Bosetto A, Santoro A: Hemoscan™: a dialysis machine-integrated blood volume monitoring. Int J Artif Organs 1995;18:487–494.
9   Santoro A, Mancini E, Basile C, Amoroso L, Di Giulio S, Usberti M, Colasanti G, Verzetti G Rocco A, Imbasciati E, Panzetta G, Bolani R, Grandi F, Polacchini M: Blood volume controlled hemodialysis in hypotension-prone patients: a randomized, multicenter controlled trial. Kidney Int 2002;62:1034–1045.
10 Basile C, Giordano R, Vernaglione L: Efficacy and safety of hemodialysis treatment with the Hemocontrol biofeedback system: a prospective medium-term study. Nephrol Dial Transplant 2001;16:328–334.

11 Ronco C, Brendolan A, Milan M, Rodeghiero M, Zanella M, La Greca G: Impact of biofeedback-induced cardiovascular stability on hemodialysis tolerance and efficiency. Kidney Int 2000;58: 800–808.

12 Maggiore Q, Pizzarelli F, Zoccali C: Influence of blood temperature on vascular stability during hemodialysis and isolated ultrafiltration. Int J Artif Organs 1985;8:175–178.

13 Rosales LM, Schneditz D, Morris AT, Rahmati S, Levin NW: Isothermic hemodialysis and ultrafiltration. Am J Kidney Dis 2000;36:353–361.

14 Maggiore Q, Pizzarelli F, Santoro A, Panzetta G, Bonforte G, Hannedouche T, de Lara MA, Tsouras I, Loureiro A, Ponce P, Solkovà S, Van Roost G, Brink H, Kwan JT: The effects of control of thermal balance on vascular stability in hemodialysis patients: results of the European randomized clinical trial. Am J Kidney Dis 2002;40:280–290.

15 Santoro A, Mancini E, Canova C, Mambelli E: Thermal balance in convective therapies. Nephrol Dial Transplant 2003;18(suppl 7):vii41–vii45.

16 Mancini E, Mambelli E, Santoro A: An automatic system based on fuzzy logic for the control of intradialytic hypotension. Nephrol Dial Transplant 2003;18(suppl 4):418.

Antonio Santoro, MD
Malpighi Division of Nephrology, Dialysis, Hypertension
Policlinico S. Orsola-Malpighi, Via P. Palagi, 9
IT–40138 Bologna (Italy)
Tel. +39 051 6362430, Fax +39 051 6362511, E-Mail antonio.santoro@aosp.bo.it

Ronco C, Cruz DN (eds): Hemodialysis – From Basic Research to Clinical Trials.
Contrib Nephrol. Basel, Karger, 2008, vol 161, pp 210–214

....

Calcium and Phosphorus Kinetics in Hemodialysis Therapy

Frank Gotch

Renal Research Institute, New York, N.Y., USA

Abstract

The kinetics of interdialytic calcium (Ca) absorption and intradialytic flux are examined with particular emphasis on achievement of near zero Ca mass balance over complete dialysis cycles. It is concluded that a rational approach to management of mineral metabolism in hemodialysis consists of: (1) appropriate doses of vitamin D_3 analogs to facilitate now normal Ca absorption and avoid both Ca overload and depletion; (2) adequate phosphorus (P) binder to normalize serum calcium and the Ca•P product; (3) in most instances modest reduction of dialysate Ca to the level of 2.00–2.25 are appropriate to assure zero Ca balance, and (4) use of a calcimimetic to control secondary hyperparathyroidism.

Patients undergoing hemodialysis (HD) frequently develop calcification of the media of their arteries which is strongly associated with adverse cardiovascular outcomes and is widely considered to be associated with excess body content of calcium (Ca) and phosphorus (P) [1–5]. It is recognized that body overload of Ca can occur in the absence of elevated serum Ca [1, 2], which emphasizes the need to quantify Ca balance in these patients which in turn requires reliable estimates of net Ca absorption (or loss) between dialyses and net Ca removal (or accumulation) during dialyses. Thus rational management of mineral metabolism in HD must be based on quantitative evaluation of the following aspects of therapy: (1) intake of Ca and P; (2) absorption of Ca and P; (3) removal of Ca and P during dialysis, and (4) inhibition of secondary hyperparathyroidism (sHPT).

Intake of Ca and P

All patients should have diet prescriptions which limit Ca intake to 500 mg/day and P intake to <1,000 mg/day as per DOQI guidelines. Patients with hyperphosphatemia and a need for high doses of P binders will often have high PCRs [6] and substantial ingestion of dairy products. Diet recalls and urea kinetic modeling can be very helpful in assessing these aspects of control.

Absorption of Phosphorus

Approximately 85–90% of dietary P is passively absorbed. It is not strongly influenced by vitamin D analogs so the only effective way to limit P uptake is control of dietary intake.

Absorption of Calcium

Ca absorption is strongly dependent on the active forms of vitamin D. A series of Ca absorption studies was performed some 25 years ago at Baylor University [7–9] showing that the bulk of Ca absorption is vitamin D dependent. An analysis of one of these studies [8] is shown in figure 1. Figure 1a shows the authors' data expressed as fractional absorption for two levels of Ca intake (120 and 300 mg) at three different levels of calcitriol (C_3). The mean values of these points at the two levels of intake form virtually perfect logarithmic regressions which are strongly dependent on the level of C_3 and indicate a C_3-mediated active transport system for Ca absorption. In figure 1b the curves in figure 1a are used to compute a family of Ca absorption values as a function of C_3 and the two levels of diet intake. A third point is shown (y = x) at very low level of intake where active absorption can be considered complete. The family of points in figure 1b can be used to develop the family of logarithmic absorption curves depicted in figure 1c. Finally, the same authors extended the measurements of Ca absorption in normal subjects to include 1,000 mg of Ca as calcium acetate ($CaAc_2$) [9] with results shown as curve for $C_3 = 40$ in figure 1c. Both the efficacy of P binding by $CaAc_2$ and the magnitude of Ca absorption have been extensively studied [9] and hence well known which makes it an attractive binder in terms of estimating mass balance.

Figure 1c graphically depicts the need to target low-dose C_3 to avoid excessive absorption in the case of both Ca-based and non-Ca-based binders. Note that the absorption curves are quite flat over the range of 500–2,000 mg/day intake but that they increase sharply as C_3 increases. The dose of C_3 required to

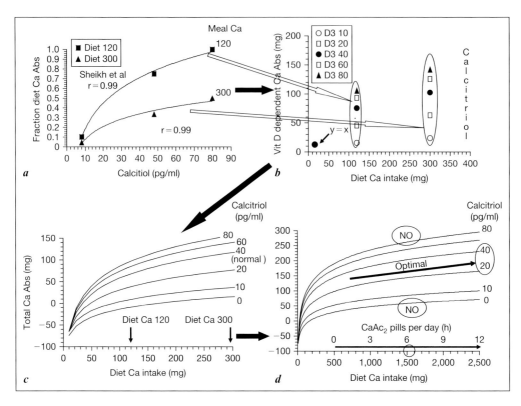

Fig. 1. A series of Ca absorption studies showing that the bulk of Ca absorption is vitamin D dependent (see text for details).

achieve plasma concentrations of 20–40 mg/ml is in the range of 0.50–0.75 μg/day. Note that with both non-Ca-containing and Ca-based binders high doses of C_3 are to be avoided. The absorption curve for $C_3 = 80$ indicates that with total intake only 500 mg/day, the absorption can reach 200 mg/day.

Kinetics of P Flux during HD

We have previously reported on the kinetics of P removal during HD [6]. Figure 2c depicts the reported characteristics of the plasma P concentration as a function of spKt/V_P. Note that the normalized TAC falls during the first hour to a level about 40% of the initial concentration and then remains stable as spKt/V_P increases. It can be estimated from this profile of diffusion gradient

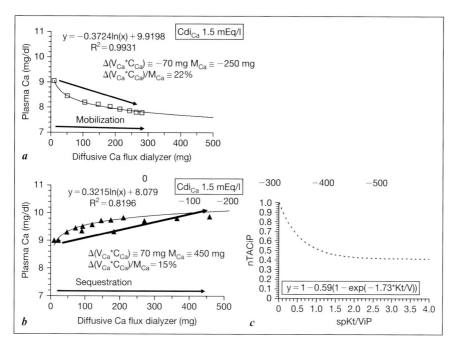

Fig. 2. Intradialytic kinetics of Ca and P flux (see text for details).

that only a modest fraction of the total absorbed P can be removed by the dialyzer except with greatly prolonged weekly treatment time such as in long nocturnal HD. The bulk of P must be removed by binders.

Kinetics of Ca Flux during Dialysis

We have also previously reported a kinetic model of intradialytic Ca flux [10]. Mathematical analysis of literature data indicated that the extracellular Ca pool is very effectively buffered against change in concentration induced by concentration gradients between blood and dialysate across the dialyzer. This buffering effect is thought to reside in the miscible calcium pool (MCP) [10]. Figure 2a depicts removal of 320 mg Ca with $C_{di}Ca$ 1.5 mEq/l. Analysis of this data indicated that only 70 mg came from the plasma and extracellular fluid while 300 mg were calculated to be mobilized from the MCP. Figure 2b depicts accumulation of 520 mg of Ca during dialysis with $C_{di}Ca$ 3.5 mEq/l. Only 15% of this accumulated in plasma and extracellular fluid while 450 mg were sequestered in the MCP. These analyses showed that large amounts of both removal and sequestration of Ca can occur during dialysis with relatively small effect on the extracellular concentration. The behavior of this MCP needs to be studied over a wide range clinical parameters with the goal of predicting its behavior quantitatively.

Inhibition of sHPT

The Ca mass balance and kinetic relationships discussed above strongly suggest that large doses of C_3 and its analogs should be avoided and hence not used for their suppressive effect on PTH with large doses. It would seem more appropriate to return vitamin D_3 metabolism to normal and use a calcimimetic agent such as Cinacalcet to control sHPT. Since substantial quantities of Ca removal during dialysis may be required in some instances, this may also be a stimulus for sHPT which would be most rationally managed with a calcimimetics agent.

References

1   Goodman W, London G, et al: Vascular calcification in chronic kidney disease. Am J Kidney Dis 2004;43:672–579.
2   Goodman W, Goldin J, Kuizon B, et al: Coronary calcification in young adults with end-stage renal disease who are undergoing dialysis. N Engl J Med 2000;342:147801483.
3   Block G, Klassen P, lazarus J, Ofsthun N, Lowrie E, Chertow G: Mineral metabolism, mortality and morbidity in maintenance hemodialysis. J Am Soc Nephrol 2004;8:2208–2218.
4   Cozzolino M, Brancaccio D, Galleni M, Slatopolsky E: Pathogenesis of vascular calcification in chronic kidney disease. Kidney Int 2006;68:429–426.
5   Sigrist M, McIntyre C: Calcium exposure and removal in chronic hemodialysis in chronic hemodialysis patients. J Ren Nutr 2006;16:41–46.
6   Gotch F, Panlilio F, Sergeyva O, Rosales L, Folden T, Kaysen G, Levin N: A kinetic model of inorganic phosphorus mass balance in hemodialysis therapy. Blood Purif 2003;21:51057.
7   Ramirez J, Emmett M, White M, et al: The absorption of dietary phosphorus and calcium in hemodialysis patients. Kidney Int 1986;30:752–759.
8   Sheikh M, Ramirez J, Emmett M, Santa Ana C, et al: Role of vitamin D dependent and vitamin D independent absorption of food calcium. J Clin Invest 1988;81:126–136.
9   Sheikh M, Maguire J, Emmett M, Santa Ana C, et al: Reduction of dietary phosphorus absorption by phosphorus binders. J Clin Invest 1989;83:66–73.
10 Gotch F, Kotanko P, Handelman G, Levin N: A kinetic model of calcium mass balance during dialysis therapy. Blood Purif 2007;25:139–149.

Frank Gotch, MD
144 Belgrave Ave.
San Francisco, CA 94117 (USA)
Tel. +1 415 661 6191, Fax +1 415 731 7876, E-Mail frank.gotch.md@fmc-na.com

Ronco C, Cruz DN (eds): Hemodialysis – From Basic Research to Clinical Trials.
Contrib Nephrol. Basel, Karger, 2008, vol 161, pp 215–221

....

Impact of Ca/P Disorders on Risks and Comorbidities

Piergiorgio Messa

Nephrology, Dialysis, and Renal Transplant Unit, Ospedale Maggiore-Policlinico-IRCCS, Milan, Italy

Abstract

Cardiovascular morbidity and the mortality rate are manifoldly greater in chronic kidney disease (CKD) patients. Mineral metabolism (MM) derangements and particularly changes in calcium (Ca) and phosphate (P) metabolism have been included among the large array of putative causal factors of this poor clinical outcome due to their possible negative effects on the vascular calcification process. However, these opinions are mainly based on experimental in vitro studies or retrospective association studies which cannot be considered definitive demonstrations for a cause-effect link between MM changes and the observed increased mortality rate. Furthermore, there is some evidence that Ca and/or P changes appear in later stages of CKD, in contrast with the observation of a very early increase in the mortality rate over the course of CKD. Finally, no evidence has been as yet produced that the correction of the MM parameters might be followed by an improvement in clinical outcome. In conclusion, even if many experimental and retrospective clinical studies strongly suggest a possible involvement of Ca and P derangements as causal factors in the increased mortality rate of CKD patients, there is still not any convincing clinical data giving evidence that the correction of the MM parameters may, at least in part, improve the clinical outcome of these patients.

Copyright © 2008 S. Karger AG, Basel

Cardiovascular morbidity and the mortality rate are manifoldly greater in renal patients as compared with the general population from the very early stages of chronic kidney disease (CKD) [1].

It is widely recognized that calcium (Ca) and phosphate (P) disorders, either as due to secondary hyperparathyroidism per se or to the therapeutic interventions undertaken for controlling secondary hyperparathyroidism, are associated with increased cardiovascular morbidity and mortality risk. However a clear-cut demonstration of a cause-effect relationship between mineral metabolism (MM) disorders and major adverse outcomes in renal patients is far from having being reached.

In general terms, in order to establish an unequivocal cause-effect relationship between any two series of events, it is necessary to fulfill at least the following four main criteria: (1) a pathophysiological plausibility of the cause-effect relationship; (2) the availability of epidemiological evidence supporting the causal relationship; (3) a time-related plausibility between hypothetical causal factor(s) and the secondary events, and (4) a demonstration that correcting causal factor(s) would make it possible to prevent the occurrence of the secondary events.

In the following paragraphs the above four main points specifically related to the possible cause-effect relationship between MM disorders and adverse clinical outcome in renal patients will be addressed.

Pathophysiologic Plausibility

Ca and P salts, even if with a very variable biochemical composition, are the main constituents of the mineral phase of both orthotopic (bone) and etherotopic (visceral, stone) calcifications. So it would follow that a preliminary condition for the calcification process to occur is that at least the local concentration of these elements should overcome the formation product of their salts. In fact, several in vitro studies have provided evidence that, increasing either Ca or P concentration, a proportional increment of Ca deposition in the vascular wall is observed [2]. However, the possibility that Ca-P product might play a direct role in the vascular calcification process also in vivo has been, at least in part, questioned [3].

There is now general agreement that either the physiological and the pathological calcification processes are mainly dependent on the cellular activity of specialized cells in the bone (osteoblasts) or of cells which acquire the osteoblast lineage characteristics outside the bone (e.g., mesenchymal vascular cells) [4]. These cells, through the production of a huge array of specialized proteins, trigger the calcification process and induce its progression. The above complex biochemical and metabolic events are controlled by either physiological endocrine systems (parathyroid hormone, calcitonin, vitamin D metabolites, phosphatonins, etc.) and a great number of other physiologically and pathologically activated systems (fetuin, MGP, lipids, cytokines, AGE products, ROS, etc.) which can increase or reduce the propensity for the calcification process to occur [5].

Even though the physicochemical mechanism of elevated Ca-P product on vascular calcification has been challenged, overwhelming evidence has been produced which demonstrates that both Ca and P can directly induce osteogenic differentiation of smooth muscle cells [4, 6], at least in in vitro models.

Furthermore, the destiny of the amount of Ca and P which might accumulate in the body of patients on dialysis treatment remains an unanswered question, particularly when vitamin D metabolites and/or high Ca-based P binders are utilized. In these conditions, a positive global balance for both these elements is expected, due to the insufficiently negative and null/positive dialysis balance of P and Ca respectively, in spite of their increased intestinal absorption and null renal excretion.

On the grounds of these considerations, it seems at least plausible that an overall positive Ca and/or P balance might play a role in the vascular calcification process.

Epidemiological Evidence

A great number of papers dealing with the association between MM-related parameters and morbidity and mortality rate in either dialysis patients or in predialysis patients have been published in the last decade [7–12]. Some of these studies, performed on large cohorts of dialysis patients, where the biochemical variables entered into the statistical analysis were recorded only at the beginning of the observational period, concluded that an almost linear increase in mortality risk was observed along with the progressive increase in Ca concentration [7, 8]. On the other hand, an increased mortality odds ratio was recorded either when high or very low P levels were recorded, underlining that the contemporary increase in Ca and P levels were associated with an even higher mortality risk [7, 8]. Further studies, using an adjusted model for the time-dependent exposition to the same biochemical variables recorded over a longer period of time, gave substantially the same results [9–11].

However, it is worth stressing that all these studies were based on the analysis of retrospective data which, in addition to the well-known limitations of any retrospective study, have some particular drawbacks related to the specific topic. First, at least as far as P is concerned, whose serum levels are highly dependent on dietary intake, it should be taken into account that its higher intake is almost invariably matched with also higher sodium, fat, and animal protein consumption. Second, since P concentrations in dialysis patients are also greatly affected by the overall efficiency of the dialysis treatment, it is easy to speculate that a lower dialysis dose might contemporarily affect the clearance of many other known and unknown substances which might affect patient survival: this limitation cannot be fully overcome by correcting for Kt/V for urea, which usually is just a spot measurement of dialysis efficiency for a molecule which only roughly correlated with P clearance. Finally, it is also common experience that higher P levels are often due to a lower patient compliance to P binders and this should be expected to be associated with a lower compliance to other drugs too (e.g. antihypertensive drugs) which might contribute to overall increased mortality.

For at least all these reasons, even if these association studies strongly suggest a possible link between derangements of MM and mortality risk in dialysis patients, they cannot be considered a definitive demonstration for establishing a cause-effect link.

Time-Related Plausibility

An additional requested criterion for establishing a possible cause-effect relationship relies on the observation that the potential causal factor(s) need to be present and active before the occurrence of the putative caused effects.

The literature provides us with many data which suggest that mortality rate increases from the very early stages of the CKD process and it is mainly due to cardiovascular disease [1]. Furthermore, there are also studies which found an association between the increased mortality rate and MM changes also in pre-dialysis patients [12]. However, when the time course of the metabolic changes is compared with the time course of the increased mortality risk through the different stages of CKD, it becomes evident that the increase in the mortality rate precedes by far the changes of the main MM-related parameters [1, 13]. In fact, Go et al. [1] reported that already in stage 3 CKD patients, the mortality rate was about fivefold greater than in patients with normal renal function. On the other hand, it has been widely demonstrated that, at these levels of GFR, when the mortality rate is already increased, either Ca and P levels are often still within the normal range [13, 14]. These observations cast some doubt about a causal role for the MM-associated factors playing a major role in the increased mortality rate of kidney patients. However, it cannot be completely excluded that, in spite of normal serum concentrations of the main MM-related parameters, some more subtle and not evident metabolic change might be directly or indirectly related to the increased mortality in this clinical set.

Correction of Hypothetical Causal Factors and Prevention of Secondary Events

Independently of the presence or not of the conditions satisfying the first three listed criteria, the final and definitive demonstration of a causal-effect relationship should anyway rely on the possibility to prevent the occurrence of the secondary clinical events by correcting the putative causal factors. However, it is necessary to preliminarily underline the fact that the topic we are discussing lends itself little to be the object of such a demonstration for many reasons. First, to demonstrate that the correction of any involved MM factor is effective in preventing the secondary clinical events, we should have available means for correcting the specific putative factor, without any contemporary change of the other parameters: this condition is very difficult to be obtained, at least in the usual clinical set. Second, most of the tools used for correcting Ca and/or P also affect PTH levels, which have been suggested to have some impact on mortality rate [7–11]. Third, some of the utilized drugs, namely vitamin D metabolites, have been claimed to be directly involved in affecting mortality rates or to interfere, either positively or negatively, with the vascular calcification process, which is strictly related to cardiovascular morbidity and mortality [9–11, 15]. Finally, a study which would address such a difficult topic should be designed as a prospective, double-blinded, randomized study, performed on a large cohort of patients, followed up in the long term: all these conditions are not easy to be achieved in a non-sponsored study. For all these reasons, and not only, in the literature there are mainly company-driven studies designed to explore the effect of a single drug mostly on the control of biochemical parameters and only occasionally directed to explore the clinical bone and cardiovascular outcomes.

Taking into consideration only the latter ones, most of these studies compared the effect of two kinds of P binders, sevelamer versus Ca salts. These studies explored not only the effects of these different types of P binders on biochemical parameters, but also on some main clinical outcomes, such as vascular calcification progression, overall and cardiovascular mortality. All these studies have been recently reviewed by Tonelli et al. [16] and the main conclusions were that, even if sevelamer is associated with an almost equivalent control of P and a slightly better control of Ca levels, there was no clear evidence for any significant difference in all-cause or cardiovascular mortality, in the frequency of symptomatic bone disease or health-related quality of life.

Some more recent studies have been planned which will in part provide an answer to the topic we are dealing with in this paragraph. The design of a double-blind, randomized, placebo-controlled trial has been recently published, which will explore the effects of cinacalcet therapy on some main clinical outcomes: all-cause mortality and first non-fatal cardiovascular event. The study will be event-driven and was programmed to be terminated at 1,882 events, with an anticipated duration of approximately 4 years [17].

Even if this study should add some very important information, probably it will not completely answer our questions about the role of Ca and P on the increased mortality rate of patients with renal failure. In fact, it has been shown that cinacalcet can affect at the same time, Ca, P, and PTH levels and can also allow modifications in either vitamin D and P binders doses [18] and this will make it almost impossible to determine which of these effects, if any, could play a role as a causal factor of the observed clinical events.

In conclusion, though there are many experimental and epidemiological data which suggest a possible link between Ca and P metabolism with the high mortality rate observed in CKD patients, there is no conclusive demonstration that a cause-effect relationship unequivocally exists between the MM derangements and the negative outcome in renal patients.

Acknowledgement

This study was supported by the grant 'Project Glomerulonephritis' in memory of Pippo Neglia.

References

1   Go AS, Chertow GM, Fan D, McCulloch CE, Hsu CY: Chronic kidney disease and the risks of death, cardiovascular events, and hospitalization. N Engl J Med 2004;351:1296–1305.
2   Lomashvili K, Garg P, O'Neill WC: Chemical and hormonal determinants of vascular calcification in vitro. Kidney Int 2006 69:1464–1470.
3   O'Neill WC: The fallacy of the calcium-phosphate product. Kidney Int 2007;72:792–796.
4   Johnson RC, Leopold JA, Loscalzo J: Vascular calcification: pathobiological mechanisms and clinical implications. Circ Res 2006;99:1044–1059.
5   Moe SM, Chen NX: Mechanisms of vascular calcification in chronic kidney disease. J Am Soc Nephrol 2008;19:213–216.
6   Ketteler M, Schlieper G, Floege J: Calcification and cardiovascular health: new insights into an old phenomenon. Hypertension 2006;47:1027–1034.
7   Block GA, Klassen PS, Lazarus JM, Ofsthun N, Lowrie EG, Chertow GM: Mineral metabolism, mortality, and morbidity in maintenance hemodialysis. J Am Soc Nephrol 2004;15:2208–2218.
8   Slinin Y, Foley RN, Collins AJ: Calcium, phosphorus, parathyroid hormone, and cardiovascular disease in hemodialysis patients: the USRDS waves 1, 3, and 4 study. J Am Soc Nephrol 2005;16: 1788–1793.
9   Melamed ML, Eustace JA, Plantinga L, Jaar BG, Fink NE, Coresh J, Klag MJ, Powe NR: Changes in serum calcium, phosphate, and PTH and the risk of death in incident dialysis patients: a longitudinal study. Kidney Int 2006;70:351–357.
10 Kalantar-Zadeh K, Kuwae N, Regidor DL, Kovesdy CP, Kilpatrick RD, Shinaberger CS, McAllister CJ, Budoff MJ, Salusky IB, Kopple JD: Survival predictability of time-varying indicators of bone disease in maintenance hemodialysis patients. Kidney Int 2006;70:771–780.
11 Tentori F, Hunt WC, Rohrscheib M, Zhu M, Stidley CA, Servilla K, Miskulin D, Meyer KB, Bedrick EJ, Johnson HK, Zager PG: Which targets in clinical practice guidelines are associated with improved survival in a large dialysis organization? J Am Soc Nephrol 2007;18:2377–2384.
12 Voormolen N, Noordzij M, Grootendorst DC, Beetz I, Sijpkens YW, van Manen JG, Boeschoten EW, Huisman RM, Krediet RT, Dekker FW, PREPARE Study Group: High plasma phosphate as a risk factor for decline in renal function and mortality in pre-dialysis patients. Nephrol Dial Transplant 2007;22:2909–2916.

13 Levin A, Bakris GL, Molitch M, Smulders M, Tian J, Williams LA, Andress DL: Prevalence of abnormal serum vitamin D, PTH, calcium, and phosphorus in patients with chronic kidney disease: results of the study to evaluate early kidney disease. Kidney Int 2007;71:31–38.

14 Messa P, Vallone C, Mioni G, Geatti O, Turrin D, Passoni N, Cruciatti A: Direct in vivo assessment of parathyroid hormone-calcium relationship curve in renal patients. Kidney Int 1994;46: 1713–1720.

15 Teng M, Wolf M, Lowrie E, Ofsthun N, Lazarus JM, Thadhani R: Survival of patients undergoing hemodialysis with paricalcitol or calcitriol therapy. N Engl J Med 2003;349:446–456.

16 Tonelli M, Wiebe N, Culleton B, Lee H, Klarenbach S, Shrive F, Manns B, Alberta Kidney Disease Network: Systematic review of the clinical efficacy and safety of sevelamer in dialysis patients. Nephrol Dial Transplant 2007;22:2856–2866.

17 Chertow GM, Pupim LB, Block GA, Correa-Rotter R, Drueke TB, Floege J, Goodman WG, London GM, Mahaffey KW, Moe SM, Wheeler DC, Albizem M, Olson K, Klassen P, Parfrey P: Evaluation of cinacalcet therapy to lower cardiovascular events (EVOLVE): rationale and design overview. Clin J Am Soc Nephrol 2007;2:898–905.

18 Messa P, Macário F, Yaqoob M, Bouman K, Braun J, von Albertini B, Brink H, Maduell F, Graf H, Frazão JM, Bos WJ, Torregrosa V, Saha H, Reichel H, Wilkie M, Zani VJ, Molemans B, Carter D, Locatelli F: The OPTIMA study: assessing a new cinacalcet (Sensipar/Mimpara) treatment algorithm for secondary hyperparathyroidism. Clin J Am Soc Nephrol 2008;3:36–45.

Dr. Piergiorgio Messa
Nephrology, Dialysis, and Renal Transplant
Ospedale Maggiore-Policlinico, Pad. Croff- Via Commenda 15
IT–20122 Milan (Italy)
Tel. +39 025 50345512, Fax +39 025 5034550, E-Mail pmessa@policlinico.mi.it

Ronco C, Cruz DN (eds): Hemodialysis – From Basic Research to Clinical Trials.
Contrib Nephrol. Basel, Karger, 2008, vol 161, pp 222–233

························

Diagnostic Procedures and Rationale for Specific Therapies in Chronic Kidney Disease-Mineral and Bone Disorder

Jordi Bover[a], *Cristina Canal*[a], *Helena Marco*[a], *P. Fernandez-Llama*[a], *R.J. Bosch*[b], *J. Ballarín*[a]

[a]Fundació Puigvert, Universitat Autònoma de Barcelona and [b]Universidad de Alcalá de Henares, REDinREN, Instituto de Investigación Carlos III, Barcelona, Spain

Abstract

Chronic kidney disease (CKD) is associated with increased mortality. Non-traditional risk factors, such as mineral metabolism disturbances, seem to contribute to the unexpected high mortality rate. A *chronic kidney disease-mineral bone disorder* (CKD-MBD) has recently been defined as a systemic disorder manifested by one or a combination of abnormalities in bone biopsy, laboratory parameters, and/or vascular or other soft tissue calcifications. Recent research developments and new available treatments have all contributed to move the former treatment paradigm beyond the control of PTH. Thus, despite much of the advice given by different societies being just opinion-based evidence, the effect of different drugs on laboratory parameters, vascular calcification (VC) or survival may steer the choice of specific treatments. Aluminum and calcium-based phosphorus binders have been associated either with metal toxicity or progression of VC. Sevelamer hydrochloride has been related to an attenuation of the progression of VC and it has also been associated with improved survival at least in certain subgroups of dialysis patients. Lanthanum carbonate decreases phosphorus levels but its impact on surrogate or hard outcomes is not known. Selective vitamin D-receptor activators may have differential effects on VC, are associated with a survival advantage and thereby may have a best-fitted profile for CKD patients. On the other hand, calcimimetics markedly help to achieve current guidelines and ongoing clinical trials are evaluating hard outcomes. It is likely that a regimen combining several drugs might improve individual results. However, the utility of any new approach to CKD-MBD will need to be evaluated in prospective trials including thorough pharmacoeconomic analysis.

Supported by REDinREN (Red renal de investigación española 16/06, de la RETICS, Instituto de Investigación Carlos III).

Table 1. Non-traditional risk markers associated with morbidity and mortality in patients with CKD and/or maintenance dialysis

---

Anemia and hypercoagulability state
Albuminuria
Chronic volume overload
Arteriovenous fistula
Reduction of renal and cardiac capillaries
Activation of the renin-angiotensin system and sympathetic nervous system
Altered nitric oxide/endothelin balance
Decreased number of endothelial progenitor cells
Chronic inflammation-malnutrition-inflammation-atheromatosis syndrome
(C-reactive protein, interleukins, tumor-necrosis factor, cytokines…)
Adipokines
Hyperhomocysteinemia
Oxidative (free oxygen radicals, asymmetric dimethylarginine…) and carbonyl stress
Accumulation of advanced end-glycation products
Sleep disturbances
Early menopause
Therapeutic nihilism (infrequent use of β-blockers, statins, aspirin…)
Late nephrology referral
Biocompatibility of dialysis membranes
Immunosuppressors in kidney transplantation
Phosphorus, calcium, Ca×P product and parathyroid hormone
Vitamin D deficiency or insufficiency (serum 25-OH-vitamin D levels)
Excessive vitamin D therapy
Increased vascular and valvular calcification
Arterial stiffness
Pulse wave velocity and pulse pressure

In italics, disturbances directly related to mineral-bone disorders.

Several epidemiologic studies have demonstrated that chronic kidney disease (CKD), even at early stages, is associated with increased mortality, mainly from cardiovascular origin. Early detection by laboratory reports of the estimated glomerular filtration rate is currently recommended [1, 2]. Despite the high prevalence of *classical* cardiovascular risk factors in renal patients, other *non-traditional* risk factors, including several mineral metabolism disturbances, seem to contribute to the unexpected high cardiovascular mortality rate of this population [3] (table 1). In the present article, we will review current trends on diagnostic procedures of CKD-associated mineral and bone disorders which may potentially influence the use of specific therapies.

From Renal Osteodystrophy to Chronic Kidney Disease-Mineral and Bone Disorder and Its Evaluation

Renal osteodystrophy is the term usually used to describe the abnormalities in bone morphology which develop in CKD [4, 5]. In clinical practice, the invasive bone biopsy is used infrequently. The international KDIGO initiative (Kidney Disease: Improving Global Outcomes) recently suggested a new definition and classification system [5]. It is now advised that *renal osteodystrophy* should exclusively define just the bone pathology related to CKD, becoming *one component* of the new syndrome *chronic kidney disease-mineral and bone disorder* (CKD-MBD). It is defined as a systemic disorder manifested by either one or a combination of the following: (1) abnormalities in bone turnover, mineralization, volume, linear growth or strength; (2) abnormalities of calcium (Ca), phosphorus (P), parathyroid hormone (PTH) or vitamin D metabolism, and/or (3) vascular or other soft tissue calcification [5].

Bone Biopsy and the 'TMV' System

Although biopsy is *not* recommended as part of the routine evaluation of CKD-MBD, it remains as an important diagnostic tool in selected patients [4, 5]. In order to help with the interpretation of bone biopsy results, it was recently agreed to use three main histological parameters – bone *Turnover*, *Mineralization* and *Volume* (the TMV system), with any combination of each of the descriptors possible in any given sample [5].

Laboratory Abnormalities-Biomarkers of CKD-MBD

Parathyroid Hormone

The initial evaluation of CKD-MBD should include PTH, ionized or corrected calcium, phosphorus, alkaline phosphatase and bicarbonate.

Despite some controversy, biomarkers such as 'intact' circulating PTH levels remain the best surrogate indicator of bone turnover, mainly because nearly all the currently available information on bone histomorphometry and clinical outcomes has been correlated with 'intact' PTH assays. Variability among different assays is extremely high [5, 7], and knowledge of the local PTH assay used is clinically important. National and international initiatives [5, 7] are underway to bypass this important problem. Furthermore, the specificity of PTH seems to be poor, especially for intermediate values [8]. 'Whole'

1-84 PTH assays will probably gain increasing acceptance but their use is not routinely recommended yet.

Although there is not a direct and unequivocal causal relationship between PTH and cardiovascular lesions, different studies have shown increased mortality in patients with either very *high* or *low* PTH values [3, 9]. PTH has classically been related to many systemic effects beyond bone [4].

Calcium and Phosphorus

Serum calcium concentration and total-body calcium balance are independent variables. Moreover, normality of calcium and phosphorus levels does not preclude the presence of important mineral and bone disturbances. Both Ca and P are also associated with higher mortality rates in several observational studies [3, 9].

Other Biomarkers

Alkaline phosphatase (total or bone-specific), in conjunction with PTH, may be helpful in predicting bone turnover or even mortality [5, 9]. Several other biomarkers such as osteoprotegerin, FGF-23 or fetuin-A, among others, have been examined in CKD patients but their use only meets research purposes. Some societies recommend the determination of *25-OH-vitamin D* (*calcidiol*) [6, 7] since it has been associated with survival even in dialysis patients [10]. Plasma bicarbonate serial measurements are recommended, but targets may not be a clear as initially thought. Calciuria and phosphaturia may be helpful to monitor a potential calcium and phosphorus loading.

Imaging Techniques for Soft Tissue Calcification

Imaging techniques, according to local availability, should be included in the initial evaluation of CKD-MBD [5, 7]. They had been important to evaluate bone disease, but the ongoing development of sensitive imaging techniques is leading to their more widespread use in clinical diagnosis and may influence decision-making in the near future.

Bone Radiology

Beyond children, plain radiographs of hands, pelvis and lateral abdominal X-rays represent nowadays a valuable and low-cost screening tool for the detection

---

of extraskeletal calcifications, especially vascular calcifications (VC) [11–13]. The semiquantitative evaluation of these radiological tests is predictive of the presence and extension of VC in the coronaries [12]. Moreover, a positive correlation has been described between these VC and an increased risk of mortality [11, 13]. Thus, the Spanish Society of Nephrology currently considers that at least a plain X-ray should be taken in all patients with CKD to evaluate VC [7]; however, their sensitivity is low.

Bone Densitometry

We do not recommend the routine evaluation of bone mineral density (BMD) except in adult transplant patients. Correlation of BMD with fracture risk in CKD populations is inconsistent, and BMD without a full consideration of the underlying bone pathology may be very misleading since the same BMD may be caused by somehow 'opposite' diseases. Moreover, BMD measurements may result in the inappropriate administration of anti-osteoporotic therapy [5]. Nevertheless, several studies have shown that BMD measured at the distal radius site is predictive of fracture risk and correlates well with PTH levels [5]. BMD measurement by quantitative computed tomography is valuable in differentiating cortical from trabecular bone. Femoral BMD is inversely associated with VC but vertebral BMD is unreliable in CKD patients with aortic VC.

Non-Invasive Detection and Quantification of Vascular Calcifications

Multislice computed tomography scans and *electron-beam computed tomography* are much more precise and sensitive for the qualitative and quantitative assessment of VC as compared to plain X-rays, and currently represent the gold standard [12]. Despite a poor correlation with angiographic findings, calcium scores appear to be predictive of unfavorable outcomes in dialysis patients [14]. However, their availability is very limited, they provide substantial exposure to ionized radiation, and they add a substantial supplementary cost. Thus, their use is not currently justified as a screening tool but they are useful in monitoring VC progression and to assess the effect of different therapeutic strategies on VC [15, 16].

Other Imaging Techniques

Echocardiography, a readily available moderately expensive tool, can be easily employed to detect *valvular* calcifications [12]. *2D ultrasound* reveals calcifications at atheromatous plaques and the measurement of carotid intima-media thickness. Increases in carotid intima-media thickness, carotid calcification and plaques and an increased risk of valvular calcification have all been related, and an association has also been described between valvular and coronary VC [12]. Finally, the importance of the measurement of arterial stiffness, by *pulse wave velocity* or *central vessel pressure* profiles, has been increasingly recognized [17]. Increased *pulse pressure* is also a sign of increased vascular stiffness. It seems clear that arterial stiffness increases as glomerular filtration rate declines, and that it is not only associated with VC but it is also an independent predictor of all-cause and cardiovascular mortality [17]. A thorough review of techniques and technologies to assess VC has been recently presented by Bellasi et al. at http://cin2007.uninet.edu/en/trabajos/show/30.html.

Rationale for Specific Therapies in CKD-MBD

Recent research developments and new available treatments have all contributed to shift the former paradigm of CKD-MBD treatment beyond PTH control. According to many big cross-sectional studies, bone and mineral abnormalities including VC impact heavily on morbidity and mortality in dialysis patients [3, 9, 14]. VCs and their progression are not exclusive of CKD patients, since they have been related to older age, diabetes mellitus and gender, among others, but important associations have been described with CKD stage, dialysis vintage as well as several abnormalities and treatments of mineral metabolism. Thus, despite much of the advice given by different societies being just opinion-based evidence, the effect of different drugs on laboratory parameters, VC and survival may steer the choice of specific treatments.

Control of Hyperphosphatemia

Aluminum and calcium-based phosphorus binders decrease plasma P levels but they are not absent of potential problems. Even oral aluminum has been related to toxicity. The dose of Ca-based phosphorus binders has been related to an increased risk of hypercalcemia, excessive PTH suppression and progression of VC [14–16]. *Sevelamer hydrochloride* has been widely studied and it has been shown to be effective in reducing P, Ca×P, and LDL cholesterol levels among other pleiotropic effects [18]. In both the Treat to Goal [15] and the RIND (Renagel in New Dialysis patients) studies [16], a significant progression of VC was observed at different times in the Ca-based P binders group as compared to sevelamer. A contribution of the proacidic effect of sevelamer (and the decrease of calcium carbonate or acetate), cannot be ruled out [19, 20]. Importantly enough, no patients with a zero calcium score as measured by electron-beam computed tomography progressed, whereas patients with a baseline calcium score >30 progressed in both arms [16], albeit more rapidly and showing a more severe progression in those receiving Ca-based P binders. These studies confirm previous recommendations that Ca-based P binders should be avoided at least in patients with evidence of *severe* calcification [6]. Some consider that it may not be reasonable to wait until 'severe' calcifications are present to limit Ca-based P binders. Non-calcium, non-aluminum P binders should also be recommended as first-line treatment options for patients with hypercalcemia and/or low PTH [6, 8]. In the recently completed CARE-2 study, Qnibi et al. have reported in abstract form that no significant difference in progression of VC between patients treated with calcium acetate or sevelamer was observed when equivalent control of LDL cholesterol was achieved with atorvastatin in the calcium arm in a highly prevalent diabetic population. These results are somehow contradictory, especially considering that some prospective studies with atorvastatin did not attenuate VC.

The effect of sevelamer on survival is also controversial [18]. In hemodialysis patients, there were no differences in all-cause mortality between sevelamer and Ca-based P binders treated groups in the large 3-year DCOR (Dialysis Clinical Outcomes Revisited) trial [21], as well as in a recent systematic review mainly based on DCOR results. Nevertheless, in a subgroup of DCOR patients >65 years (a prespecified variable but not a primary endpoint) sevelamer was associated with a significant reduction in all-cause mortality as well as it was seen in those treated for more than 2 years (post-hoc analysis) [21]. In the smaller RIND trial, data suggest that there is an overall survival benefit with sevelamer [16]. Multivariate analysis are not adjusted to vitamin D treatment, despite in some studies sevelamer groups receive more frequently vitamin D. Consequently, reported survival benefits as well as the cost-effectiveness of sevelamer remain a matter of dispute [18].

Recent clinical studies have described that *lanthanum carbonate* effectively decreases P levels, decreasing the incidence of significant hypercalcemia and without an excessive suppression of PTH. Chewable and a lower number of tablets as compared to sevelamer may improve patient's compliance. However, impact on surrogate markers such as VC or hard cardiovascular or global outcomes are not known. Combination of several P binders may be needed to achieve newer P-goals <5 mg/dl [7]. New formulations and new P-binders are going to be available soon, also in the predialysis setting, where disorders in mineral metabolism may not only influence survival but also CKD progression [19].

Control of Secondary Hyperparathyroidism and Beyond

Vitamin D Derivatives and Selective Vitamin D-Receptor Activators (sVDRA)

Calcidiol levels have been related to survival benefits in both the general population and dialysis patients [10]. We and others have seen that vitamin D deficiency is very common in CKD patients [22]. Classic forms of hydroxylated vitamin D, such as calcitriol or α-calcidol, have shown to be helpful suppressing PTH, but they may also improve patient survival, at least in retrospective studies [23]. Important pleiotropic effects have been attributed to vitamin D compounds [22]. However, vitamin D causes frequent episodes of hypercalcemia and hyperphosphatemia due to its narrow therapeutic window [4]. Some experimental models and few clinical reports have shown increased VC with the use of vitamin D derivatives [24]. Selective VDRA (most of the available information is from paricalcitol) are more selective for parathyroid glands but paricalcitol also seems to induce less VC than equipotent doses of calcitriol or doxercalciferol [22, 24]. Moreover, intravenous paricalcitol was associated with improved survival in hemodialysis patients [9, 25] even compared with calcitriol [25]. Vitamin D derivatives may improve albuminuria and progression of experimental CKD. Thus, sVDRA seem to have a best fitted profile for CKD patients at the expense of higher prices than classical compounds.

Calcimimetics

Cinacalcet is a calcimimetic agent which helps to achieve K-DOQI guidelines, even in patients who were not controlled by conventional therapy, by suppressing PTH, decreasing serum calcium and, at least in some patients, phosphorus levels [26]. Calcimimetics are effective in different degrees of secondary hyperparathyroidism but achievement of KDOQI goals improves when they are started early [27]. Nausea and vomiting are frequent and dose-dependent, but we have observed that the administration with the first meal after dialysis may at least in some cases improve these symptoms, and that less than 3% of patients withdrew the study for this reason [27]. Hypocalcemia <7.5 mg/dl is unusual and hypocalcemic episodes are transient and rarely associated with symptoms. However, calcimimetics are expensive drugs. In addition to a higher rate of goal achievements with calcimimetics, we and others have described in preliminary reports that a decrement in the need on expensive P-binders may at least partially compensate its acquisition cost.

In post-hoc analysis of several prospective studies, the risks of parathyroidectomy, fractures and cardiovascular hospitalization significantly decreased with cinacalcet [28]. A calcimimetic has also been recently shown to be beneficial on progression of experimental renal damage. There are two ongoing clinical prospective trials evaluating hard endpoints in dialysis patients (EVOLVE: 'EValuation Of cinacalcet therapy to Lower cardioVascular evEnts' and ADVANCE: A randomizeD VAscular calcificatioN study to evaluate the effects of CinacalcEt). These studies should be applauded since important resources are being invested to find out whether a drug initially dedicated to bone disease has an effect on hard outcomes.

Combination of Calcimimetics and Vitamin D Derivatives

Several clinical studies demonstrate the ability of calcimimetics to decrease PTH levels and normalizing Ca×P product, allowing decrements of vitamin D dosage. Whereas it is not known whether some patients may benefit preferentially by the use of a calcimimetic or a sVDRA, there is the potential to use low doses of both. This 'mixed' approach has been extensively used by nephrologists in other pathologies such as hypertension or immunosuppression in kidney transplantation, maximizing the beneficial effects of drugs, acting in different pathways, and limiting their secondary effects. The rationale behind this clinical approach is experimentally supported since calcimimetics and vitamin D may respectively increase VDR and the calcium receptor, or that some calcimimetics may protect against untoward effects of vitamin D [29]. An additional benefit is that treatment of severe hyperparathyroidism with calcimimetics may require high doses, which may be less tolerated and economically unsustainable, whereas a regimen combining lower doses of a calcimimetic with vitamin D or a sVDRA might decrease secondary effects and be more cost-effective.

Other Therapies

Bisphosphonates, as well as other drugs, have been shown to influence the progression of VC [1]. Most of this evidence is obtained in experimental studies where it has been demonstrated that VC (ossification, 'fossification') is an actively regulated, cell-mediated process, thereby potentially subjected to medical interference. Therapies which may influence VC are listed in table 2.

Table 2. Therapeutic aspects which may influence VC (alphabetical order)

Acidosis
Bone morphogenetic proteins (BMP-7/BMP-2)
Bisphosphonates
Calcimimetics
Calcium channel blockers
Dialysis technique
EDTA (ethylenediaminetetraacetic acid)-tetracycline long-term chemotherapy
Endothelin antagonists (i.e. bosentan)
Osteoprotegerin and antireceptor activator of nuclear factor-κβ ligand
Parathyroidectomy
Phosphorus binders
Teriparatide (1–34 human PTH)
Transplantation
Vitamin D dosage/selective activators of vitamin D receptors
Warfarin/vitamin K

Conclusion

The knowledge that bone and mineral abnormalities impact heavily on morbidity and mortality, and that VC is uniformly associated with cardiovascular complications in patients with CKD, emphasizes the need for a better monitoring, earlier detection and control of these disturbances. Whereas the cost/benefit of the new therapies is under strong debate, several drugs such as sevelamer, lanthanum, sVDRA and/or calcimimetics seem to offer clinically important advantages over classical therapies with narrower therapeutic windows. Depending on economical resources, it is possible that the most expensive drugs should be used preferentially in patients with certain biochemical patterns or those with VC detected by different means. Nonetheless, the diagnostic utility and prognostic significance of any new approach to CKD-MBD will need to be evaluated in future prospective trials including thorough pharmacoeconomic studies.

References

1   Bover J, Canal C, Pérez SG, Bosch RJ, Ballarín JA: Slowing the progression of vascular calcification in chronic kidney disease patients. Eur Renal Dis 2007;1:18–23.
2   Gracia S, Montañés R, Bover J, Cases A, Deulofeu R, Martín de Francisco AL, Orte LM, on behalf of the Spanish Society of Nephrology: Recommendations for the use of equations to estimate glomerular filtration rate in adults. Nefrologia 2006;26:658–665.
3   Block GA, Klassen PS, Lazarus JM, Ofsthun N, Lowrie EG, Chertow GM: Mineral metabolism, mortality, and morbidity in maintenance hemodialysis. J Am Soc Nephrol 2004;15:2208–2218.

4   Llach F, Bover J: Renal osteodystrophies; in Brenner BM (ed): The Kidney. Philadelphia, Saunders, 2000, pp 2103–2186.

5   Moe S, Drüeke T, Cunningham J, Goodman W, Martin K, Olgaard K, Ott S, Sprague S, Lameire N, Eknoyan G, Kidney Disease: Improving Global Outcomes (KDIGO): Definition, evaluation, and classification of renal osteodystrophy: a position statement from KDIGO. Kidney Int 2006;69:1945–1953.

6   National Kidney Foundation: K/DOQI clinical practice guidelines for bone metabolism and disease in chronic kidney disease. Am J Kidney Dis 2003;42(suppl 3):S1–S201.

7   Torregrosa V, Cannata J, Bover J, et al: Recommendations of the Spanish Society of Nephrology for the treatment of mineral and bone metabolism disorders in patients with chronic kidney disease. Nefrologia 2008 (in press).

8   Ferreira A, Frazão JM, Monier-Faugere MC, Gil C, Galvao J, Oliveira C, Baldaia J, Rodrigues I, Santos C, Ribeiro S, Hoenger RM, Duggal A, Malluche HH, Sevelamer Study Group: Effects of sevelamer hydrochloride and calcium carbonate on renal osteodystrophy in hemodialysis patients. J Am Soc Nephrol 2008;19:405–412.

9   Kalantar-Zadeh K, Kuwae N, Regidor DL, Kovesdy CP, Kilpatrick RD, Shinaberger CS, McAllister CJ, Budoff MJ, Salusky IB, Kopple JD: Survival predictability of time-varying indicators of bone disease in maintenance hemodialysis patients. Kidney Int 2006;70:771–780.

10 Wolf M, Shah A, Gutierrez O, Ankers E, Monroy M, Tamez H, Steele D, Chang Y, Camargo CA Jr, Tonelli M, Thadhani R: Vitamin D levels and early mortality among incident hemodialysis patients. Kidney Int 2007;72:1004–1013.

11 Adragao T, Pires A, Lucas C, Birne R, Magalhaes L, Gonçalves M, Negrao AP: A simple vascular calcification score predicts cardiovascular risk in hemodialysis patients. Nephrol Dial Transplant 2004;19:1480–1488.

12 Bellasi A, Ferramosca E, Muntner P, Ratti C, Wildman RP, Block GA, Raggi P: Correlation of simple imaging tests and coronary artery calcium measured by computed tomography in hemodialysis patients. Kidney Int 2006;70:1623–1628.

13 London GM, Guérin AP, Marchais SJ, Métivier F, Pannier B, Adda H: Arterial media calcification in end-stage renal disease: impact on all-cause and cardiovascular mortality. Nephrol Dial Transplant 2003;18:1731–1740.

14 Block GA, Raggi P, Bellasi A, Kooienga L, Spiegel DM: Mortality effect of coronary calcification and phosphate binder choice in incident hemodialysis patients. Kidney Int 2007;71:438–441.

15 Chertow GM, Burke SK, Raggi P, Treat to Goal Working Group: Sevelamer attenuates the progression of coronary and aortic calcification in hemodialysis patients. Kidney Int 2002;62: 245–252.

16 Block GA, Spiegel DM, Ehrlich J, Mehta R, Lindbergh J, Dreisbach A, Raggi P: Effects of sevelamer and calcium on coronary artery calcification in patients new to hemodialysis. Kidney Int 2005;68:1815–1824.

17 Guérin AP, Pannier B, Marchais SJ, London GM: Cardiovascular disease in the dialysis population: prognostic significance of arterial disorders. Curr Opin Nephrol Hypertens 2006;15:105–110.

18 Goldsmith DR, Scott LJ, Cvetković RS, Plosker GL: Sevelamer hydrochloride: a review of its use for hyperphosphataemia in patients with end-stage renal disease on haemodialysis. Drugs 2008; 68:85–104.

19 Cozzolino M, Staniforth ME, Liapis H, Finch J, Burke SK, Dusso AS, Slatopolsky E: Sevelamer hydrochloride attenuates kidney and cardiovascular calcifications in long-term experimental uremia. Kidney Int 2003;64:1653–1661.

20 Mendoza FJ, Lopez I, Montes de Oca A, Perez J, Rodriguez M, Aguilera-Tejero E: Metabolic acidosis inhibits soft tissue calcification in uremic rats. Kidney Int 2008;73:407–414.

21 Suki WN, Zabaneh R, Cangiano JL, Reed J, Fischer D, Garrett L, Ling BN, Chasan-Taber S, Dillon MA, Blair AT, Burke SK: Effects of sevelamer and calcium-based phosphate binders on mortality in hemodialysis patients. Kidney Int 2007;72:1130–1137.

22 Andress DL: Vitamin D in chronic kidney disease: a systemic role for selective vitamin D receptor activation. Kidney Int 2006;69:33–43.

23 Marco MP, Craver L, Betriu A, Fibla J, Fernández E: Influence of vitamin D receptor gene polymorphisms on mortality risk in hemodialysis patients. Am J Kidney Dis 2001;38:965–974.

24 Cardús A, Panizo S, Parisi E, Fernandez E, Valdivielso JM: Differential effects of vitamin D analogs on vascular calcification. J Bone Miner Res 2007;22:860–866.

25 Teng M, Wolf M, Lowrie E, Ofsthun N, Lazarus JM, Thadhani R: Survival of patients undergoing hemodialysis with paricalcitol or calcitriol therapy. N Engl J Med 2003;349:446–456.

26 Moe SM, Chertow GM, Coburn JW, Quarles LD, Goodman WG, Block GA, Drüeke TB, Cunningham J, Sherrard DJ, McCary LC, Olson KA, Turner SA, Martin KJ: Achieving NKF-K/DOQI bone metabolism and disease treatment goals with cinacalcet HCl. Kidney Int 2005; 67:760–771.

27 Schaefer RM, Bover J, Dellanna F, Sanz D, Asensio C, Sánchez González MC, Gross P, Zani V, Carter D, Jehle PM. Efficacy of cinacalcet administered with the first meal after dialysis: the SENSOR study. Clin Nephrol 2008 (submitted).

28 Cunningham J, Danese M, Olson K, Klassen P, Chertow GM: Effects of the calcimimetic cinacalcet HCl on cardiovascular disease, fracture, and health-related quality of life in secondary hyperparathyroidism. Kidney Int 2005;68:1793–1800.

29 Lopez I, Mendoza FJ, Aguilera-Tejero E, Perez J, Guerrero F, Martin D, Rodriguez M: The effect of calcitriol, paricalcitol, and a calcimimetic on extraosseous calcifications in uremic rats. Kidney Int 2008;73:300–307.

Dr. Jordi Bover
Fundació Puigvert, C./Cartagena 340
ES–08025 Barcelona (Spain)
E-mail jbover@fundacio-puigvert.es

Ronco C, Cruz DN (eds): Hemodialysis – From Basic Research to Clinical Trials.
Contrib Nephrol. Basel, Karger, 2008, vol 161, pp 234–239

···················

Preventive Measures and New Pharmacological Approaches of Calcium and Phosphate Disorders

Mario Cozzolino, Andrea Galassi, Sabina Pasho, Guditta Fallabrino, Maurizio Gallieni, Diego Brancaccio

Chair and Division of Nephrology, University of Milan, S. Paolo Hospital, Milan, Italy

Abstract

Abnormalities of bone mineral parameters (calcium, phosphate, vitamin D, and parathyroid hormone) are nearly omnipresent in patients with advanced chronic kidney disease (CKD). These typically consist of hypocalcemia, hyperphosphatemia, abnormalities of vitamin D metabolism, and secondary hyperparathyroidism (SHPT). Currently, several lines of evidence suggest that these abnormalities may have consequences beyond the typical consequence of renal bone disease, with a major role in determining cardiovascular disease, including arterial calcification. The 'classical' treatment of SHPT and hyperphosphatemia in HD patients consists of phosphate binders, vitamin D receptor activators (VDRAs), and/or calcimimetics. Calcium- or aluminum-based phosphate binder prescriptions and calcitriol administration are therapeutic tools not free of complications, increasing the risk of cardiovascular calcification in the HD population. New calcium- and aluminum-free phosphate binders, such as lanthanum carbonate and sevelamer hydrochloride, new VDRA (paricalcitol), and cinacalcet hydrochloride can be used to treat SHPT, slow down the atherosclerotic process, and prevent vascular calcification in HD patients.

Copyright © 2008 S. Karger AG, Basel

Physiopathology of Secondary Hyperparathyroidism

The modern strategies to prevent and treat secondary hyperparathyroidism (SHPT) in chronic kidney disease (CKD) patients give great relevance to understand the molecular mechanisms involved into the pathogenesis of parathyroid hyperplasia and PTH synthesis and secretion. In fact, normal parathyroid cells are characterized by a low turnover and rarely undergo mitoses. However, in the presence of the SHPT features, such as low calcium, high phosphorus, vitamin D deficiency, and uremia, parathyroid cells leave quiescence [1].

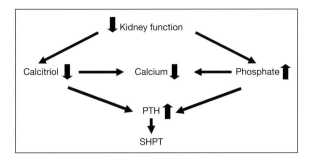

Fig. 1. Physiopathology of secondary hyperparathyroidism.

Elevated serum phosphate levels induce SHPT through indirect and direct mechanisms [1]. In addition, hyperphosphatemia indirectly inhibits calcitriol production [2], with subsequent hypocalcemia. In contrast to the mitogenic effects of hyperphosphatemia, dietary phosphorus restriction appears to counteract the proliferative signals induced by uremia, thus preventing parathyroid cell replication and the increase in parathyroid gland size [2].

Calcium is a key regulator factor in SHPT progression. Low serum calcium levels decrease the activation and the expression of the calcium-sensing receptor (CaSR), a plasma membrane G-protein-coupled molecule that allows parathyroid cells to sense calcium ions in the extracellular fluid, thus greatly promoting PTH synthesis and secretion [3]. In contrast, hypercalcemia activates the CaSR, rapidly suppressing SHPT. Recent evidence suggests that signaling through the CaSR plays an important role in parathyroid hyperplasia [3].

In the 5/6 nephrectomized rats, calcitriol suppresses uremia-induced parathyroid cell proliferation both in vitro and in vivo [4]. Many studies have been conducted to assess whether supplementation with vitamin D sterols can prevent or ameliorate SHPT in CKD. Serum concentrations of calcitriol start to decrease at values of creatinine clearance near 70 ml/min. Therefore, a sound approach to SHPT prevention and treatment requires taking into account many factors, including stage of CKD, underlying renal disorder, levels of circulating PTH, bone status, vitamin D deposits, and serum calcium and phosphate levels (fig. 1).

Phosphate Binders in Dialysis Patients

Calcium-Based Phosphate Binders

During the end of the 1980s and the following decade [5], calcium carbonate was introduced as first-choice drug, at high dosage, because there was a general consensus that, in addition to phosphate binding, high serum calcium levels were helpful to ameliorate the control of PTH secretion. Many reports however indicate that this strategy was associated with persistent hypercalcemia [6]. Furthermore, a simultaneous treatment with calcium carbonate and calcitriol may increase intestinal absorption of calcium and phosphorous leading to an oversuppression of PTH production and low-turnover bone disease [6]. Clearly, hypercalcemia is a major concern in hemodialysis (HD) patients. In several studies conducted in this population, coronary calcification was related to serum phosphorus concentration, calcium-phosphate product and the dose of calcium contained in the phosphate binders [7]. These data indicate that calcium overload is associated with a greater prevalence and progression of vascular calcification and that normal serum calcium levels are not representative of a present or past exposure to calcium overload [8].

Sevelamer Hydrochloride

Sevelamer hydrochloride belongs to a new generation of phosphate binders. This compound is a quaternary amine anion exchange resin that binds phosphate ions and releases protons. Experimental observations in uremic rats [9] and in dialysis patients [10] indicate that this calcium and aluminum-free phosphate binder reduces the progression of cardiovascular calcifications observed in control groups treated with calcium-based phosphate binders. In addition, reduction in total serum cholesterol and low-density lipoprotein is a further, peculiar, advantage of this phosphate binder [10]. However, the limited hypophosphatemic effect demanding the use of several pills in many patients hinders compliance thus making the management of hyperphosphatemia problematic in HD patients. Recently, a randomized comparison of sevelamer and calcium-based phosphate binders was performed in HD patients treated up to 45 months. The primary endpoint of this study was mortality. Overall mortality was not significantly reduced by sevelamer, even if among patients ≥65 years of age, sevelamer reduced the risk of death [11].

Lanthanum Carbonate

Lanthanum carbonate is an aluminum- and calcium-free salt with a high phosphate-binding capacity. Although lanthanum is a metal cation, it is not comparable to aluminum in its side effects: in fact there is no increased deposition of lanthanum in HD patients compared to controls with normal renal function. The phosphate-binding efficacy of lanthanum carbonate was compared in vitro with those of aluminum hydroxide, calcium carbonate and calcium acetate at pH of 3, 5 and 7 [12]. Importantly, lanthanum carbonate had a strong phosphate-binding capacity, at each pH value, similar to that of aluminum hydroxide, but greater than those of calcium salts. Several studies have shown that lanthanum carbonate is a highly effective phosphate binder in HD patients and is well tolerated with a demonstrated safety profile [12]. Lanthanum significantly reduced serum phosphorus levels when administered at doses between 2,250 and 3,000 mg daily over 4–6 weeks. The efficacy of lanthanum salts was studied in a double-blind and randomized fashion by Finn et al. [13]. In this study, 145 patients were randomized to receive either lanthanum carbonate versus placebo for 6 weeks. The intention-to-treat analysis showed a dose-dependent reduction of serum phosphorous levels documenting the efficacy and the safety of lanthanum carbonate, demanding a low pill burden compared to the other phosphate binders.

Vitamin D Receptor Activators

Prevention and treatment of SHPT commonly requires administration of vitamin D receptor activators (VDRAs). In fact, active vitamin D analogs effectively suppress PTH production and improve bone histology in HD patients [1]. VDRAs with a lower hypercalcemic and hyperphosphatemic activity are now available as an efficient alternative to calcitriol treatment. Between them, 1,25-dihydroxy-19-norvitamin D_2 (paricalcitol) was the first analog approved for use in HD patients and is available for intravenous administration, commonly three times a week after HD. Clearly, several studies established that paricalcitol rapidly suppresses PTH with no significant difference in the incidence of hyperphosphatemia or hypercalcemia compared to placebo. Paricalcitol has also been directly compared to calcitriol in an international study involving 263 HD patients. This study showed that paricalcitol reduced iPTH 50% or more from baseline, and did so significantly faster than calcitriol. Patients receiving paricalcitol had significantly fewer sustained episodes of hypercalcemia and/or increased calcium- phosphate product [14]. In addition, a historical study examined the records of 67,399 patients who had been treated exclusively with calcitriol or paricalcitol. Patients were evaluated over a 2-year period until one of the following occurred: death, a switch to another vitamin D formulation, renal transplantation, or transfer to another facility. This study showed a statistically significant difference in survival rate in favor of paricalcitol over calcitriol [15]. Furthermore, in patients taking paricalcitol a reduced hospitalization rate was observed. These findings will need to be supported by prospective trials before definitive conclusions can be made.

During the last 5 years, more studies analyzed new potential effects of paricalcitol on cardiovascular disease in renal patients. In experimental animal models, the limited hypercalcemic effect of paricalcitol results from a lower affinity for vitamin D receptor in intestine and bone. In addition, paricalcitol causes a selective vitamin D deficiency and a reduction in intestinal calcium absorption [1, 2]. Recently, in a very elegant in vivo study, Mizobuchi et al. [16] demonstrated that both calcitriol and doxercalciferol significantly increased the serum calcium-phosphate product and aortic calcium content in uremic rats. In contrast, paricalcitol had no effect on vascular calcification.

Cinacalcet Hydrochloride

The CaSR located on the surface of chief cells in the parathyroid gland is the principal regulator of PTH secretion and therefore is an ideal target for therapies to treat SHPT [3]. Calcimimetics are positive allosteric modulators of the CaSR that increase its sensitivity to extracellular calcium by lowering the threshold for activation by extracellular calcium ions. This causes a shift to the left in the sigmoidal curve that describes the relationship of blood-ionized calcium to PTH, lowering the calcium set point and resulting in reductions of PTH secretion. In clinical trials of HD patients with SHPT, oral administration of the calcimimetic cinacalcet hydrochloride decreased PTH with concurrent reductions in calcium-phosphate product, calcium, and phosphorus [17]. Because cinacalcet is not associated with elevations in calcium and phosphorus, treatment strategies that include cinacalcet may allow better achievement of the K/DOQI targets and possibly reduce complications associated with SHPT. In addition, lowering calcium and phosphorus levels with cinacalcet may allow the use of physiologic doses of VDRAs with a reduced risk for occurrence of hypercalcemia and hyperphosphatemia. Further studies to evaluate vascular calcification and cardiovascular outcomes will be needed to determine whether reductions in these parameters are associated with improved cardiovascular health.

Conclusions

The therapeutic strategies for SHPT are now changing. The availability of new calcium- and aluminum-free phosphate binders, paricalcitol and cinacalcet, warrants inhibition of parathyroid glands with a lower effect on calcium and phosphate levels, and perhaps reduces mortality of dialysis patients. Since cardiovascular disease is the leading cause of morbidity and mortality in HD patients, these data suggest that the beneficial effect associated with this 'new generation' treatment on HD patients survival is at least partially related to their effects on the cardiovascular system.

References

1   Cozzolino M, Brancaccio D, Gallieni M, et al: Pathogenesis of parathyroid hyperplasia in renal failure. J Nephrol 2005;18:5–8.
2   Denda M, Finch J, Slatopolsky E: Phosphorus accelerated the development of parathyroid hyperplasia and secondary hyperparathyroidism in rats with renal failure. Am J Kidney Dis 1996;28:596–602.
3   Brown EM: Calcium receptor and regulation of parathyroid hormone secretion. Rev Endocr Metab Disord 2000;1:307–315.
4   Szabo A, Merke J, Beier E, et al: 1,25(OH)$_2$ vitamin D$_3$ inhibits parathyroid cell proliferation in experimental uremia. Kidney Int 1989;35:1049–1056.
5   Slatopolsky E, Weerts C, Lopez-Hilker S, et al: Calcium carbonate as a phosphate binder in patients with chronic renal failure undergoing dialysis. N Engl J Med 1986;315:157–161.
6   Block GA, Klassen PS, Lazarus JM, et al: Mineral metabolism, mortality, and morbidity in maintenance hemodialysis. J Am Soc Nephrol 2004;15:2208–2218.
7   Cozzolino M, Brancaccio D, Gallieni M, Slatopolsky E: Pathogenesis of vascular calcification in chronic kidney disease. Kidney Int 2005;68:429–436.
8   Brancaccio D, Cozzolino M: The mechanism of calcium deposition in soft tissues. Contrib Nephrol. Basel, Karger, 2005, vol 149, pp 279–286.
9   Cozzolino M, Staniforth ME, Liapis H, et al: Sevelamer hydrochloride attenuates kidney and cardiovascular calcifications in long-term experimental uremia. Kidney Int 2003;64:1653–1661.
10   Chertow GM, Burke SK, Lazarus JM, et al: Poly[allylamine hydrochloride] (Renagel): a noncalcemic phosphate binder for the treatment of hyperphosphatemia in chronic renal failure. Am J Kidney Dis 1997;29:66–71.
11   Suki WN, Zabenh R, Cangiano JL, et al: Effects of sevelamer and calcium-based phosphate binders on mortality in hemodialysis patients. Kidney Int 2007;72:1130–1137.
12   Cozzolino M, Brancaccio D: Hyperphosphatemia in dialysis patients: the therapeutic role of lanthanum carbonate. Int J Artif Organs 2007;30:293–300.
13   Finn WF, Joy MS, Hladik G; Lanthanum Study Group: Efficacy and safety of lanthanum carbonate for reduction of serum phosphorus in patients with chronic renal failure receiving hemodialysis. Clin Nephrol 2004;62:193–201.
14   Sprague SM, Llach F, Amdhal M, et al: Paricalcitol versus calcitriol in the treatment of secondary hyperparathyroidism. Kidney Int 2003;63:1483–1490.
15   Teng M, Wolf M, Lowrie E, et al: Survival of patients undergoing hemodialysis with paricalcitol or calcitriol therapy. N Engl J Med 2003;349:446–456.
16   Mizobuchi M, Finch JL, Martin DR, Slatopolsky E, Cardus A, Panizo S, Parisi E, et al: Differential effects of vitamin D receptor activators on vascular calcification in uremic rats. Kidney Int 2007;72:709–715.
17   Block GA, Martin KJ, de Francisco ALM: Cinacalcet for secondary hyperparathyroidism in patients receiving hemodialysis. N Engl J Med 2004;350:1516–1525.

Mario Cozzolino, MD, PhD
Renal Division, S. Paolo Hospital, University of Milan
Via A. di Rudinì, 8, IT–20142 Milan (Italy)
Tel. +39 02 8184 4381, Fax +39 02 8912 9989, E-Mail mariocozzolino@hotmail.com

Ronco C, Cruz DN (eds): Hemodialysis – From Basic Research to Clinical Trials.
Contrib Nephrol. Basel, Karger, 2008, vol 161, pp 240–246

....

Insights in Anemia Management

Angel L.M. de Francisco, Celestino Piñera

Servicio de Nefrología, Hospital Universitario Valdecilla, Santander, Spain

---

Abstract

After almost 20 years, anemia in chronic kidney disease (CKD) and its treatment remain the focus of multiple questions for clinicians and investigators. The optimal hemoglobin (Hb) for patients with CKD is controversial and different targets are probably required for different populations. The current literature does not support an upper Hb target $>12\,g/dl$ and there is a clear demonstration of increased risk with Hb targets $>13\,g/dl$. With this narrow target of $11–12\,g/dl$, fluctuations in Hb concentration are commonly observed in patients being treated with erythropoiesis-stimulating agents (ESAs). Studies to date provide a suggestion of an association between Hb cycling and mortality, but they have been primarily exploratory in nature and clinical trials comparing treatment strategies leading to different degrees of Hb variability are needed. The great majority of incidences of pure red cell aplasia (PRCA) was associated with ESA therapy and was first recognized several years ago after a change in the formulation in which human serum albumin was eliminated and replaced by polysorbate-80 in patients on epoetin alfa (Eprex®). Years later, a registry (PRIMS) was established by the health authorities as part of a reapproval of the subcutaneous route to confirm that the cause of PRCA has been eliminated. The ongoing PRIMS study is a 3-year observation period prospective multicenter and international (Europe and Australia) registry that could serve as a model for assessment of the immunogenicity profiles of currently marketed and future ESAs. The association with a change in formulation makes PRCA of interest to the biotechnology industry as well as the medical community because it raises the broader question of the potential immunogenicity of biopharmaceuticals in general.

Copyright © 2008 S. Karger AG, Basel

Both anemia and erythropoietin deficiency in chronic kidney disease (CKD) patients are associated with adverse consequences in both cardiac and vascular structure and function. Epoetin therapy was introduced as a therapeutic agent in 1989, and treatment with recombinant human erythropoietin (rHuEPO) to partially correct anemia has greatly improved patients' lives and substantially reduced requirements for blood transfusion. After 19 years, anemia in CKD and its treatment remain the focus of multiple questions for clinicians and investigators.

Target Hemoglobin

The optimal target Hb level for anemic patients with CKD is controversial and different targets are probably required for different populations. KDOQI clinical practice guidelines and clinical practice recommendations for anemia in CKD in adults were published in May 2006 and recommended some changes to an effective target range of 11–13 g/dl. A specific upper limit was not defined but these guidelines include that there is insufficient evidence to recommend routinely maintaining Hb at ≥13.0 g/dl in erythropoiesis-stimulating agents (ESA)-treated patients [1]. Observational studies have found that lower levels of Hb are associated with worse outcomes, higher mortality risk, and an increased rate of hospitalizations, although no favorable effect on mortality was observed beyond a Hb level of 13.0 g/dl [2].

Four randomized control trials with adequate sample sizes have been published. The Normal Hematocrit Study [3] was a randomized controlled study of hemodialysis patients with established heart disease comparing a hematocrit target of 42–30%. The study was stopped because of concern for increased mortality in the patients randomized to the higher hematocrit group. Supplemental data, including endpoint events that occurred after the dataset was analyzed, have been reported recently. These additional data show no further evidence of detrimental outcomes associated with a normal hematocrit and the authors maintain their original conclusion that a target hematocrit value of 42% cannot be recommended in patients with cardiac disease who are undergoing hemodialysis [4]. The Canada-Europe study also randomized hemodialysis patients (excluding patients with symptomatic heart disease as well as those with left ventricular dilatation) to a higher versus lower Hb (Hb values of 13.0 vs. 11.0 g/dl, respectively). No significant benefit in either of the cardiac structural or functional parameters was observed in the high versus low Hb groups [5].

Two important randomized studies were performed in CKD patients in the USA (CHOIR) and Europe (CREATE). The CHOIR study [6] was an open-label, randomized trial that studied 1,432 patients with CKD: 715 patients were randomized to receive epoetin alfa targeted to achieve a Hb of 13.5 g/dl, and 717 were randomized to receive epoetin alfa targeted to achieve a Hb of 11.3 g/dl. Neither death nor congestive hospitalization were statistically significantly higher in the higher versus lower Hb group. The CREATE study [7] enrolled approximately 600 patients who were randomized to an early anemia correction or a late anemia correction group. The early anemia correction group received epoetin beta therapy immediately for a target Hb of 13–15 g/dl. The late anemia correction group did not receive treatment until their Hb was <10.5 g/dl; the target Hb was 10.5–11.5 g/dl. The study showed that 'complete correction' was not associated with a statistically significantly higher rate of the first cardiovascular event. Unlike CHOIR, in CREATE a quality-of-life benefit, at least in year 1 of the study, was observed for the higher versus lower Hb group.

A critical review has been published by Levin [8]. CREATE and CHOIR have helped to focus attention on the need for randomized clinical trials, but have not yet sufficiently answered the key question as to what and if there is an optimal Hb for patients with CKD: 'High doses of ESA are known to have vascular effects, the dosing regimen itself rather than the Hb values per se drove the results. It may be that there really is harm to targeting higher Hb in patients with significant co-morbidity, especially those who have had ischemic cardiac events. CHOIR cannot and should not be overinterpreted, given the multiple problems with the dropout and analytic issues raised earlier.'

The most accepted conclusion at the moment is that the current literature does not support an upper Hb target >12 g/dl. There is a clear demonstration of increased risk with Hb targets >13 g/dl, and an area of uncertainty, at which increased risk cannot be excluded between 12 and 13 g/dl. Targeting Hb levels 12–13 g/dl might be acceptable, despite the possibility of increased risk, if there was a clear tradeoff with treatment benefit [9].

Hemoglobin Cycling

Maintenance of Hb concentrations within current target ranges in clinical practice is complicated by large fluctuations in Hb concentration that are commonly observed in patients being treated with ESAs [10]. Variability in Hb levels over time is very common, with almost 90% of patients experiencing Hb level changes during a 6-month period, in part as a result of intercurrent illness, infections, bleeding complications, hospitalizations, and epoetin-dosing changes. A change in ESA dose appears to be the most important of these factors. Fishbane and Berns [11] found that increases in Hb concentration of ≥ 1.5 g/dl were most frequently associated with increases in rHuEPO dose (84% of cases), whereas decreases in Hb concentration were most frequently associated with holds or decreases in rHuEPO dose (15 and 62% of cases, respectively).

The question to be answered is whether these Hb oscillations are associated with an increased mortality risk. Gilbertson et al. [12] studied in a retrospective study of 159,720 hemodialysis patients receiving epoetin therapy the associations between the degree of Hb level variability in the first 6 months of 2004 and subsequent mortality rates in the following 6 months. They conclude that the number of months with Hb values below the target range, rather than Hb variability itself, may be the primary driver of increased risk of death.

Yang et al. [13] used a Fresenius Medical Care database to retrospectively examine a cohort of 34,963 hemodialysis patients from 1996. They demonstrated that Hb variability, defined by residual standard deviation, was significantly associated with mortality, even after accounting for a number of potential confounders.

Studies to date however have been primarily exploratory in nature and only provide a suggestion of an association between Hb cycling and mortality. In addition, studies have been confined to hemodialysis patients alone. This phenomenon requires more investigation. We have observed that Hb variability is also common in renal transplant patients treated with ESA due to dose changes and inflammatory status and independently of the ESA used [14]. Clinical trials comparing treatment strategies leading to different degrees of Hb variability will be needed to clarify the true causal nature of this association, to distinguish cause from effect, to understand the underlying mechanism of Hb variability cause from effect and to understand the underlying mechanism of Hb variability.

Pure Red Cell Aplasia – Where Are We?

Pure red cell aplasia (PRCA) associated with ESA therapy was first recognized in 2002. Most of the initial cases, reported by Casadevall et al. [15], were in patients who were treated with epoetin manufactured by Ortho Biotech outside the USA (Eprex®, Erypo®), but cases have since been reported with all commercially available ESAs. The hallmark of ESA-induced PRCA is the absence of erythroblasts from an otherwise normal bone marrow and the presence of neutralizing antierythropoietin antibodies.

Almost all patients with PRCA require regular packed red cell transfusions until the PRCA resolves and the antierythropoietin antibodies disappear. Early recognition of PRCA and withholding of ESA therapy are essential, but cessation of ESA treatment alone generally will not cure ESA-induced PRCA. In patients with CKD and ESA-induced PRCA, immunosuppressive treatment is usually required to induce disappearance of antierythropoietin antibodies. Recovery rates from PRCA of 2% have been reported without immunosuppressive therapy, 52% after immunosuppressive treatment(s) outside the renal transplantation setting, and 95% after kidney transplantation. A recent animal study suggested that a possible alternative strategy may be to administer a novel peptide-based erythropoietin receptor agonist called Hematide that does not cross-react with antierythropoietin antibodies, and will allow ongoing stimulation of erythropoiesis; this is the subject of a clinical trial with excellent results [16].

The great majority of incidences occurred in patients who received epoetin alfa (Eprex®/Erypo®), between 1998 and 2002, after a change in the formulation in which human serum albumin was eliminated and replaced by polysorbate-80 to avoid the risk for virus or previous transmission. The exact mechanism that leads to the development of antibody-induced PRCA remains unknown. It has been proposed that leachates released from rubber stoppers used only in syringes from Ortho Biotech could act as adjuvants and induce an immune response against erythropoietin, but experimental data substantiating this claim are controversial.

In 2002, the subcutaneous route for Eprex®/Erypo® was contraindicated in the European Union and Switzerland, and in 2006 the European health authorities reapproved subcutaneous administration (with coated stoppers) in CKD patients. A registry was established by the health authorities as part of a reapproval to confirm that the cause of PRCA has been eliminated and to estimate the incidence rate of erythropoietin antibody-mediated PRCA in patients with CRF (established CKD) after subcutaneous exposure to Eprex® (epoetin alfa) or any other ESAs marketed at registry initiation (e.g., NeoRecormon® (epoetin beta) and Aranesp® (darbepoetin alfa)). The ongoing PRIMS study is a 3-year observation period prospective multicenter and international (Europe and Australia) registry that could serve as a model for assessment of the immunogenicity profiles of currently marketed and future ESAs.

Biosimilars

The association with a change in formulation makes PRCA of interest to the biotechnology industry as well as the medical community because it raises the broader question of the potential immunogenicity of biopharmaceuticals in general. The number of biological/biotechnology-derived proteins used as therapeutic agents is steadily increasing. These products may induce an unwanted immune response in treated patients, which can be influenced by various factors, including patient-/disease-related factors and product-related factors.

Recombinant proteins are associated with a number of issues which distinguish them from traditional chemical drugs and their generics. Recombinant proteins are highly complex at the molecular level, and biological manufacturing processes are highly elaborate involving cloning, selection of a suitable cell line, fermentation, purification and formulation.

Generics may be introduced when the patent of an innovative drug expires. Clinical trials required for the approval of new products to demonstrate safety and efficacy are not necessary for the approval of conventional generics, so the clinical data generated with the original product can be extrapolated to the generic [17]. However, results of appropriate preclinical tests or clinical trials must be provided in the case of biosimilars. Guidelines on immunogenicity assessment of biotechnology-derived therapeutic proteins are finalized by EMEA and in the context of immunogenicity assessment, biosimilars have to be considered on the same basis as innovative products [18].

Reducing health costs is a strong political issue in the majority of countries. A potential opportunity for price reductions versus the originator biopharmaceuticals remains to be determined, as the advantage of a slightly cheaper price may be outweighed by the hypothetical increased risk of side effects from biosimilar molecules that are not exact copies of their originators.

References

1   KDOQI: National Kidney Foundation. II. Clinical practice guidelines and clinical practice recommendations for anemia in chronic kidney disease in adults. Am J Kidney Dis 2006;47:S16–S85.
2   Regidor DL, Kopple JD, Kovesdy CP, Kilpatrick RD, McAllister CJ, Aronovitz J, Greenland S, Kalantar-Zadeh K: Associations between changes in hemoglobin and administered erythropoiesis-stimulating agent and survival in hemodialysis patients. J Am Soc Nephrol 2006;17:1181–1191.
3   Besarab A, Bolton WK, Browne JK, Egrie JC, Nissenson AR, Okamoto DM, Schwab SJ, Goodkin DA: The effects of normal as compared with low hematocrit values in patients with cardiac disease who are receiving hemodialysis and epoetin. N Engl J Med 1998;339:584–590.
4   Besarab A, Goodkin DA, Nissenson AR; Normal Hematocrit Cardiac Trial Authors: The normal hematocrit study – follow-up. N Engl J Med 2008;358:433–434.
5   Parfrey PS, Foley RN, Wittreich BH, Sullivan DJ, Zagari MJ, Frei D: Double-blind comparison of full and partial anemia correction in incident hemodialysis patients without symptomatic heart disease. J Am Soc Nephrol 2005;16:2180–2189.
6   Singh AK, Szczech L, Tang KL, Barnhart H, Sapp S, Wolfson M, Reddan D; CHOIR Investigators: Correction of anemia with epoetin alfa in chronic kidney disease. N Engl J Med 2006;355:2085–2098.
7   Drueke TB, Locatelli F, Clyne N, Eckardt KU, Macdougall IC, Tsakiris D, Burger HU, Scherhag A; CREATE Investigators: Normalization of hemoglobin level in patients with chronic kidney disease and anemia. N Engl J Med 2006;355:2071–2084.
8   Levin A: Understanding recent haemoglobin trials in CKD: methods and lesson learned from CREATE and CHOIR. Nephrol Dial Transplant 2007;22:309–312.
9   Singh AK, Fishbane S: The optimal hemoglobin in dialysis patients – a critical review. Semin Dial 2008;21:1–6.
10 Berns JS, Elzein H, Lynn RI, Fishbane S, Meisels IS, Deoreo PB: Hemoglobin variability in epoetin-treated hemodialysis patients. Kidney Int 2003;64:1514–1521.
11 Fishbane S, Berns JS: Hemoglobin cycling in hemodialysis patients treated with recombinant human erythropoietin. Kidney Int 2005;68:1337–1343.
12 Gilbertson DT, Ebben JP, Foley RN, Weinhandl ED, Bradbury BD, Collins AJ: Hemoglobin level variability: associations with mortality. Clin J Am Soc Nephrol 2008;3:133–138.
13 Yang W, Israni RK, Brunelli SM, Joffe MM, Fishbane S, Feldman HI: Hemoglobin variability and mortality in ESRD. J Am Soc Nephrol 2007;18:3164–3170.
14 Fernandez-Fresnedo G, De Francisco A, Ruiz JC, Rodrigo EG, Alamillo C, Pinera C, Arias M: Hemoglobin variability in renal transplant patients treated with erythropoiesis stimulant agents (abstract). American Society of Nephrology Annual Meeting, San Francisco 2007.
15 Casadevall N, Nataf J, Viron B: Pure red-cell aplasia and antierythropoietin antibodies in patients treated with recombinant erythropoietin. N Engl J Med 2002;346:469–475.

16   Macdougall I: Epoetin-induced pure red cell aplasia: diagnosis and treatment. Curr Opin Nephrol
      Hypertens 2007;16:585–588 and personal communication.
17   Schellekens H: The first biosimilar epoetin: but how similar is it? Clin J Am Soc Nephrol 2008
      3:174–178.
18   http://www.emea.europa.eu/pdfs/human/biosimilar/1432706enfin.pdf

Prof. Angel L.M. de Francisco
Servicio de Nefrologia, Hospital Universitario Valdecilla
ES–39008 Santander (Spain)
Tel. +34 942 202738, Fax +34 942 320415, E-Mail martinal@unican.es

Ronco C, Cruz DN (eds): Hemodialysis – From Basic Research to Clinical Trials.
Contrib Nephrol. Basel, Karger, 2008, vol 161, pp 247–254

....

Red Blood Cell Lifespan, Erythropoiesis and Hemoglobin Control

Anja Kruse[a], Dominik E. Uehlinger[b,c], Frank Gotch[a],
Peter Kotanko[a], Nathan W. Levin[a]

[a]Renal Research Institute, New York, N.Y., USA; [b]Division of Pharmacokinetics and
Drug Therapy, Uppsala University, Uppsala, Sweden; [c]Department of Nephrology and
Hypertension, Inselspital, University of Bern, Switzerland

Abstract

Erythropoietin (EPO) and iron deficiency as causes of anemia in patients with limited renal function or end-stage renal disease are well addressed. The concomitant impairment of red blood cell (RBC) survival has been largely neglected. Properties of the uremic environment like inflammation, increased oxidative stress and uremic toxins seem to be responsible for the premature changes in RBC membrane and cytoskeleton. The exposure of antigenic sites and breakdown of the phosphatidylserine asymmetry promote RBC phagocytosis. While the individual response to treatment with EPO-stimulating agents (ESA) depends on both the RBC's lifespan and the production rate, uniform dosing algorithms do not meet that demand. The clinical use of mathematical models predicting ESA-induced changes in hematocrit might be greatly improved once independent estimates of RBC production rate and/or lifespan become available, thus making the concomitant estimation of both parameters unnecessary. Since heme breakdown by the hemoxygenase pathway results in carbon monoxide (CO) which is exhaled, a simple CO breath test has been used to calculate hemoglobin turnover and therefore RBC survival and lifespan. Future research will have to be done to validate and implement this method in patients with kidney failure. This will result in new insights into RBC kinetics in renal patients. Eventually, these findings are expected to improve our understanding of the hemoglobin variability in response to ESA.

Copyright © 2008 S. Karger AG, Basel

While erythropoietin (EPO) and iron deficiency as causes of anemia in patients with limited renal function or end-stage renal disease are well addressed, the loss of erythrocytes is still a relevant but less recognized part of the problem. In addition to frank bleeding, such loss occurs to a substantial extent because of premature cell death. The impaired red blood cell (RBC) survival (contributing to what is called 'EPO resistance' and thus treatment costs) has been considered as an important factor for many years, yet little is known today about the natural history and the pathogenesis nor the possibilities of influencing this condition. The subject has been largely neglected.

The Erythrocyte Lifespan

Cell death in human hematopoietic cells is regulated by signals from cell surface receptors that can either promote apoptosis or protect from cell death through transcriptional protein regulation. Human mature erythrocytes are terminally differentiated cells possessing neither mitochondria nor nucleolus through which death is considered to be controlled in other hematopoietic cells. The regulation of the RBC's lifespan is to a great extent unknown. The erythrocyte normally circulates in the blood for about 120 days; thereafter it is phagocytized by resident macrophages. Physiological mechanisms leading to changes in cytoskeleton and cell membrane and finally to the erythrocyte's death as well as signals enabling the macrophages to recognize specifically senescent RBCs are subject to ongoing research.

During their life, erythrocytes experience a decrease in diameter and corpuscular volume due to a release of membrane segments as vesicles containing only small amounts of hemoglobin. Loss of size, surface area as well as higher plasma density and viscosity contribute to impaired deformation capability when RBCs pass the capillary bed and splenic cord and increase their susceptibility to phagocytosis [1].

Aging RBCs increase exposure of antigenic sites in the RBC membrane, such as senescent cell antigen due to band 3 modification. Binding of IgG autoimmune antibodies leads to phagocytosis [2].

An alternative pathway of particular interest is the loss of the lipid asymmetry of the RBC membrane in senescent or injured RBCs. Phosphatidylserine (PS), of which in healthy erythrocytes 96% is located in the inner leaflet, triggers macrophage recognition when exposed at the outside [3]. The breakdown of the membrane asymmetry is initiated by the Ca^{2+}-sensitive enzyme scramblase, which is activated by an increase of cytosolic Ca^{2+} through activation of a Ca^{2+} permeable cation channel in the RBC membrane.

As a carrier of oxygen, erythrocytes are permanently exposed to oxygen-derived free radicals and other reactive oxygen species. Mature RBCs lack a nucleolus and cannot produce new proteins in response to stress. In senescent erythrocytes, activities of protective enzymes such as superoxide dismutase or the glutathione system are decreased. This leads to time-dependent changes in the lipid organization of the cell membrane and cytoskeleton. Scavenger receptors of the macrophages recognize oxidative damaged cells in an antibody-independent manner and induce cell death and phagocytosis by binding [4].

Erythrocyte Survival in Renal Failure

EPO is essential for differentiation and survival of the red blood precursor cells. A suppressed bone marrow response to signals of erythropoiesis despite EPO levels in the (high) normal range suggests the presence of toxic compounds or cytokines in uremic blood leading to EPO resistance. Besides lower production, a distinct shorter RBC lifespan (45–85 days compared to 120 days in healthy subjects) contributes to the anemia of renal disease and seems to be unchanged during the last decades. Erythrocytes from uremic patients show an almost normal survival when transfused into healthy subjects. This points towards specific properties of the uremic environment resulting in a shortened RBC lifespan [5]. It is speculated that higher molecular weight uremic toxins are at least in part causal since methods removing a greater amount of them reduce the capability of uremic serum to induce loss of PS asymmetry and patients on peritoneal dialysis show less PS exposure compared to hemodialysis [6].

Although the effect of EPO on RBC survival is limited in the mature compared to the progenitor cell, EPO can inhibit Ca^{2+} channels on the RBC membrane and thus reduce the lethal breakdown of PS asymmetry [7]. This observation is in accordance with clinical reports of prolonged RBC survival in patients on EPO therapy [8].

The capability to respond to oxidative stress is crucial for RBC survival. Several authors suggest an imbalance between the greater amount of oxidative stress in the uremic state and the capability of the RBC to deal with it. Decreased glutathione plasma levels in uremic patients as well as a defect in antioxidant forces outside the glutathione system could attenuate the RBCs defense mechanism and lead to cell damage [9]. Clinical studies showing a RBC lifespan prolongation with glutathione infusion or vitamin-E-coded dialysis membranes support this concept [10].

As in patients suffering from anemia of chronic disease, the state of chronic inflammation of hemodialysis patients contributes to anemia not only because of a decreased RBC production (due to direct inhibition of erythropoiesis or indirectly due to an altered iron metabolism), but also due to decreased RBC survival [11, 12].

Influence of the RBC Lifespan on Therapy Management and Dosing Algorithms of EPO-Stimulating Agents

The total number of RBC at any time point is given by the RBC production rate and lifespan. During steady-state conditions, RBC production rate equals the RBC death rate. Increasing the RBC production rate with the introduction of a therapy with EPO-stimulating agents (ESA) will lead to a rise in hematocrit since none of the additionally produced erythrocytes have yet died. After reaching one lifespan, the RBCs start dying at the increased rate they were produced and a new steady state is achieved. The time to this new steady state depends only on the lifespan of the erythrocytes (or exogenous blood loss), whereas the increase in hematocrit depends on both the increase in RBC production and the RBC lifespan.

Observed changes in hematocrit induced by ESA can be modeled by summing up all the produced RBC generations still alive at any time point. A simplified model accounting for multiple ESA dose changes has previously been described [13]:

$$Hct(t) = Hct_0 + \sum_{i=1}^{n} \delta(t - T_i) \cdot (\beta_i - \beta_{i-1}) \cdot \int_0^{t-T_i} S(x)dx$$

where $Hct(t)$ is the hematocrit at time t, Hct_0 is the baseline hematocrit, T_i is the time of the i-th dose change, β_i is the change in RBC production rate induced by the i-th dose, $S(x)$ is the RBC survival function and

$$\delta(x) = \begin{bmatrix} 1 & \text{if} & x \geq 0 \\ 0 & \text{otherwise} \end{bmatrix}$$

Theoretically, any survival function definition can be used for the model described above. A simple survival function assuming RBC death from aging only would be:

$$S(x) = \frac{1}{1 + e^{\alpha(x-\tau)}}$$

where τ is the finite RBC lifespan and α is an empiric value to describe the dispersion of RBC lifespans around a mean lifespan τ.

The use of this model is successful if sufficient observations over a long time period are available [13]. When a new ESA therapy is started, neither prior information on the individual dose-response relationship nor on the individual RBC lifespan are usually available. It will therefore take one or two dose changes and a minimum observation period of one RBC lifespan after the last dose change before sufficient information is gathered to derive an optimal dosage of ESA (fig. 1).

Kruse/Uehlinger/Gotch/Kotanko/Levin

250

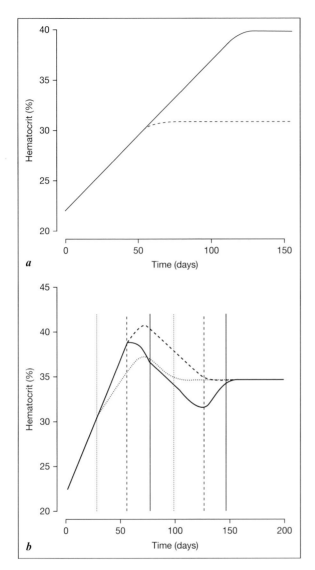

a

b

Fig. 1. Influence of RBC lifespan or changes in RBC production rate on the expected course of hematocrit during treatment with ESA. *a* The influence of two different lifespans, i.e. 120 days (——) or 60 days (– – –) on the course of hematocrit during a constant dose of ESA. *b* The expected courses of hematocrit after a decrease of the ESA to a lower, constant dose assuming a constant RBC lifespan of 70 days. The ESA dose is either decreased after 4 weeks (···) or after 8 weeks (– – –) or it is stopped after 8 weeks and recommenced at the lower constant dose as soon as the hematocrit starts falling (1 week after reaching the RBC lifespan, i.e. at week 11). The vertical lines represent the times of the last dose changes (at 4, 8 and 11 weeks) and the reaching of the steady-state conditions one RBC lifespan later (at 14, 18 and 21 weeks, respectively).

The use of the model described above might be greatly improved if independent estimates of RBC production rate or lifespan were available and the concomitant estimation of both parameters became unnecessary. Numerous models describing the influence of ESA on reticulocyte distribution and survival are available. A recently published model describing reticulocyte and mature RBC distribution and survival concomitantly has shown that small misjudgments of the reticulocyte age distribution will lead to a large error in the estimation of the RBC lifespan [14]. For the clinical use of such models and the derivation of future ESA-dosing algorithms, an independent measure of the RBC lifespan is therefore of utmost importance.

Determination of the RBC Lifespan

In order to study alterations in the erythrocytes survival, reliable and simple methods of lifespan estimation are crucial. While estimation of RBC survival using reticulocyte percentage and hematocrit is simple, it is of limited accuracy and different direct and indirect methods have been employed.

RBC Lifespan Estimation by [51]Cr Labeling

The most frequent used method is random labeling with ^{51}Cr where a sample of the subject's own RBCs is incubated with a ^{51}Cr chloride solution. After reinjection the ^{51}Cr remaining in the circulation is measured in intervals to determine ^{51}Cr half-life.

Interpretation of the results is complicated by the fact that ^{51}Cr is eluted from the erythrocytes to an amount that differs from patient to patient and can exceed the clearance of RBCs. Thus, the observed half-time is shorter than the theoretical value (55–60 days), in the range of 28–37 days for healthy adults. Besides ^{51}Cr labeling tagging of the RBC with ^{14}C-cyanate, DF[32]P or biotin has been used.

Hemoxygenase Carbon Monoxide Pathway

When RBCs are dying, the heme contained is converted to bilirubin by the hemoxygenase pathway. The resulting carbon monoxide (CO) is exhaled in the breath where it can be detected using a gas chromatograph or infrared absorption technology.

As hemoglobin breakdown represents the majority of heme turnover, the CO amount in the alveolar breath depends on heme turnover and therefore RBC survival and production and the RBC lifespan can be calculated with the formula [15]:

$$\text{RBC lifespan (days)} = \frac{\text{hemoglobin (g/ml)} \cdot 22400 \cdot 4 \cdot \text{blood volume}}{0.7 \cdot \text{endogenous pCO} \cdot 64000 \cdot 1440 \cdot \text{alveolar ventilation}}$$

where 22400 is the volume (ml) of 1 mol CO; 4 mol of CO are bound to 1 mol of Hb; 0.7 is the approximate fraction of CO derived from circulating hemoglobin; 64400 is the molecular weight of hemoglobin and 1440 are minutes per day.

Blood volume and alveolar ventilation can be cancelled out in this equation because of roughly similar magnitudes when expressed in ml and ml/min. This leads to:

$$\text{RBC lifespan} = \text{Hb} \cdot \text{K/endogenous CO (ppm)} \quad (\text{K} = 1380\,\text{ml} \cdot \text{day/g})$$

Future research will have to be done to validate and implement this method in patients with kidney failure. This will result in new insights into RBC kinetics in renal patients. Eventually, these findings are expected to improve our understanding of the hemoglobin variability in response to ESA.

References

1   Bratosin D, Mazurier J, Tissier JP, Estaquier J, Huart JJ, Ameisen JC, et al: Cellular and molecular mechanisms of senescent erythrocyte phagocytosis by macrophages. A review. Biochimie 1998;80:173–195.
2   Arese P, Turrini F, Schwarzer E: Band 3/complement-mediated recognition and removal of normally senescent and pathological human erythrocytes. Cell Physiol Biochem 2005;16:133–146.
3   Kuypers FA, de Jong K: The role of phosphatidylserine in recognition and removal of erythrocytes. Cell Mol Biol (Noisy-le-Grand) 2004;50:147–158.
4   Sambrano GR, Parthasarathy S, Steinberg D: Recognition of oxidatively damaged erythrocytes by a macrophage receptor with specificity for oxidized low density lipoprotein. Proc Natl Acad Sci USA 1994;91:3265–3269.
5   Bonomini M, Sirolli V: Uremic toxicity and anemia. J Nephrol 2003;16:21–28.
6   Sirolli V, Cappelli P, Amoroso L, Di Liberato L, Muscianese P, Santarelli P, et al: Online HFR and removal of uremic toxins inducing the loss of phospholipidic asymmetry of the erythrocyte membrane (in Italian). G Ital Nefrol 2004;21(suppl 30):S208–S211.
7   Myssina S, Huber SM, Birka C, Lang PA, Lang KS, Friedrich B, et al: Inhibition of erythrocyte cation channels by erythropoietin. J Am Soc Nephrol 2003;14:2750–2757.
8   Polenakovic M, Sikole A: Is erythropoietin a survival factor for red blood cells? J Am Soc Nephrol 1996;7:1178–1182.
9   Weinstein T, Chagnac A, Korzets A, Boaz M, Ori Y, Herman M, et al: Haemolysis in haemodialysis patients: evidence for impaired defence mechanisms against oxidative stress. Nephrol Dial Transplant 2000;15:883–887.

10   Usberti M, Gerardi G, Micheli A, Tira P, Bufano G, Gaggia P, et al: Effects of a vitamin E-bonded membrane and of glutathione on anemia and erythropoietin requirements in hemodialysis patients. J Nephrol 2002;15:558–564.

11   Stenvinkel P: The role of inflammation in the anaemia of end-stage renal disease. Nephrol Dial Transplant 2001;16(suppl 7):36–40.

12   Mitlyng BL, Singh JA, Furne JK, Ruddy J, Levitt MD: Use of breath carbon monoxide measurements to assess erythrocyte survival in subjects with chronic diseases. Am J Hematol 2006;81: 432–438.

13   Uehlinger DE, Gotch FA, Sheiner LB: A pharmacodynamic model of erythropoietin therapy for uremic anemia. Clin Pharmacol Ther 1992;51:76–89.

14   Krzyzanski W, Perez-Ruixo JJ: An assessment of recombinant human erythropoietin effect on reticulocyte production rate and lifespan distribution in healthy subjects. Pharm Res 2007;24: 758–772.

15   Strocchi A, Schwartz S, Ellefson M, Engel RR, Medina A, Levitt MD: A simple carbon monoxide breath test to estimate erythrocyte turnover. J Lab Clin Med 1992;120:392–399.

Dr. Nathan W. Levin
Renal Research Institute, 207 East 94th Street, Suite 303
New York, NY 10128 (USA)
Tel. +1 646 672 4002, Fax +1 212 996 5905, E-Mail nlevin@rriny.com

Ronco C, Cruz DN (eds): Hemodialysis – From Basic Research to Clinical Trials.
Contrib Nephrol. Basel, Karger, 2008, vol 161, pp 255–260

....

New Erythropoiesis-Stimulating Agents: How Innovative Are They?

Lucia Del Vecchio, Francesco Locatelli

Department of Nephrology, Dialysis and Renal Transplant,
Ospedale A. Manzoni, Lecco, Italy

Abstract

Recombinant human erythropoietin (rHuEPO) has revolutionized the management of anemia in patients with chronic kidney disease. However, being similar to the naturally occurring molecule, rHuEPO is not a perfect pharmaceutical. Given its relatively short half-life, it requires a relatively frequent administration schedule. Moreover, it can be administered only subcutaneously or intravenously and it is unstable at room temperature, making necessary a strict cold chain. Pharmacological research has focused on the development of new agents in order to circumvent these relative disadvantages. New-generation erythropoietin-stimulating agents containing increased carbohydrate content (i.e. darbepoetin-α) or a large water-soluble polyethylene glycol moiety (continuous erythropoiesis receptor activator) are already available or nearly for clinical use and allow less frequent administration schedules than rHuEPO. Hematide, which is a dimeric peptide with chemical structure unrelated to EPO, is undergoing phase III clinical trials. Other possible strategies currently under research include fusion EPO proteins, gene therapy, hypoxia-inducible transcription factor stabilizers, GATA inhibition and hematopoietic cell phosphatase inhibition.

Copyright © 2008 S. Karger AG, Basel

Anemia, resulting primarily from insufficient production of erythropoietin to support erythropoiesis, is a common complication of chronic kidney disease (CKD). Left untreated, it may significantly impair quality of life, increase cardiovascular risk, and reduce long-term survival. Previously, treatment options were essentially limited to blood transfusions; however, since the late 1980s the availability of recombinant human erythropoietin (rHuEPO) has revolutionized the management of anemia in patients with CKD. Today, erythropoiesis-stimulating agents (ESA) are the main tool to achieve anemia correction in CKD patients.

Is There Any Room for New Erythropoietin-Stimulating Agents?

Since its synthesis in 1986, rHuEPO has been proven effective and relatively safe in correcting anemia and maintaining stable hemoglobin levels in CKD patients. However, naturally occurring proteins rarely make perfect pharmaceuticals. This is also true for rHuEPO, which cannot be considered the ideal ESA for a number of reasons. First, it requires a relatively frequent administration schedule that may increase the workload to caregivers when the drug is not self-administered. Second, it can be administered only subcutaneously or intravenously, but the intravenous route increases dose needs compared to the subcutaneous one. This implies that in the setting of hemodialysis, where the intravenous route is more convenient, physicians have to balance increased costs due to extra dose needs with patient discomfort related to subcutaneous injections for months or years. Moreover, the subcutaneous use of epoetin-α may have had a causal role in the upsurge of pure red cell aplasia cases observed in the last years. The oral or nasal administration of ESAs would be more easy and comfortable for patients, but the bioavailability of rHuEPO by the oral route is insufficient and the burden of the number of pills to be taken is relevant. Another important limitation of rHuEPO is that it is unstable at room temperature. A strict cold chain is thus necessary, starting from the manufacturer till the moment of administration; an inadequate handling of the drug may increase the risk of immunization in patients self-administering the drug at home. At present the treatment of anemia with rHuEPO is quite expensive, given that its synthesis, as that of other biomolecules, is complex. New ESAs are or will be more expensive than rHuEPO, because of the high costs of pharmacological research not yet covered by years of selling. However, the synthesis of simpler molecules not related to ESA structure may lead to the creation of cheaper ESAs that would revolutionize the market.

High-Molecular-Weight Erythropoietins

In order to improve pharmodynamics and pharmacokinetics of rHuEPO and allow a reduction in the frequency of administration, in the last decade pharmacological research has made a great effort in modifying the EPO molecule. Darbepoetin-α is the first EPO analogue with prolonged survival in the circulation and greater biological activity; like epoetin-α and -β, it is produced in Chinese hamster ovary cells but it differs from EPO in the amino acid sequence at five positions and contains five N-linked carbohydrate chains instead of three [1]. As a result, it has increased molecular weight, increased negative charge, sialic acid content and increased negative charge than EPO.

These characteristics cause a longer circulating half-life (~25 h when given intravenously and ~48 h by the subcutaneous route), counterbalancing a lower relative affinity for the EPO receptor than that of rHuEPO. Given its longer half-life, darbepoetin-α can be administered less often than rHuEPO [2]. Data from secondary analyses [2] and from one prospective and randomized crossover study [3] suggest that dose requirements are independent of the administration route.

Another possibility is the adding of a large water-soluble polyethylene glycol moiety to the EPO molecule in order to increase half-life. Continuous erythropoiesis receptor activator was obtained. This agent has a nearly double molecular weight than that of EPO and a longer half-life (~130 h when administered either i.v. or s.c). Moreover, it has a reduced binding affinity for the erythropoietin receptor, which is ~45-fold lower than that of epoetin-β, mainly due to a much slower association rate. These receptor-binding properties may contribute to distinct pharmacological characteristics. Results of phase II and III clinical trials suggest that this agent is effective in maintaining hemoglobin levels after switching from rHuEPO therapy or darbepoetin-α when administered up to once a month [4]. As for darbepoetin-α, the dose does not need to be modified according to the administration route.

Other EPO Derivates

In order to increase EPO half-life, a number of fusion polymers have been created. One approach is the production of a multivalent molecule consisting of two EPO molecules linked by small flexible peptides [5] or the fusion the carboxyl-terminal peptide of human chorionic gonadotropin β-subunit to human EPO [6].

Another approach includes increasing the molecular weight of the protein of interest by fusion to the Fc part of an antibody [7]. Interestingly, this approach has recently been used to create an Fc fusion protein that can be administered by aerosol inhalation [8].

CNTO 530 is an EPO-mimetic antibody fusion peptide with no homology to EPO [9]. In vitro CNTO 530 activated the EPO receptor, rescued cells from apoptosis and mediated proliferation. In vivo data obtained in mice showed a mean half-life of approximately 40 h and a long-lived stimulation of erythropoiesis after a single subcutaneous dose.

As already underlined, rHuEPO is produced through an expensive and complicated process requiring recombinant DNA technology. The research has attempted to circumvent this disadvantage by synthesizing artificially a glycoprotein similar to EPO, called synthetic erythropoiesis protein. This is a 51-kDa protein polymer consisting of a 166-amino-acid polypeptide chain and two covalently attached polymer moieties that are negatively charged [10].

All these EPO-modified proteins rise some concerns about immunogenicity, as testified by the induction of antibodies and severe anemia in monkeys receiving a dimeric fusion protein of EPO.

Small-Molecule Erythropoiesis-Stimulating Agents

Near a decade ago a number of isolate small peptides that bind to and activate the EPO receptor were isolated with no sequence homology to EPO; covalent dimerization was found to improve characteristics of selected peptides. Among these, hematide was selected for clinical development. This is a pegylated synthetic dimeric peptide with no sequence homology to EPO. Differing from rHuEPO, darbepoetin-α and continuous erythropoiesis receptor activator, it has longer half-life in the presence of renal insufficiency consistent with the hypothesis that hematide is cleared, at least partially, via the kidney [11]. Phase II trials ended and preliminary results were presented: the drug given either intravenously or subcutaneously was effective in both the correction and maintenance phase of anemia treatment at dose ranges between 0.025 and 0.05 mg/kg. Antibodies against hematide have been found in patients receiving the drug. However, they do not seem to cross-react with EPO [12]. Potential advantages of this new class of agents are that their manufacturing process is simpler and cheaper than that of current ESAs and that they have higher stability at room temperature.

Gene Therapy

EPO gene therapy has been explored in animal studies and in trials on CKD patients. This approach has the theoretical advantage of releasing small but continuous amounts of EPO into the circulation. A number of different techniques have been tried, such as the delivering of naked plasmid DNA into skeletal muscles, the subcutaneous implantation of EPO-secreting genetically engineered autologous bone marrow stromal cells, viral transfection or use of artificial human chromosome.

While gene therapy could be more economical and more convenient for long-term management of anemic patients than conventional ESA treatment, its major problem is immunogenicity of ex vivo transfected implanted cells and of the recombinant protein produced after ex vivo or in vivo EPO cDNA transfer. Another technical problem related to gene therapy is the difficulty to exactly tune the exact amount of EPO needed to correct anemia, maintaining a level of expression that sufficiently promotes erythropoiesis in the long term but avoids the development of polycythemia.

Other Strategies to Increase Erythropoiesis

EPO gene expression is modulated by a number of transcription factors. Their inhibition or activation may be thus an alternative option for stimulating erythropoiesis to agents activating the EPO receptor.

The hypoxia-inducible transcription factors (HIFs) are central components in the cellular responses to hypoxia; under normoxic conditions, EPO gene expression is suppressed as a result of HIF inactivation because of O_2-dependent enzymatic hydroxylation. 2-Oxoglutarate analogues, which prevent HIF-α hydroxylation, have emerged as promising tools for stimulation of erythropoiesis and angiogenesis (the so-called HIF stabilizers). Unfortunately the clinical development of the first candidate molecule, FG-2216, which is orally administrable, was stopped after the occurrence of a fatal case of hepatic necrosis.

In addition to HIF inactivation, EPO expression is regulated by other transcription factors. Oral administration of K-7174, which is a GATA-specific inhibitor, was found effective in a in vitro and in vivo experimental model [13].

Inhibition of the hematopoietic cell phosphatase is another possible strategy to increase erythropoiesis. This protein, also known as *src* homology domain 2-containing tyrosine phosphatase-1, binds and activates the negative regulatory domain of the EPO receptor, inhibiting is transduction inside the cell; HCF inhibitors may be a novel target molecule to treat renal anemia and/or sensitize patients to EPO action.

Conclusions

The development of new strategies for stimulating erythropoiesis is a rapidly evolving field with important implication in our knowledge about physiology and pathophysiology of EPO and its receptor. The creation of new, simpler molecules, which can be administered orally and would be easily synthesized appears feasible in the short term. We hope this will not only improve significantly the management of anemia in CKD patients, but also reduce the costs of treatment. In an era in which biosimilars of epoetin-α are entering the market at reduced costs than the originator molecule or other available ESAs, improved pharmacological properties, such as decreased administration frequency or oral administration, would be appreciated only if not too expensive.

References

1 Egrie JC, Browne KJ: Development and characterisation of novel erythropoiesis stimulating protein. Nephrol Dial Transplant 2001;16(suppl 3):3–13.
2 Locatelli F, Canaud B, Giacardy F, et al: Treatment of anaemia in dialysis patients with unit dosing of darbepoetin alfa at a reduced dose frequency relative to recombinant human erythropoietin. Nephrol Dial Transplant 2003;18:362–369.
3 Aarup M, Bryndum J, Dieperink H, et al: Clinical implications of converting stable haemodialysis patients from subcutaneous to intravenous administration of darbepoetin alfa. Nephrol Dial Transplant 2006;21:1312–1316.
4 Levin NW, Fishbane S, Cañedo FV, et al, MAXIMA Study Investigators: Intravenous methoxy polyethylene glycol-epoetin-β for haemoglobin control in patients with chronic kidney disease who are on dialysis: a randomised non-inferiority trial (MAXIMA). Lancet 2007;370:1415–1421.
5 Sytkowski AJ, Lunn ED, Risinger MA, et al: An erythropoietin fusion protein comprised of identical repeating domains exhibits enhanced biological properties. J Biol Chem 1999;274: 24773–24778.
6 Fares F, Ganem S, Hajouj T, et al: Development of a long-acting erythropoietin by fusing the carboxyl-terminal peptide of human chorionic gonadotropin β-subunit to the coding sequence of human erythropoietin. Endocrinology 2007;148:5081–5087.
7 Schriebl K, Trummer E, Lattenmayer C, et al: Biochemical characterization of rhEpo-Fc fusion protein expressed in CHO cells. Protein Expr Purif 2006;49:265–275.
8 Dumont JA, Bitonti AJ, Clark D, et al: Delivery of an erythropoietin-Fc fusion protein by inhalation in humans through an immunoglobulin transport pathway. J Aerosol Med 2005;18:294–303.
9 Bugelski PJ, Capocasale RJ, Makropoulos D, et al: CNTO 530: molecular pharmacology in human UT-7 (EPO) cells and pharmacokinetics and pharmacodynamics in mice. J Biotechnol 2007;134: 171–180.
10 Kochendoerfer GG, Chen SY, Mao F, et al: Design and chemical synthesis of a homogeneous polymer-modified erythropoiesis protein. Science 2003;299:884–887.
11 Fan Q, Leuther KK, Holmes CP, et al: Preclinical evaluation of Hematide, a novel erythropoiesis stimulating agent, for the treatment of anemia. Exp Hematol 2006;34:1303–1311.
12 Woodburn KW, Fan Q, Winslow S, et al: Hematide is immunologically distinct from erythropoietin and corrects anemia induced by antierythropoietin antibodies in a rat pure red cell aplasia model. Exp Hematol 2007;35:1201–1208.
13 Nakano Y, Imagawa S, Matsumoto K, et al: Oral administration of K-11706 inhibits GATA binding activity, enhances hypoxia-inducible factor-1 binding activity, and restores indicators in an in vivo mouse model of anaemia of chronic disease. Blood 2004;104:4300–4307.

Lucia Del Vecchio
Department of Nephrology, Dialysis and Renal Transplant
Ospedale A. Manzoni, Via dell'Eremo 9
IT–23900 Lecco (Italy)
Tel. +39 034 148 9862, Fax +39 034 148 9860, E-Mail luciadelvecchio@yahoo.com

Ronco C, Cruz DN (eds): Hemodialysis – From Basic Research to Clinical Trials.
Contrib Nephrol. Basel, Karger, 2008, vol 161, pp 261–270

....

Is the Advent of Biosimilars Affecting the Practice of Nephrology and the Safety of Patients?

Claudio Ronco

Dipartimento Interaziendale ULSS4-5-6 di Nefrologia Dialisi e Trapianto Renale,
Ospedale San Bortolo, Vicenza, Italy

Abstract

Low-molecular-weight drugs are classical medicinal pharmaceutical products. Generic drugs are the chemical and therapeutic equivalent of low-molecular-weight drugs whose patent has expired. Biopharmaceuticals are medicinal products developed by means of biotechnological processes such as recombinant DNA, controlled gene expression, antibody methods. Biosimilar or similar biological medicinal products are those that are referenced to an existing product and submitted to regulatory authorities for marketing authorization by an independent applicant after the time of protection of the data has expired for the original product. The terms 'biogeneric', 'second entry biological', 'subsequent entry biological', 'non-patented biological product' and 'multisource product' have also been used for these substances but the EMEA (European Agency for the Evaluation of medicinal products) prefers the term 'biosimilar' (the FDA coined the term 'follow-on biologic'). For nephrologists, who are used to prescribing biopharmaceuticals such as erythropoietin to their patients, the issue of emerging biosimilars is of particular importance. Responsibility exists, therefore, at the highest level to review the safety profile of the biopharmaceutical products and the emerging biosimilar products in terms of efficacy, immunological response and tolerance.

Biopharmaceuticals (biotechnology-derived drugs) have been available for over 20 years, and the patents for several of these drugs have now either expired or are about to expire. This opens the way for the manufacture of similar (generic) versions of these products, known as biosimilars. The potential market for biosimilars is huge, not least because of pressures to reduce healthcare costs. However, biopharmaceuticals and biosimilars have unique characteristics that set them apart from low-molecular-weight drugs and their generic versions.

The concern that has been generated in the scientific community by the imminent arrival of biosimilars is reflected not only in the efforts of the regulatory authorities in Europe to provide an appropriate framework for their evaluation, but also in the plethora of literature on biosimilars and generic drugs that has appeared in recent years.

Many of the issues related to biopharmaceuticals are unique because of their high molecular weights, their structural complexity, the dependence of their biological activity on structural integrity, the complexity of their manufacturing processes, the inadequacy of current analytical techniques to fully characterize them, and their potential for immunogenicity [1, 2]. The principle of essential similarity, as defined by the European Union (EU) regulatory agencies, requires a generic low-molecular-weight drug to have the same active substance in the same physicochemical form as the originator product with bioequivalence demonstrated in healthy volunteers. This established principle for evaluating generic drugs cannot therefore be applied to biosimilars [3].

The issue of emerging biosimilars is of importance to nephrologists, who routinely prescribe biopharmaceutical products, in particular, epoetins. As nephrologists will be involved in deciding whether the originator biopharmaceutical or a biosimilar is to be used to treat patients, it is timely to review the issues related to evaluation and approval of biosimilars in the context of nephrology.

Differences between Biosimilars and Low-Molecular-Weight Generic Drugs

Product Differences

Generally, biopharmaceuticals not only have molecular weights that are very much larger than low-molecular-weight drugs, but they are also much more structurally complex (fig. 1). Their three-dimensional structure is stabilized by a variety of relatively weak covalent and non-covalent bonds and is further modified by the addition of other chemical groups, as for example in glycosylation of epoetin alfa, to produce different isoforms of the molecule. This complex protein structure is very sensitive to its environment, and if a biopharmaceutical is not stored and handled correctly, it can denature and form aggregates [3].

The biological activity of a biopharmaceutical depends on its interaction with other molecules, such as cell surface receptors and binding proteins, and these interactions require very precise three-dimensional structures [4]. The pharmacokinetic and pharmacodynamic profiles (including biological activity),

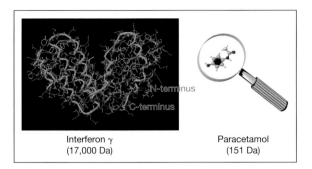

Fig. 1. Examples of the molecular structures of a biopharmaceutical and a low-molecular-weight drug.

clinical efficacy, and safety of a biopharmaceutical are thus intimately related to its structure, its isoform profile, and the degree of aggregation. All of these characteristics, in addition to the primary (chemical) structure, must be identical for a biosimilar to be considered the same product as the originator biopharmaceutical [1].

Manufacturing Differences

While low-molecular-weight drugs are made from known reagents in controlled and predictable chemical reactions, biopharmaceuticals are produced by harvesting proteins secreted by genetically engineered cells. The manufacturing process may take months and comprises many stages, including developing the host cell, establishing the master cell bank, producing the biopharmaceutical protein, purifying and analyzing the protein, and formulating, storing, and distributing the product [1]. Changes at any of these stages, even if minor, can affect the structure and identity of the biopharmaceutical, and hence its clinical efficacy and safety. It is therefore very unlikely that a biosimilar, which is manufactured using a different production process, will be identical to the originator. The total dependence of the end product on the precise details of the manufacturing process is well summarized by the phrase: 'the process is the product'.

Immunogenicity

Another feature distinguishing biopharmaceuticals from low-molecular-weight drugs is their capacity to elicit an immune response [2]. For many biopharmaceuticals, this has no clinical consequences, but for some it may lead to clinical inefficacy and/or generalized immune effects (allergy, anaphylaxis, serum sickness). If the biopharmaceutical is similar to an endogenous protein and elicits production of neutralizing antibodies that inhibit the endogenous protein, the consequences may be very severe.

Immunogenicity may be related to differences in primary sequence from the endogenous protein [5] (though this may not always enhance immunogenicity [6]), variation in the extent of glycosylation of the recombinant molecule depending on the host cell used for its manufacture [7, 8], the presence of contaminants [2, 9, 10], changes in formulation, or inappropriate storage or handling that causes protein denaturation and/or aggregation [1]. Immunogenicity may also be related to the route of administration of the biopharmaceutical, the dose and duration of treatment, immunosuppression in the recipient, and congenital lack of an endogenous protein (which leads to a predisposition to an immune response to its 'replacement') [1, 2]. Although some important factors that contribute to immunogenicity have been identified, others remain unknown. The predictive ability of current analytical methods for immune reactions in humans is limited, and standardized assays to determine immunogenicity do not exist. In addition, as immune-mediated reactions are usually rare, immunogenic safety can only be thoroughly assessed on the basis of clinical data, including robust post-marketing data [1]. Taking all of this into account, it is clear that biosimilars are not identical to the originator biopharmaceuticals and consequently they cannot be assumed that they have the same immunogenicity profiles.

Comparative Studies of Epoetin Biosimilars with the Originator Product

A number of biosimilar epoetins are available outside Europe and the USA, and preclinical as well as clinical studies of these products have been reported. In a study of 11 epoetin alfa biosimilars from 8 manufacturers in Korea, Argentina, India and China, several of the biosimilars studied showed not only deviations from the reference European pharmacopoeia standard in both chemical properties and biological activity, but also differences between separate batches of the same biosimilar epoetin (table 1) [11]. Of particular concern was the fact that the epoetin content exceeded specifications in 3 samples (121–158%), while in vivo bioactivity was markedly higher than specifications in 4 samples (137–226%) and below specifications in 2 samples (71–75%). A Brazilian study of 12 biosimilar epoetins from 5 manufacturers also revealed potencies of 68–119% of that stated on the label, variations in

Table 1. Preclinical comparisons of biosimilar epoetins. Data from Schellekens presented as in Combe et al. [14]

Biosimilar IU/ml	Osmolality mosm/kg	Human serum albumin	Protein mg/ml	Isoforms	Immuno-assay IU/ml	In vitro bioassay IU/ml	In vivo bioassay (activity index)
Specifications	215–260[1] 225–275[†]	Conforms to standard	2.0–3.0	Conforms to standard	80–120%	80–120%	0.80–1.20
IA (2,000)	268	Complies	1.1	Additional isoform	2,427 (1,800–2,400)	3,900[3] (1,600–2,500)	1.84[3]
IB (4,000)	269	Complies	1.2	Additional isoform, intensity deviation	6,302[3] (3,600–4,800)	7,870[3] (3,200–5,000)	1.05
IIA (2,000)	305	Complies	3.0	Complies	2,080 (1,800–2,400)	1,890 (1,600–2,500)	1.19
IIB (10,000)	303	Complies	3.0	Additional isoform	10,145 (9,000–12,000)	9,080 (8,000–12,500)	1.37[3]
IIIA (2,000)	279	Complies	3.2	Complies	2,392 (1,800–2,400)	2,190 (1,600–2,500)	1.89[3]
IIIB (10,000)	278	Complies	3.2	Additional isoform	12,457[3] (9,000–12,000)	9,900 (8,000–12,500)	2.26[3]
IV (2,000)	260	Complies	1.3	Additional isoform, intensity deviation	2,045 (1,800–2,400)	2,130 (1,600–2,500)	0.99
V (10,000)	314	Complies[4]	2.9	Additional isoform, intensity deviation	11,607 (9,000–12,000)	11,430 (8,000–12,500)	1.15
VI (4,000)	277	Complies	1.2	Additional isoform, intensity deviation	5,936[3] (3,600–4,800)	11,580[3] (3,200–5,000)	0.98

Table 1. (continued)

Biosimilar IU/ml	Osmolality mosm/kg	Human serum albumin	Protein mg/ml	Isoforms	Immuno-assay IU/ml	In vitro bioassay IU/ml	In vivo bioassay (activity index)
VII (10,000)	293	Complies[4]	2.5	Additional isoform, intensity deviation	10,237 (9,000–12,000)	13,690[3] (8,000–12,500)	0.71[5]
VIII (6,000)	227	Complies[4]	3.2	Additional isoform, intensity deviation	5,966 (5,400–7,200)	6,640 (4,800–7,500)	0.75[5]

[1]Specification of Eprex® (Johnson & Johnson) phosphate buffered.
[2]Specification of Eprex® new stabilizer.
[3]Markedly exceeds specifications for epoetin alfa.
[4]Additional compound detected.
[5]Fails to meet specifications for epoetin alfa.

isoform patterns between manufacturers, and unacceptable levels of bacterial endotoxins in 3 products [12].

In another study, however, a direct comparison of epoetin alfa with a biosimilar epoetin available in Cuba showed that the pharmacokinetic and pharmacodynamic characteristics of the two products were similar, with similar increases in reticulocyte count over 216 h [13].

Unfortunately, no robust well-controlled randomized clinical trials with the biosimilars shown in table 1 have yet been reported in the peer-reviewed literature [14]. However, the above studies show that several of the biosimilar epoetins available outside Europe and the USA display clear differences from the original epoetin alfa product. These differences may potentially lead to undesired effects on efficacy and patient safety.

The Current Regulatory Situation Relating to Evaluation and Approval of Biosimilars

Regulatory authorities in the EU and the USA have recognized that biosimilars differ from generic low-molecular-weight drugs in many important ways, and have concluded that the established legal and regulatory principle of 'essential similarity' (EU) or 'bioequivalence' (USA) that is applied to standard generics cannot be applied to biosimilars.

In 2005 and 2006, the European Medicines Agency Committee for Medicinal Products for Human Use (EMEA/CHMP) issued general guideline documents on biosimilars (which consist of an overarching guideline and other guidelines on quality, non-clinical and clinical issues for the development of biosimilars) and four product-class-specific annexes on the development of biosimilars of recombinant granulocyte colony-stimulating factor, insulin, human growth hormone, and erythropoietin. Draft guidelines on biosimilars (follow-on biologicals) from the US Food and Drug Administration have been delayed.

The overarching biosimilars guideline [15] indicates that EMEA/CHMP will decide on a case-by-case basis what kind of tests and data will be required to assess the safety and efficacy of biosimilars. The key aspects, however, are that a biosimilar must be evaluated in the same pharmaceutical form, strength and route of administration as the originator product, and that the same reference product should be used in all studies during the development of the biosimilar. Importantly, this reference product must be licensed in the EU and must have similar molecular and biological properties to the product under development. For example, a biosimilar interferon alfa-2a must be compared with an EU-licensed interferon alfa-2a, not with interferon alfa-2b.

The other EMEA/CHMP biosimilars guidelines cover quality issues and non-clinical and clinical issues during development of recombinant DNA-derived biosimilars. The quality guideline [16] lays down the basis for an extensive comparability exercise, using a clearly identified EU reference product rather than comparison with official, published data. State-of-the-art analytical techniques must be used to characterize both the biosimilar and the reference products, and formulation studies may be needed to demonstrate the suitability of the proposed formulation in terms of stability, compatibility and integrity of the active substance for its intended use. Finally, the product used in non-clinical studies and clinical trials should be produced using the final manufacturing process, which represents the quality profile of future (commercial) batches.

The guideline on non-clinical and clinical issues [17] focuses on safety and efficacy studies, again with comparability firmly in mind. As far as safety is concerned, non-clinical studies must include in vitro and in vivo pharmacodynamic comparisons of the biosimilar with the EU reference product and limited toxicological studies. The efficacy data required include comparative pharmacokinetic and pharmacodynamic studies and efficacy trials to demonstrate clinical comparability. Recognizing that pre-licensing studies are usually insufficient to identify all potential differences between a biosimilar and the reference product, the guideline also requires a risk management plan in accordance with current EU legislation and pharmacovigilance guidelines. Potential immunogenicity must be closely monitored, using state-of-the art assays with appropriate sensitivity and specificity. In view of the unpredictability of onset and incidence of immunogenicity, long-term results of antibody monitoring will be required post-marketing, and in the case of chronic administration, 1-year follow-up data are required pre-licensing.

The four product-class-specific annexes go into even further detail. For example, for recombinant erythropoietins [18], the annex defines not only the exact types of in vitro and in vivo pharmacodynamic assay systems that must be used, but also the type and duration of toxicology data that are required. To demonstrate comparable clinical efficacy, at least two randomized, parallel-group clinical trials are required with the reference product, preferably in patients with renal anemia, and in both correction of anemia (previously untreated patients) and maintenance of hemoglobin level in patients previously stable on the reference product. It is mandatory to provide at least 12-month comparative immunogenicity data pre-submission. Retention of samples for both the correction and the maintenance phases is recommended. For detection of anti-erythropoietin antibodies, a validated highly sensitive assay should be used. In addition, the intravenous and subcutaneous routes must be investigated separately. Finally, if efficacy and safety are demonstrated in renal anemia, it may be possible, if appropriate justification is provided, to extend the biosimilar indications to other indications of the reference product.

The Nephrology Perspective

The patents for several of the biopharmaceuticals used by nephrologists to treat their patients recently expired or are about to expire. Eprex® (epoetin alfa), for example, lost its patent protection in December 2004, and the patent for NeoRecormon® (epoetin beta) expired in 2005.

Very recently Biosimilars of epoetin alfa have been introduced in some European countries (Germany for example), so that nephrologists will soon be faced with the challenge of deciding whether to switch to biosimilar versions of off-patent biopharmaceuticals.

Although many of the biosimilar epoetins evaluated in the studies described above are unlikely to gain regulatory approval in Europe, the data presented emphasize the difficulty in replicating and consistently producing a biopharmaceutical protein. Those biosimilars that will be allowed on the market by the EMEA will need to be closely monitored by using robust risk management programs. Nephrologists need to be aware of the potential differences in efficacy and safety between the biosimilar and the original biopharmaceutical and alert regulatory authorities when unexpected adverse events occur. A tracking system to identify which product(s) is given to each patient is essential, as it is a key instrument for effective post-marketing pharmacovigilance monitoring. Patient safety depends on regulatory authorities, physicians, and pharmacists ensuring that safe, effective and high-quality biosimilars reach the patient.

References

1   Crommelin D, Bermejo T, Bissig M, et al: Pharmaceutical evaluation of biosimilars: important differences from generic low-molecular-weight pharmaceuticals. Eur J Hosp Pharmacy 2005;11: 11–17.
2   Schellekens H: Bioequivalence and the immunogenicity of biopharmaceuticals. Nat Rev Drug Discov 2002;1:457–462.
3   Crommelin D, Bermejo T, Bissig M, et al: Biosimilars, generic versions of the first generation of therapeutic proteins: do they exist? Contrib Nephrol. Basel, Karger, 2005, vol 149, pp 287–294.
4   Crommelin DJA: Differences between biopharmaceuticals and low-molecular-weight pharmaceuticals. Eur J Hosp Pharmacy 2003;8:74–76.
5   Vanderschueren SM, Stassen JM, Collen D: On the immunogenicity of recombinant staphylokinase in patients and in animal models. Thromb Haemost 1994;72:297–301.
6   Melian EB, Plosker GL: Interferon alfacon-1: a review of its pharmacology and therapeutic efficacy in the treatment of chronic hepatitis C. Drugs 2001;61:1661–1691.
7   Gribben JG, Devereux S, Thomas NSB, et al: Development of antibodies to unprotected glycosylation sites on recombinant human GM-CSF. Lancet 1990;335:434–437.

8   Karpusas M, Whitty A, Runkel L, et al: The structure of human interferon-β: implications for activity. Cell Mol Life Sci 1998;54:1203–1216.
9   Rosendaal FR, Nieuwenhuis HK, van den Berg HM, et al: A sudden increase in factor VIII inhibitor development in multitransfused hemophilia patients in The Netherlands. Blood 1993; 81:2180–2186.
10 Ryff JC: Clinical investigation of the immunogenicity of interferon-α2a. J Interferon Cytokine Res 1997;17(suppl 1):S29–S33.
11 Schellekens H: Biosimilar epoetins: how similar are they? Eur J Hosp Pharmacy 2004;3:43–47.
12 Schmidt CA, Ramos AS, da Silva JEP, et al: Activity evaluation and characterization of recombinant human erythropoietin in pharmaceutical products. Arq Bras Endocrinol Metabol 2003;47: 183–189.
13 Pérez-Oliva J, Casanova-González M, García-García I, et al: Comparison of two recombinant erythropoietin formulations in patients with anemia due to end-stage renal disease on hemodialysis: a parallel, randomized, double-blind study. BMC Nephrol 2005;6:5–15.
14 Combe C, Tredree R, Schellekens H: Biosimilar epoetins: an analysis based on recently implemented European Medicines Evaluation Agency guidelines on comparability of biopharmaceutical proteins. Pharmacotherapy 2005;25:954–962.
15 EMEA Committee for Medicinal Products for Human Use: Guideline on similar biological medicinal products. CHMP/437/04, 30 October 2005. http://www.emea.eu.int/pdfs/human/biosimilar/043704en.pdf
16 EMEA Committee for Medicinal Products for Human Use: Guideline on similar biological medicinal products containing biotechnology-derived proteins as active substances: quality issues. EMEA/CHMP/BWP/49348/2005, 22 February 2006. http://www.emea.eu.int/pdfs/human/biosimilar/4934805en.pdf
17 EMEA Committee for Medicinal Products for Human Use: Guideline on similar biological medicinal products containing biotechnology-derived proteins as active substances: non-clinical and clinical issues. EMEA/CHMP/BMWP/42832/2005, 22 February 2006. http://www.emea.eu.int/pdfs/human/biosimilar/4283205en.pdf
18 EMEA Committee for Medicinal Products for Human Use: Annex to guideline on similar biological medicinal products containing biotechnology-derived proteins as active substances: non-clinical and clinical issues. Guidance on similar medicinal products containing recombinant erythropoietins. EMEA/CHMP/BMWP/94526/2005 Corr, 22 March 2006. http://www.emea.eu.int/pdfs/human/biosimilar/9452605en.pdf

Prof. Claudio Ronco, Director
Dipartimento Interaziendale ULSS5-ULSS6 di Nefrologia Dialisi e Trapianto Renale
Ospedale San Bortolo, Viale Rodolfi 37, IT–36100 Vicenza (Italy)
Tel. +39 0444 753 650, Fax +39 0444 753 949
E-Mail claudio.ronco@ulssvicenza.it

Author Index

Subject Index

chromium-51 labeling 252
effects on erythropoietin-stimulating
agent therapy 250–252
overview 248, 249
pure red cell aplasia with erythropoiesis-
stimulating agents 243, 244
survival in renal failure 249
Renal osteodystrophy, definition 224
RISCAVID Study 187, 188

Secondary hyperparathyroidism (SHPT)
control 214, 229, 230, 235–238
pathophysiology 234, 235
Sevelamer
hyperphosphatemia control 227, 228
secondary hyperparathyroidism control
236
Sodium
consequences of sodium excess and
overhydration 102–104
dialysate
concentration 7, 8
conductivity kinetic modeling 8, 9
modulation of overhydration 104–106
Soy, diet effects on inflammation 80, 81
Statins, Dialysis Outcomes and Practice
Patterns Study findings 51, 52

Thrombectomy, vascular access stenosis
33, 34
Treatment time, *see* Hemodialysis treatment
time

Ultrafiltration (UF) rate, treatment time
considerations 156–158
Ultrasonography
arteriovenous fistula blood flow
surveillance 18, 19
preoperative fistula evaluation
arterial assessment 25, 26
venous assessment 27
vascular calcification 226, 227
Urea distribution volume, body mass index
relationship 112, 113
Uremia, definition 125
Uremic retention
complexity 126, 127
solutes 125

Uremic syndrome, definition 125
Uremic toxicity
assessment in vitro 127, 128
definition 125
HEMO Study 128, 129

Vascular access, *see also* Arteriovenous
fistula; Central venous catheter
online hemodiafiltration 193
percutaneous balloon angioplasty for
stenosis 31–33
thrombectomy 33, 34
tunneled hemodialysis catheter
procedures 34, 35
Vascular calcification, *see* Cardiovascular
disease; Chronic kidney disease-mineral
and bone disorder
Vitamin C, diet effects on inflammation 79
Vitamin D
analogs in secondary
hyperparathyroidism control 229, 230,
237, 238
calcidiol as chronic kidney disease-mineral
and bone disorder biomarker 225
deficiency in insulin resistance and
chronic kidney disease 140, 141
Vitamin E
anemia studies 93–95
dialysis membrane coating
clinical studies 92
mechanisms of action 92, 93
synthetic membrane biocompatibility
96
dietary supplementation 90–92
low-density lipoprotein oxidation
inhibition 90

Water treatment
clinical benefits 4, 5
contaminant limits 2
distribution loop 2–4
prospects 5
technology 2, 5
Whole-body impedance spectroscopy
(BCM)
dry weight assessment 117, 118
model description and validation
115–117